Health Authorities and Av  P9-BIP-633
Alike are Raving about NHE!

"Having read *Natural Hormonal Enhancement* cover-to-cover (twice), **I definitely agree with the doctors, scientists, and bodybuilders who are calling it the most important and revolutionary book ever written** on the topic of health and fitness. Powerful and comprehensive, this may truly be the closest we will ever get to 'steroid-like' results from exercise and diet."

Dan Gallapoo, Editor, "Bodybuilding for the Genetically Average Joe"

"*Natural Hormonal Enhancement* is a book of immeasurable significance and value. It belongs in every household and **should be required reading for every health professional**. Never has there been a book of such sweeping scope and penetrating insight, which advances so many original ideas and holds such potential to help so many people improve their lives."

Kay Lachowski, Book Review Editor, Online USA

"*Natural Hormonal Enhancement* is **the bible of health and fitness**. I have benefited tremendously both in terms of my own health and fitness and from the new perspective I have gained from this fascinating book. It is great to see that there are people who want to make the world healthier, not just fill their pockets with money made from phony information."

Brian Plowman, Certified U.S. Olympic Weightlifting Coach

"*Natural Hormonal Enhancement* brings together in a unified way many loose threads that have made the rounds of both the research establishment and the general hearsay conduits. **A marvelous synthesis** - congratulations to Rob Faigin for shouldering the task."

Bob Gallo, Great Mills, MD

"Superbly written and researched, *Natural Hormonal Enhancement* is **must-reading** for anyone interested in super-health and optimal performance."

Rick Hughes, LLB, MFS, ND, former Mr. New Zealand, author of Fat Attack

"Thank you for writing NHE and having the visceral **fortitude to stand by the truth** when so many powerful others are contradicting and attacking your views. As someone who is very much a part of the medical establishment, I can tell you that things are changing, just very slowly."

Michael D. Ringler, National Institutes of Health, Bethesda, MD

"NHE explains the way that exercise and nutrition work together to build fit and healthy human bodies. The author does so with expert articulation, a good sense of humor, and a no-holds-barred, 'tell the truth and damn the torpedoes' style. NHE provides **detail and clarity with practical application** to sports, fitness, bodybuilding, and health in general, for everyone."

Udo Erasmus, author, Fats That Heal Fats That Kill

"I have tried all kinds of fat loss programs over the years, and they all have one thing in common – they don't work. Money spent on books, weight loss supplements, energy bars, sports drinks – and nothing to show for it except a skinnier wallet. How long can you stick to a diet or exercise program when you are not seeing results? At the peak of frustration, I found *Natural Hormonal Enhancement*. I can describe NHE in one word – different. Different in concept, different in results. The first change was greater energy levels. Then, just a few weeks after beginning the program, **I could see my abs for the first time!** Everyone around me noticed and started asking questions. I have more motivation now than ever because of the excellent results. NHE is the best. "

Luke Buckley, Sydney, Australia

"It is hard speaking out against the majority's way of thinking, and I must confess at first I was a little embarrassed to mention NHE because it is so different from the conventional view. That is, . . . until I started **feeling better**, **losing body fat**, **my sugar cravings stopped**, **and my energy levels increased**. I think NHE is great!"

Debbie Virts, Fitness Instructor, Baltimore, MD

"*Natural Hormonal Enhancement* is phenomenal. What it preaches is absolutely true. **I am living proof** of the principles of this book."

Chris Berger, #4 Ranked U.S. Amateur Bodybuilder, Middleweight Division
(featured in Muscle and Fitness 6/99, pages 60-66)

"With all the hype out there, Rob Faigin is front-and-center with **the best advice I've heard** and, more importantly, with what my OWN body tells me about how it responds to different regimes."

Valerie Bishop, Atlanta, GA

"*Natural Hormonal Enhancement* is **the most fascinating book I have ever read**. I actually sat down and read continuously for 5 hours a night until I finished a few days later (and I'm not a big reader). I have read a lot about exercise and health, and NHE is the most informative and well-researched book I have seen."

Jon Barrett, Champaign, IL

"I will be contacting you in the near future about a volume discount as I plan to give *Natural Hormonal Enhancement* as a gift to all my friends and family members. As far as comparing the book to others, there is NO COMPARISON. I've read books by Sears (*The Zone*), Eades & Eades (*Protein Power*), Atkins (*New Diet Revolution*), and Peskin (*Beyond the Zone*). All of these authors and books are ahead of their time and present profound pieces of the big picture, but they all left me with the sense that something was missing. A 'Grand Unified Theory' if you will. Well, after reading *Natural Hormonal Enhancement*, I have no doubt whatsoever that **NHE is the Grand Unified Theory of Health**. At last, I have found the 'Big Picture.' Thank you."

Steve Mink, Dallas, TX

"I loved NHE. It was revolutionary for me. I have been a brown rice, wheatgrass juice, and aerobics geek for 30 years, and I had the potbelly to prove it. Since reading your book, **I have lost lots of fat and gained lots of muscle** and willpower. Thanks so much."

Roger Bird, Colorado Springs, CO

"*Natural Hormonal Enhancement* is a masterpiece of research combined with honest, intelligent thought. I believe it will be seen as **a landmark in health and fitness literature**. Sacred, long established dogmas are challenged and demolished with argument and experience backed by scientific reference. But much more than a theoretical work, *Natural Hormonal Enhancement* shows how to maximize health and fitness simply by working within the body's own hormonal systems, naturally, safely, and effectively.

You should read and act upon this book - **it will quite simply change your life** for the better."

Richard J. Marsh, MD., MA, BM., BCh.(Oxon), MRCGP. - Churchill Fellow

"As an anti-aging specialist, I have read many of the popular health and longevity books. Very few have impressed me. For this reason, I probably never would have read *Natural Hormonal Enhancement* had my associate not insisted, after reading it himself. Admittedly, I picked-up the book with a negative predisposition, assuming it would be more of the same. I couldn't have been more wrong in that assumption. *Natural Hormonal Enhancement* is exceptionally well-written and well-researched and it **contains revolutionary information that even many of my peers don't understand or don't recognize**. I highly recommend this book."

Dr. Rashid Buttar, founder,
Institute of Advanced Concepts in Alternative and Preventative Medicine

"NHE is fabulous, an excellent collection of information. I can't say enough about it. Since beginning the program, **my health has improved and I have lost 25 pounds of fat!** You should see the reaction of people when they see me and ask, "What pills are you taking?" to lose the weight. We are blessed to have this information."

Ronnetta Lee, Cleveland, OH

"*Natural Hormonal Enhancement* is **a brilliant book**. I have read many fitness books and many recommend various routines and diets but none so completely explain the reasoning behind it and none are backed by so much evident scientific knowledge."

Tim Humble, Newcastle-Upon-Tyne, England

"*Natural Hormonal Enhancement* is a truly great book with **more knowledge packed into it than any book I have ever seen**---congratulations on an honest, intelligent and revolutionary book."

Bob Berger, Ph.D., Ft. Lauderdale, FL

"I have read *Natural Hormonal Enhancement* twice, and want to read it again. Not because it is hard to understand, but that there is SO much info and it is so inter-related that it's **like suddenly finding you have x-ray vision and you're able to see through the human body**... and it's overwhelming!!!!"

Linda Hinson, Eldon, MO

"*Natural Hormonal Enhancement* is **the best resource in the world**. I personally recommend you read this book."

Peter Klein, CEO, Sports One Inc.

"Two and a half weeks ago, I started the NHE program and I am delighted to say that have **never felt so energetic!** My mood is better and I am shedding bodyfat withou effort."

John Thompson, Rochester, NY

"I've been an avid bodybuilder and fitness enthusiast for nearly two decades. As incredibl as it may sound, **I have made more progress towards achieving a lean muscular physique in just over 2 months since applying NHE, than have in the previous 20 years** (embarrassing but true). Specifically, hydrostati bodyfat testing indicates that since beginning the NHE program, my bodyfat has droppe from 22% to 14% while I have actually gained muscle mass! I am finally developing th "chiseled look" I've always wanted thanks to this program, and I feel confident as I prepar for my first bodybuilding competition. Based on the astounding results I have achieved i such a short period of time, I recommend *Natural Hormonal Enhancement* with unequivoca enthusiasm."

Jon Ayling, Tasmania, Australia

"To be a good trainer, one must first be a good student. NHE cleared-up a lot of th missing pieces of what I knew from experience was right, but did not know why. In my opinion, Rob Faigin is the Grand Champion of health and fitness authors, and his book i truly a masterpiece. I have learned from the best teachers and studied from the best books and *Natural Hormonal Enhancement* is in a class by itself. It is cutting-edge fitnes technology presented in a format that the average person can easily understand, follow, an apply instantly. There you have it: "The World's Best Personal Trainer's" recommendatio for what he feels is **The World's Best Book for building a better body**. "

George Baselice, Grand Champion, Met-Rx World's Best Personal Trainer Contest

"When I received NHE, I read it cover to cover. **It was like a John Grisham novel**; the information was so compelling that I couldn't put it down. Finally, I had a crysta clear picture of what I needed to do. I've turned a half-dozen friends on to NHE, an everybody is experiencing fantastic results. Thanks again for opening my eyes. You have a NHE convert for LIFE!!!"

Steven M. Kip, Senior Director of Corporate Marketing, Tampa Bay Lightning, Tampa, FL

"*Natural Hormonal Enhancement* is, by far, **the most extensively researched well thought-out, and beautifully presented health and fitness book I have ever read**. Mr. Faigin has quite the gift of the pen, and the 1700 research reference are absolutely mind-boggling. A real credit to him for being able to assemble all of these different sources of information into a book that I simply could not put down. As a persona trainer, I am especially grateful because *Natural Hormonal Enhancement* not only benefit me and my wife, but also my present and future clients. Many thanks."

Trevor Beairsto, personal trainer, Toronto, Canada

"I love NHE because it explains everything clearly and cites specific references. have already told many people about the book and have urged them to buy it. I believe i to be very beneficial and crucial for everyone's health. I cannot say enough about NHE **all fitness books should be written like this**. Rob Faigin has done an incredibl job and a service to us all."

Bryan Eckhardt, Cornell University, Cornell, NY

"Thanks for a fantastic book! I've read *Natural Hormonal Enhancement* cover to cover and have learned more about fitness in a few days than in my entire life."

Ruben A. Matos, Captain, United States Air Force

"I have read NHE and incorporated it into my life over the last month with amazing results. I thought I was fit, but the information in NHE put me in touch with an unprecedented physical, emotional and psychological well-being and strength. NHE is simply the most profound, cutting edge information that I have come into contact with in years. I am deeply grateful for what Mr. Faigin has contributed toward my own health and the health of the country."

Arthur Giacalone, Ph.D., Walnut Creek, CA

"Like many women, weight and appearance have been serious issues for me since I stumbled into puberty. I always had a tendency to be a little on the chunky side. My junior year in high school, I tipped the scales at 150 pounds. Here began a lifelong battle with overeating, starving, and emotional upheaval.

A few years later, at 18, I became pregnant with my oldest son, Zachary, and my weight ballooned up to 172 pounds (I'm 5'2"). My weight became a constant reminder for me of a lack of control in my life. I started running four miles a day five days a week, working out with weights five days a week, and restricting fat and calories. I lost weight, but I was exhausted, nervous, always hungry, and my knees were killing me. NHE changed all this, and improved my life.

I have been on the NHE program for over a year and have achieved great success. My triglycerides have dropped all the way down to 70, and my HDL/LDL cholesterol ratio has improved remarkably. Though I've had three children, I am in my best shape ever. I weigh between 115 and 118 pounds, my bodyfat is low and my muscle tone is excellent. Thanks to NHE, I spend much less time working-out and get better results. I'm finally healthy, with a healthy attitude about food instilled in me by Rob Faigin's teachings. I no longer suffer guilt when I eat nor do I suffer from the deprivation I used to with the radical diets I followed. As a Cajun, food is a huge part of our culture - a source of happiness. NHE is compatible with eating for pleasure, tailor-made for individuals like myself.

My friends are amazed at my success, and I owe it to NHE. It has made my lifelong goal of health and a physique I can be proud of, attainable with relative ease. I am resolved to teach my children what I have learned from NHE, so that they too will have the gift of health."

Carice Nolan, Lafayette, LA

The Application of Science

Natural
Hormonal
Enhancement

The Ultimate Strategy for Lifetime Youthfulness,
Physique Transformation, and Super-Health

Rob Faigin, J.D.

illustrations and cover by Kjell Anderson

www.extique.com

Natural Hormonal Enhancement by Rob Faigin ISBN 0-9675605-0-0

Copyright © 2000 by Extique

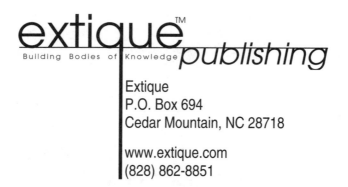

Extique
P.O. Box 694
Cedar Mountain, NC 28718

www.extique.com
(828) 862-8851

The Ultimate Strategy for Lifetime Youthfulness, Physique Transformation, and Super-Health

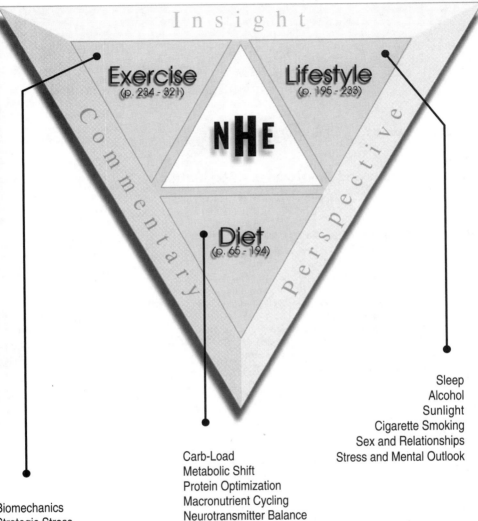

Insight

Exercise
(p. 234 - 321)

Lifestyle
(p. 195 - 233)

NHE

Commentary

Perspective

Diet
(p. 65 - 194)

Sleep
Alcohol
Sunlight
Cigarette Smoking
Sex and Relationships
Stress and Mental Outlook

Carb-Load
Metabolic Shift
Protein Optimization
Macronutrient Cycling
Neurotransmitter Balance
Glycogen Use Efficiency
Calorie Counting Prohibited
Sugar Burner vs. Fat Burner
Using Dietary Fat to Burn Bodyfat

Biomechanics
Strategic Stress
Intensity Modulation
Bioenergetic Pathways
Qualitative Progression
Duration Synchronization
Anabolic Supercompensation
Optimal Neuroendocrine Response
Pre-Workout Meal/Priming the Hormonal Environment

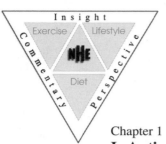

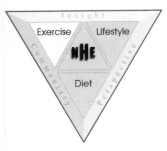

Insight
Exercise / Lifestyle
NHE
Diet
Commentary / Perspective

Chapter 21
Hormonally-Intelligent Exercise 234

"*Natural Hormonal Enhancement* is the bible of health and fitness. **It is great to see that there are people who want to make the world healthier, not just fill their pockets with money made from phony information."** Brian Plowman, Certified U.S. Olympic Weightlifting Coach

"So many thanks to Rob Faigin for standing up to the misinformation that has been pressed on average misguided people like me." Joshua Olson, Sante Fe, NM

"NHE has improved every aspect of my life... I can't stop saying thank you to Rob Faigin!" Jill Berrelli, Phoenix, AZ

"In my opinion, Rob Faigin is **the Grand Champion of health and fitness authors."** George Baselice, Grand Champion, Met-Rx World's Best Personal Trainer Contest

About the Author

Rob holds a Bachelor of Science in History from Florida Atlantic University and a Juris Doctor from the Florida State University College of Law, where he also served as teaching and research assistant. Rob has held positions in the public and private sectors as personal trainer and fitness consultant.

In 1994, greatly dismayed by the corruption, misinformation, and hypocrisy in the health and fitness industry and fiercely determined to do something about it, he founded Extique Inc., with the mission of "making honest, high-quality health and fitness information and instruction available to everyone; exposing fraudulent and deceptive practices in the health and fitness industry; and pursuing new, natural approaches to health and fitness centered upon hormonal enhancement technology."

As a drug-free bodybuilder with amateur boxing experience, Rob has sought to combine his experience and practical knowledge of sports nutrition and training with the latest research in the phenomenal field of hormonal enhancement. A landmark achievement, *Natural Hormonal Enhancement* advances a comprehensive program for harnessing the profound biological forces that reside within every human being.

Proud to be called "a new breed of health and fitness commentator," Rob is not affiliated with any fitness magazine, supplement company, or any other institutional interest. Unconstrained by the allegiances that tend to curtail objectivity, and beholden to no one except his clients and readers, Rob is free to say what needs to be said to help protect the public from a health and fitness industry tragically lacking in social responsibility and wildly out of control. In addition to being quite possibly the most important fitness instructional product ever, *Natural Hormonal Enhancement* is a broad-based and scathing attack upon the forces of misinformation that have riddled the fat loss efforts, picked the pockets, and undermined the health, of millions of Americans.

Forward

"Let the word go forth. . . that the torch has been passed."

John F. Kennedy, Inaugural Speech

I believe that once you have read this book you will share my optimistic belief that *Natural Hormonal Enhancement* heralds a new era. One in which reason and scientific truth will prevail over financially inspired misinformation propagated by snake-oil marketeers and the intellectual arrogance of a medical establishment mired in the tradition of healing sickness rather than promoting health. This book is our best hope for toppling a status quo that has produced the highest levels of obesity and degenerative disease in human history despite awesome technological advancement. We have unraveled DNA, the secret of life, but have failed to discern the secrets of health. Until now.

In terms of the revolutionary information it conveys, its meticulously cited scientific sources, and its analytical objectivity, *Natural Hormonal Enhancement* establishes a much-needed standard in a standardless industry in which contradictory half-truths compete for public acceptance. More importantly, it provides the couch potato with a realistically achievable program for physique improvement and the serious athlete with a blueprint for excellence. Moderate yet effective, cutting-edge yet practical, steeped in science yet easy to apply, *Natural Hormonal Enhancement* is both the key to unlocking human potential and a how-to manual for looking and feeling your best.

Furthermore, *Natural Hormonal Enhancement* demonstrates, more so than any other book in history, the need for an integrated, holistic approach to health and fitness. In a culture where "diet books" are all the rage, *Natural Hormonal Enhancement* is the best diet book of all, showing us how to eat for permanent fat loss and muscular enhancement without the restrictions of a low-fat or "Atkins" diet or the impracticalities of "The Zone." But at the same time, with the candor and insight that sets this book apart, Rob Faigin shows why a diet-only approach is fatally flawed. The reader will find that *Natural Hormonal Enhancement* is more than a book about using food to activate fat-burning and muscle-building hormones; or getting better results from exercise in half the time; or harnessing the power of our thoughts to influence our health; or modifying our lifestyle to reclaim the natural energy and vigor that is rightfully ours - it is all of this, and much more. At its core, *Natural Hormonal Enhancement* is a book about truth: it debunks popular misconceptions, and it illuminates the true path to optimal health and well-being.

Indeed, the torch has been passed. And with this torch of knowledge comes the enlightenment that will dispel the ignorance and greed that has plagued the health and fitness industry for far too long. The medical/pharmaceutical establishment has failed us with its narrow-minded focus on treating, rather than preventing, disease. The fad diets, the fitness contraptions, the fat loss pills, have all failed us. To quote Rob, "we must embrace scientific wisdom over conventional wisdom" and we must "discard the tried and untrue factually discredited views of old."

A new vision of health, a natural solution combining common sense with science, which produces concrete results, and which we can easily integrate into our lives, is long overdue - but finally here. Guided by a Galilean commitment to scientific truth and practical insight acquired as a trainer and athlete, Rob Faigin has produced a book of infinite value for those who desire a more attractive physique, a sharper mind, and a healthier, more youthful body.

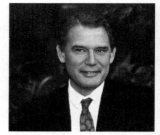

Kjell Anderson, Publisher

Note from the Author

Great care and painstaking effort were invested in the researching and writing of this book. However, no amount of care or effort can preclude the possibility of error, because no author is infallible. This is especially the case with a book of this nature, which breaks new ground and advances original ideas.

Although I have drawn heavily on the research of numerous scientists, I, alone, am responsible for the interpretations of the research presented in this book. And while the arguments advanced in this book spring from the noblest of motives and are the product of relentless effort, they will surely be disputed by equally diligent researchers with equally worthy intentions - such conflicts are inevitable in the marketplace of ideas. It is the responsibility of each reader to use reason and common sense, in conjunction with the opinion of a qualified health practitioner familiar with your medical history and current health status, to give appropriate weight to assertions made by health writers. The references that follow each chapter of this book were included to assist you in this process, by enabling you and your physician to examine the basis of the conclusions presented.

This book, necessarily, speaks in general terms and draws conclusions from scientific studies of groups. Biochemical individuality can render general principles inapplicable to a particular person. It is the role of your physician to determine the unique needs of your physiology.

Even so, I believe strongly that each individual has a responsibility for his or her own health and well-being. It is unrealistic to think that doctors - whose training and focus are directed toward curing and treating illness - can stay abreast of all the rapidly expanding developments directed toward enhancing and advancing health. Thus, while affirming the indispensable role played by your doctor as your exclusive provider of medical advice and treatment, this book seeks to assist you in fulfilling your ultimate obligation to promote your own health and well-being.

In pursuing fitness and longevity, it can be very frustrating, I know, to sort through the ocean of often-contradictory health information that we have inherited as beneficiaries, or victims, of the so-called "information age." Nonetheless, it is a duty from which we must never shrink, for the clash of ideas is our best means of ascertaining truth. And never is truth more important than when it relates to the health of human beings.

Acknowledgments

The journey from conception to completion of this book has been a lonely, soul-consuming, uphill struggle against seemingly impossible odds. While I did not have the editorial support, research assistance, or formal scientific training that would appear necessary to write a book of this nature, I did have the encouragement and support of some very special people. I wish to recognize these individuals. Each has played a constructive role in the creation and advancement of Natural Hormonal Enhancement, and I am deeply grateful to them.

First and foremost, my parents, *Michael and Michelle Faigin,* for their unfailing support, love, and counsel, throughout my life and in connection with this project.

My uncle, *Ken Faigin,* who kindled my interest in health and fitness more than twenty years ago, and has played an historic supporting role in the pioneering of *Natural Hormonal Enhancement.* A man ahead of his time, in the 1970's, long before it was fashionable, Ken was a passionate proponent of vitamin supplementation and other natural approaches to health. At the time, his ideas were viewed as radical and were dismissed by most people. But he found an attentive pupil in an inquisitive 8-year-old too naïve to be prejudiced against new and unconventional ideas. Those early lessons sparked a fascination and a sense of possibility, which have culminated in *Natural Hormonal Enhancement.* More recently, Ken remained confident in me and faithful to this project the whole way through, lending crucial support and advice. When the obstacles seemed insurmountable, and others were handing down judgment, Ken was lending a hand. I salute his longstanding commitment to the advancement of natural approaches to health, and I feel fortunate to have been influenced and assisted by someone of such rare judgment, vision, and character.

My partner *Kjell Anderson,* who, through his devotion to Extique and his commitment to the common good, has earned both my appreciation and my esteem. I met Kjell by chance - if there is such a thing - at a health food store shortly after I had completed the 300-page manuscript of NHE. I was unwilling to sell the rights to my book for any price, but less than utterly confident in my ability to market it with a net worth far below zero and cash-on-hand amounting to approximately three pennies. After he expressed an interest in reviewing and possibly marketing the book on his website, I exchanged phone numbers with the jovial Swede named "chel", not expecting much and unaware of the fateful forces afoot. I soon discovered that Kjell's easygoing charm concealed an iron-willed determination to succeed at doing what's right. We became friends, then partners - a perfect team consisting of a 44-year-old has-been and a 28-year-old never-was. He dedicated his career to advancing the unknown work of an unknown author, employing tireless effort, business acumen, technical expertise, artistic talent, and his financial resources toward this end. Although he is quick to downplay his contribution, humble disclaimers of credit cannot diminish the monumental role that Kjell has played in the publication, distribution, and marketing of *Natural Hormonal Enhancement.* I and everyone who has benefited from this book owe a debt of gratitude to Kjell Anderson.

My staunchest supporter, my most courageous defender, and unquestionably the greatest woman in the world - *my mother.*

Rick and Dave Faigin, for caring about my welfare and acting to promote it with the best of brotherly intentions.

My sister and brother-in-law, *Lisa and Ken Sharp*, for their encouragement and concern.

The Anderson children - *Kajsa, Kresten, Kjersti* - for providing their dad and "Uncle Rob" with the inspiration and perspective that only little kids can. Also, Kjell's wife *Kay*.

The Florida State University College of Law, an excellent institution that contributed to my intellectual development. In particular, *Associate Dean Ruth Witherspoon;* and *Professor John Yetter*, my mentor – he, more than anyone, helped me develop my analytical abilities.

I wish to recognize the following individuals and their indirect, but significant, influence on the development of *Natural Hormonal Enhancement.*

Dr. Michael Colgan, who, in my opinion, is the most prolific health and fitness writer of the last century. Although I believe that some of his views are refuted by the evidence presented in this book, I am grateful to him both for his immense substantive contribution to health and fitness and for his indefatigable efforts to raise public awareness of important health issues. *Mauro Di Pasquale M.D.*, who, in my opinion, is the world's foremost sports nutritionist. By virtue of his willingness to depart from the consensus of his peers when the evidence so leads, Dr. Di Pasquale represents a model for all members of the medical community to follow. *Dr. Daniel Rudman*, the visionary who began the hormonal enhancement revolution by proving the paramount role played by hormones in human aging. *Abraham Lincoln*, whose saying, "the possibility that we may fail ought not deter us from a cause we believe to be just," carried me through the periods of frustration, despair, and self-doubt that I experienced while working on this book.

Preface: My Story

If it was metal and looked like a machine part, I wanted it desperately. Since robots were made of metal parts and wires, it seemed self-evident to my 5-year-old mind that if I could gather enough metal parts and wires I could build a robot. And so as a young child I accumulated a glorious collection of discarded junk. I was aware that I was facing a challenge, but I perceived that the challenge lay in finding the right parts. I never questioned that once I had the parts, I could create a robot mighty enough to whip the school bully and durable enough to withstand a game of padless tackle football with my friends and me. Because I was so young at the time, we'll say I was naïve not stupid. But sometime around six years of age, I arrived at the disheartening realization that I would not be able to build a robot with my assorted metal parts.

My interest in robots faded and was replaced by an even greater interest in the human body. I no longer aspired to build an artificial body of metal, but rather a real body of bone and muscle – first my own, then other peoples' as well. As a teenager and young adult I no longer collected metal parts, but rather books and scientific articles. Maturity had unburderded me of the unrealistic aspiration of building a robot – and pointed me toward a different unrealistic aspiration. I firmly believed that if I read and studied everything on the subject of health and fitness and experimented on myself, I could synthesize all the information into a coherent plan that anyone could use to build an age-resistant, sick-resistant, super-body. I named my vision "Extique," a word that came to me out of nowhere, and which I later realized could be considered a contraction of "excellent" and "physique." I was so exuberantly confident that I paid a few hundred dollars of borrowed money to register "Extique" with the U.S. Patent and Trademark Office. Fortunately, I had no idea at the time of the hardship that lay ahead.

By my mid-twenties, I was facing the same disillusionment that I had encountered when I realized that I would never be able to build my robot. I had absorbed every book and article that I could find on the subject of physique enhancement and health. In so doing, I had acquired a tremendous amount of knowledge. But contrary to my central assumption, my hard-earned knowledge did not yield the understanding I needed to actualize Extique. Instead of the coherent synthesis I had envisioned, I possessed a scattered fragmentary mess of information. As hard as I tried, I couldn't pull it all together – there were too many inconsistencies and contradictions.

At this point, I was deeply in debt, forced to take a job as a waiter, and under attack from the inevitable naysayers appointed by fate to test the resolve of those who dare to dream. I was "going for broke," and getting there in a hurry. But my investment in Extique was far more than economic; and the potential rewards transcended money and promised to affect the lives of millions of people whom I had never met and never would meet. Despite such lofty ambitions, the prospects of success appeared bleak. I was serving my fellow man – the early-bird special. The Extique vision was dimming.

But unlike my error twenty years earlier in thinking I could build a robot from miscellaneous metal items, this time I felt certain that I was on the right track despite mounting evidence to the contrary. I strongly suspected that I was missing something - but what? The missing element, of course, was hormones. Like most researchers, I was aware of hormones but had vastly underestimated their importance in relation to health, aging, and body composition. Several studies published in the early 1990's provided the lead I needed.

Once I focused on hormones, everything began falling into place. My research on hormones united all that I had learned and advanced my intellectual horizon. Eleventh-hour insight had salvaged Extique from the brink of oblivion, and infused it with new purpose and potential. I became transfixed by the realization that within each of us resides enormously powerful biological forces called hormones; which literally turn boys into men, turn girls into women, and when they decline, turn strong, vigorous people into frail, feeble, weak people. And most remarkably, I came to appreciate that every day of our lives we unknowingly influence these dynamic forces. A chance meeting with a funny-named fellow (see Acknowledgments), provided the practical foundation necessary to take Extique to its fullest potential. The tide had turned - but a daunting task still lay ahead.

Having finally been granted insight and a reprieve from financial ruin, I redoubled my efforts. I dedicated every ounce of energy and intellect I possessed to learning how naturally, safely, and effectively to harness the profound biological forces that we call hormones. The result of that impassioned effort, which included reviewing more than 10,000 scientific articles from 1997 to 2000, is the book you now hold in your hands. It does not provide all the answers, and it is no more likely to be perfect than the less-than-perfect man who wrote it. But I believe that *Natural Hormonal Enhancement* can help you achieve your dreams for a long life filled with health and happiness. If it does, then I will have achieved my dream.

- Rob Faigin -

Enter a New Dimension in Fitness...

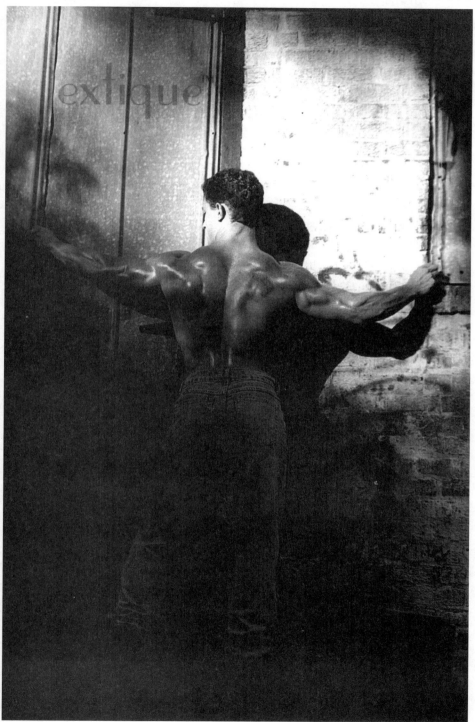

Pictured: Rob Faigin

There is a very fine line between a hopeless dreamer and a brilliant visionary.
This book is dedicated to those individuals, on either side of the line,
who have struggled against the odds and endured adversity,
to pursue their vision for a better world.

Chapter 1

Is Anti-Aging Unnatural or is Aging Unnatural

For those people who view aging negatively, it is the worst of all misfortunes;
other evils will mend, but this is every day getting worse.
Unknown

Life is pleasant. Death is peaceful. It's the transition that's troublesome.
Isaac Asimov

I think I'm starting to get old.
Gussie Faigin (Rob Faigin's great grandmother) at her 100th birthday party

It is widely accepted that aging is a part of life. However, in a sense, this is untrue. For starters, consider the fact that not all animals age in the sense that we think of aging, i.e., as a degenerative process in which physical growth ceases and physical and mental function diminish over time. Nonaging animals include lobsters, alligators, the Galapagos tortoise, and many, but not all, fish. Among fish, sturgeons and sharks do not age and neither does the female flounder.*

Nonaging animals do not experience physical maturation followed by physical decline like aging animals do, even when they are kept in captivity and thus protected from lifespan-shortening natural dangers. Rather, they continue to grow indefinitely, and if there is a decline in physical function it is so slight that scientists have been unable to detect it. What studies of these animals show is that reaction time, vital functions such as immunity, physical strength, and all other indices of aging do not change with the passage of time after sexual maturation is attained.

The obvious question that arises is why nonaging animals do not live forever and grow to monster-movie proportions. First, consider that the Galapagos tortoise has been known to live 175 years and lobsters have reached 44 pounds. But to answer the question, ask yourself this: if humans did not age, would we live forever?

The answer is no. The saying "everything happens to everyone eventually" is applicable here: every living creature is done-in by something at some point because, in the crapshoot of life, eventually everyone craps-out. So the benefit of not aging for nonaging animals is that the risk of dying from disease, accidents, or predation in any given year does not *increase* over time, but rather it remains constant from one year to the next until, eventually, every animal's number is called, including the 44-pound lobster and the 175-year-old Galapagos tortoise (which, incidentally, died from an accident when it fell through a poorly constructed platform while in captivity).

* But the male flounder does. The reason for this gender disparity is a mystery.

As you can see, aging is not as universal as people think. Given that some animals do not age, the statement "aging is a part of life" is not actually true. Now the question becomes: is aging a part of *human* life? The answer, at the present time, is yes. However, aging as we know it did not happen for the vast majority of human existence for the same reason it does not happen today to animals in the wild.

Nature imposes a very severe system of age discrimination: soon after a wild animal begins to exhibit signs of the functional impairment and weakness associated with aging, its life ends. Animals that do not see as well, run as fast, react as quickly, or leap as high have a fatal disadvantage. These deficits render the animal less successful at the competitive endeavor of obtaining food; more likely to contract diseases that disproportionately afflict faltering immune systems (but without the benefit of cures and treatments); and less capable of fending-off predators.

The natural order is such that wild animals are rarely alive to experience middle age, much less old age. The beloved, elderly, semi-blind pet dogs and cats that reside in houses across America would have been rubbed-out of existence long before reaching a state remotely approximating the doddering senility that can be attained when we provide them with sanctuary from predators and regular trips to the vet. In the same way, aging for humans is a construct of civilization.

In the scope of human history, which stretches back hundreds-of-thousands of years, aging is a very recent phenomenon. Up until we conquered our fellow creatures and asserted a measure of control over nature, we did not have to worry about such affronts to vanity as wrinkles and graying hair. We were protected from these indignities by the natural order. When viewed as a departure from the natural order, aging as we conceive it is not natural at all.

Does this mean that *anti*-aging is natural? I believe so. At the very least, anti-aging is less unnatural than aging. The only reason why aging exists today is because the technology of curing and treating disease has outpaced the technology of promoting health. Therefore, if we bring health promotion up to speed, humans today can experience a lifetime of health and youthfulness, like we did throughout most of our history, but with a much longer lifespan.

We created aging, and we can stop it. By the time you are finished reading the next chapter, you will realize that my expressed confidence in the attainability of an ageless society is neither inflated optimism nor groundless bravado. To the contrary, we have recently unlocked the key to defeating aging, and the march to battle against aging has begun.

Chapter 2

Biological Aging vs. Chronological Aging

Youth should not be presumption of vitality, nor old-age a presumption of wisdom.
John F. Kennedy

Seriously ill patient to his doctor: I've given up on being young again, but I would like to go on getting older.
Unknown

Growing old gratefully is the key to growing old gracefully. But being thankful to be alive - and therefore getting older - does not mean that aging should not be combated with every tool we have at our disposal. Rather, the war against aging is an affirmation of life, and it should be waged as aggressively and vigorously as possible. Thus, where determined resistance coexists with grateful acceptance, the ideal anti-aging mindset is achieved.

Rob Faigin

There are two kinds of aging: biological aging and chronological aging. People often confuse the two or lump them together under the term "aging." Although they are related, they are very different. Chronological age is 1) based on one factor, time, and 2) is the same for everyone. Biological age is 1) based on several factors, some controllable, others not, and 2) varies from person to person.

Chronological aging refers to how long you have been alive. The mathematical formula for determining chronological age is the same for everyone: current date minus date of birth = chronological age. In other words, chronological age is a function of time and cannot be slowed, stopped, or accelerated.*

Unlike chronological aging, biological aging, which describes the state of your body, can speed-up, slow-down, stop, or even reverse. Biological aging tracks chronological aging like a poorly trained dog follows its master. For the most part, the dog and the master move toward the same destination, and the dog never completely loses the master. But the dog may run ahead or fall behind, or do each at different times in the trip. The "destination" in this analogy is the maximum human lifespan, which most scientists agree is somewhere between 120 and 160 years. When the master (chronological aging) reaches the destination long before the dog (biological aging), a person dies young at a very old age - the ultimate victory over aging. But when the dog reaches the destination long before the master, the person dies old at a very young age - every person's nightmare. If this view of aging seems alien, it is because you harbor an outdated view of aging, a view that has been superseded by recent scientific discoveries.

Contrary to popular belief, biological aging does not pursue an inexorable downhill course. Certainly, a person who has been alive for 80 years is more likely to have wrinkles than a 20-year-old. But outside of extreme examples like this, what does years of life have to do with the biological age of your body? Not a whole lot.

* Actually, Einstein's Theory of Relativity indicates that even chronological aging is not universal; as one approaches the speed of light, time slows and so does chronological aging. But this is irrelevant for us Earthbound folks.

Evidence that biological aging and chronological aging are cousins, not twins, has been mounting for quite some time. During the Vietnam War, autopsies of soldiers in their 20's revealed 50-year-old bodies. These mens' bodies, inside and out, according to every physiological marker of "aging," were very advanced. The extreme trauma and stress of the war, which induced drastically elevated levels of catabolic hormones, literally made the soldiers old before their time.

You do not have to be a medical examiner to see evidence that biological age and chronological age do not walk in lockstep. You have probably seen 40-year-olds who look like they are 30 years old, and other 40-year-olds who look like they are 50 years old (that's a 20-year swing in appearance among individuals who have been alive for the same amount of time!). Internally and functionally, the same phenomenon is evident. Some people have the cardiovascular capacity, muscular strength, bodyfat percentage, pulse rate, blood pressure, reaction time, mental acuity, glucose tolerance, blood lipid profile, and sex drive of someone who has been alive for many fewer years, and vice versa. This is not simply a matter of health, as many people believe. Rather, biological aging goes deeper; it represents the level of degeneration of the body. This degenerative process, which is commonly referred to as "aging," can differ widely, and can speed-up, slow-down, or reverse, depending on the hormones that regulate degeneration and *regeneration* of the body at the cellular level.

Another example of how biological aging and chronological aging are only loosely related is presented by a rare disease called progeria. Victims of this cruel disease experience an extremely accelerated rate of biological aging such that they get "old" and die in their mid-to-late teens. By their teenage years, progeria victims have lost their hair, acquired wrinkles, and are at high risk for the degenerative diseases associated with old age, such as atherosclerosis and cancer. When cells from progeria victims are isolated and compared with cells from normal people, the cells from progeria victims age at a faster rate.

All this raises the following question. Who is "older": a person who was born 40 years ago with the body of a 30-year-old, or a person who was born 30 years ago with the body of a 40-year-old? Until recently, the divergence between biological and chronological aging was not fully appreciated, and thus the measure of age was simple: subtract the date on your birth certificate from the date on today's newspaper - and that's your age. As a new millennium dawns, aging is being redefined. For the first time in human history, aging is being viewed as a disease to be combated and conquered, not as an inevitable process.

As you will see in the next chapter, the hormonal revolution has rendered obsolete conventional notions of aging. It is becoming increasingly evident that biological aging is a symptom of hormonal decline; and because hormonal decline is not inevitable, neither is biological aging. If you find the concept of not merely slowing but *reversing* aging impossible to believe, it is only because you hold a view of aging that has been overtaken by science and invalidated by our newfound understanding of the profound role of hormones in the aging process. In the next chapter, you will see that a reversal of biological aging is neither impossible nor far-fetched.

Growth Hormone and the Hormonal Revolution

Incredible though it may seem, the slow decline in appearance and function that we call aging may not be fixed in our genes or part of human destiny. . . What we now call aging appears to be due in large part to the drastic decline of growth hormone in the body after adulthood [and this decline] not only can be arrested but can actually be reversed.
Dr. Ronald Klatz, President, American Academy of Anti-Aging Medicine, *Grow Young with HGH*

Doc, are all these physical ailments I'm suffering from independent of each other, or is it part of a general meltdown?
Jeff Northcutt, Lieutenant Commander U.S. Navy, struggling to make sense of age-related physical decline

Recent discoveries have yielded amazing new insights into aging, health, and fat loss. We have recently learned that these three areas are more closely interrelated than previously suspected, *and hormones are the unifying factor*. This realization lies at the heart of the hormonal revolution, and it presents the thrilling prospect of using one grand strategy to attack all three areas simultaneously - to arrest aging, while achieving super-health, while at the same time permanently eliminating excess bodyfat.

Occupying center stage in this unfolding drama is *somatotropin*, also known as human growth hormone, the most potent anti-aging force yet discovered and the most powerful fat-burning hormone in men and women. Growth hormone is produced by the pituitary gland, under direction of the hypothalamus. In addition to being a powerful *lipolytic* (fat-mobilizing)[1,2,3,4] and *anabolic* (muscle-enhancing)[5,6,7,8] hormone in both men and women, growth hormone supports immune function.[9,10,11,12] Furthermore, new research indicates that growth hormone status directly influences cholesterol and triglyceride levels,[13,14,15] and in a 1999 study published in the *Journal of Clinical Endocrinology and Metabolism* growth hormone replacement reversed early-stage atherosclerosis.[16] Unfortunately, growth hormone tends to decline with advancing age[17,18,19,20] causing adverse changes in body composition, immune function, and coronary risk factors.

Beginning in 1958, growth hormone injections were used to treat children with a condition known as growth hormone deficiency syndrome, which results in stunted growth. It was an effective treatment, but there was one problem: the only source of human growth hormone was the brains of cadavers. It took thousands of dead brains to obtain a few drops of growth hormone. What is worse, the growth hormone supply became contaminated by the deadly virus that causes Creutzfeld-Jakob or "mad cow" disease. When, consequently, three children who were taking GH extracts died, it was a no-brainer for the FDA: distribution of growth hormone was banned. With the cadaver source lost, and with no living person generous enough to donate his or her brain, growth hormone had to be created from scratch, an impossible task at the time.

In the 1980s, the impossible became possible, owing to the advent of genetic engineering. In 1985, synthetic growth hormone became the second recombinant DNA drug to be developed (insulin was the first). Having successfully cloned the growth hormone gene, the stage was set for an experiment that would make scientists gasp in astonishment.

In July 1990, the *New England Journal of Medicine*[21] published the results of one of the more important experiments of the 20th century. **It marked the first time that a therapy was proven to reverse aging**. What is meant by "proven" is that it met the gold standard of drug testing: randomized, double-blind, placebo-controlled, clinical study in human beings. (Although there are many other highly-touted anti-aging supplements and drugs - including the hormones melatonin, DHEA, and pregnenolone - none has been *proven* to alter the course of aging in *human beings*.)

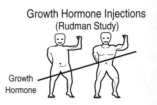

Growth Hormone Injections
(Rudman Study)

Growth
Hormone

This landmark study was conducted by an endocrinologist named Daniel Rudman, who was seeking to prove his hypothesis, published five years earlier in the *Journal of American Geriatrics Society,*[22] that hormonal decline is the root cause of the physical deterioration associated with aging. The study consisted of twelve elderly men receiving injections of growth hormone three times per week for six months. The results were breathtaking.

The subjects lost an average of 14.4% bodyfat and gained 8.8% lean body mass without diet or exercise.[23] In addition to dramatic body composition changes, which included a significant increase in bone density and muscle mass, the men experienced a measurable improvement in skin tone.[24] A follow-up study by Rudman revealed that the results of growth hormone therapy went much deeper: not only did the men *look* younger, they *became* younger internally: their organs grew back to youthful size![25]

You may be surprised (and none too pleased) to learn that, as you age, not only do your muscles shrink but so do your internal organs due to a reduction in protein synthesis.[26,27,28] Between the ages of 30 and 75, the liver, kidneys, brain, and pancreas atrophy by 30% on average.[29] As disquieting as this is, it's not the worst of it. More unsettling is the fact that organ shrinkage results in diminished functional capacity, including the ability of glands to produce hormones. Thus, a mutually aggravating cycle exists between organ atrophy and hormonal decline. However, the "chicken or the egg" question is academic here because we know, Rudman's studies and others, that hormonal enhancement can revive flagging organs. As an anti-aging strategy, Natural Hormonal Enhancement seeks to redirect this self-perpetuating cycle away from degeneration toward regeneration.

As you can see, aging is associated with functional impairments throughout the body, which herald descent into the gloomy abyss of old age. This explains why becoming older is such a horrid thought for most people. In addition to reduced hormonal output and organ atrophy, the age-related physiological downslide includes weakening of the immune system and diminished ability to metabolize sugar and cholesterol and to neutralize toxins. Fortunately, this downward spiral (or "general meltdown" as my friend Jeff Northcutt calls it) is now known to be a function of hormonal decline, *and is reversible*.

In interviews with reporters, one subject of the Rudman study, a 65-year-old man, reported that his gray hair was turning black. The wife of another man complained that she was having trouble keeping-up with her newly energized husband, even though she was fifteen years younger than him. Rudman and his colleagues wrote, in bold language reprinted in newspapers around the world, that the results were "equivalent in magnitude to the changes incurred during 10 to 20 years of aging."[30] Indeed, the invincibility of aging had been shattered. Subsequent studies in men and women have confirmed the rejuvenative effects of human growth hormone.[31,32,33]

In a sense, the men in the Rudman study had physiologically stepped back in time, morphing into their younger selves. In the wake of this landmark study, and media reports that the "fountain of youth" had been discovered, growth hormone clinics began popping-up all over the world, especially in Europe and Mexico (to avoid FDA restrictions, most of which have since been removed due to intense lobbying by drug companies). It may seem like we are on the verge of conquering aging with growth hormone injections. But are we? Are growth hormone injections the anti-aging breakthrough of the century, or in the words of Dr. Michael Colgan, "the health care farce of the century"?[34]

Several alarming and disturbing facts about this so-called "fountain of youth" exist. There is what might be called a "darker side" to this story, which has received little attention. Yes, you *can* tap into the phenomenal benefits of hormonal enhancement. But first you must understand the distinction between *exogenous* hormones and *endogenous* hormones.

Exogenous Hormones vs. Endogenous Hormones

Exogenous Hormones Exogenous hormones come into the body from outside and can cause a world of problems. (Anabolic steroids, insulin, and the growth hormone injections described above, are examples of exogenous hormones.) The problems with exogenous hormones stem from the fact that your body cannot control them - it cannot make the hormone jump back into the needle or pill bottle. All your body can do to counteract the incoming hormone is decrease or shut-off internal (endogenous) production of that particular hormone. (These natural counterregulatory mechanisms are called *feedback loops*.) If there is still too much hormone floating around after the body shuts-off internal production, a very unhealthy situation exists. In addition, no matter how carefully an exogenous hormone is administered, it cannot precisely mimic the subtle ebb and flow of naturally produced hormones. The human body is exquisitely sensitive to hormonal fluctuations. As long as your body is in control, as with Natural Hormonal Enhancement, there is no problem. But when you intake hormones, you bypass all your body's finely tuned control mechanisms; and you can upset your entire endocrine system, with potentially grave consequences.

If you take the hormone for a long enough period of time, then once you stop taking it, your body does not resume making the hormone. (Remember "use it or lose it?" - well, at this point you lost it.) When that happens, you are hooked for life on taking the hormone (a very profitable situation for the dealer of the steroids, growth hormone, etc.). Even if you do not completely lose the capacity to produce the hormone, it takes a while to come back.

And until it does, you suffer a *shortage* of that hormone, during which time all of the positive effects are reversed - just ask any ex-steroid user. As you can see, exogenous hormones are risky and have an effect *opposite* to Natural Hormonal Enhancement, by impairing, rather than enhancing, natural production of hormones.

Endogenous Hormones These are the natural hormones produced by the body. Unless you have an endocrine infirmity (like diabetes, hypogonadism, Cushing's disease or Addison's disease), your hormones can never rise too high or fall too low because your body regulates hormones in the same way a thermostat regulates temperature - it allows fluctuations within a set range. You can naturally enhance endogenous hormones from "low-normal" to "high-normal," but never above normal. **You influence endogenous hormones every day of your life.**

The Untold Story: Fountain of Youth Proves Toxic

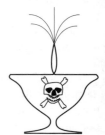

Now that you understand why *exogenous* hormones are dangerous, you should not be surprised to learn that more than half of Rudman's subjects dropped out of the experiment within a year due to side effects. (Carpel tunnel syndrome, fluid retention, high blood pressure, joint pain, hyperglycemia, and pancreatitis are some of the side effects of injected growth hormone.) In addition, when the growth hormone injections were discontinued, the mens' bodies fast-forwarded "back" to old age; they lost all the benefits of the injections. A subsequent study, entitled "Fountain of Youth Proves Toxic" also found serious side effects consequent to growth hormone administration, and the authors of this study concluded that the drawbacks outweighed the benefits.[35] Why was all this negative information unpublicized? Why are we only hearing half the story? And why are growth hormone clinics proliferating at a wild pace? Because drug companies and unscrupulous practitioners are hellbent on realizing the massive profit potential of growth hormone, and they have no intention of letting the truth get in their way.

Many of the side effects suffered by Rudman's subjects have been avoided in subsequent studies by using lower-dose regimens. Even so, as Bengtsson et. al., point-out in their 1999 study, "GH replacement therapy is well-tolerated in adults...however, it is possible that some adverse events may not become evident over the time scale covered by the present analysis."[36] Good point – especially when one considers that most of the people who suffer adverse health consequences from taking anabolic steroids (another exogenous hormone) are perfectly fine in the short term. Many toxic substances that inflict severe harm in the long term are "well-tolerated" in the short term.

The scientific literature is filled with cautionary reports of health problems associated with exogenous growth hormone[37,38,39,40,41,42,43,44] - the most troubling relating to diabetes and cancer. And while the linkage between growth hormone replacement and disease is not conclusive, there are no studies affirming its long-term safety either. To the contrary, based on 1) what we know about the physiological problems inherent in exogenous hormones (see above) 2) decades of experience with estrogen, anabolic steroids, and insulin, all of which carry significant risks 3) the research developed thus far regarding the side effects and possible long-term consequences of growth hormone injections; I must regretfully conclude that unsuspecting human beings are being used as guinea pigs in the service of the all-mighty dollar.

8

Additionally, growth hormone injections are financially costly and entail the unpleasant inconvenience of shooting-up. Therefore, and in light of the fact that the benefits disappear when you quit the injections, you are essentially looking at an expensive lifetime drug habit, fraught with a litany of undesirable side effects. *In the final analysis, enhancing growth hormone is a terrific idea with far-reaching benefits. The key is naturally to stimulate your body to upgrade growth hormone production, rather than rolling the dice with your health and incurring the lifetime expense of exogenously administering it.*

References

1. Goldman JK, Bressler R. Growth Hormone Stimulation of Fatty Acid Utilization by Adipose Tissue. *Endocrinology* 1967;81:1306.

2. Snyder DK, Underwood LE, Clemmons DR. Persistent Lipolytic Effect of Exogenous Growth Hormone during Caloric Restriction. *Am J Med* 1995;98:129.

3. Gravholt CH, et al. Effects of a Physiological GH Pulse on Interstitial Glycerol in Abdominal and Femoral Adipose Tissue. *Am J Physiol* 1999;277:E848.

4. Piatti PM, et al. Mediation of the Hepatic Effects of Growth Hormone by its Lipolytic Activity. *J Clin Endocrinol Metab* 1999;84:1658.

5. Snyder DK, Underwood LE, Clemmons DR. Anabolic Effects of Growth Hormone in Obese Diet-Restricted Subjects are Dose Dependent. *Am J Clin Nutr* 1990;52:431.

6. Welle S. Growth Hormone and Insulin-Like Growth Factor-I as Anabolic Agents. *Curr Opin Clin Nutr Metab Care* 1998;1:257.

7. Johannsson G, Bengtsson BA, Ahlmen J. Double-Blind, Placebo-Controlled Study of Growth Hormone Treatment in Elderly Patients Undergoing Chronic Hemodialysis: Anabolic Effect and Functional Improvement. *Am J Kidney Dis* 1999;33:709.

8. Ghio L, et al. Short-Term Anabolic Effects of Recombinant Human Growth Hormone in Young Patients with a Renal Transplant. *Transpl Int* 1998;11(Suppl):S69.

9. Crist DM, et al. Exogenous Growth Hormone Treatment Alters Body Composition and Increases Natural Killer Cell Activity in Women with Impaired Endogenous Growth Hormone Secretion. *Metabolism* 1987;36:1115.

10. Crist DM, Kraner JC. Supplemental Growth Hormone Increases the Tumor Cytotoxic Activity of Natural Killer Cells in Healthy Adults with Normal Growth Hormone Secretion. *Metabolism* 1990;39:1320.

11. Auernhammer CJ, Strasburger CJ. Effects of Growth Hormone and Insulinlike Growth Factor I on the Immune System. *Eur J Endocrinol* 1995;133:635.

12. Kelley KW, et al. GH3 Pituitary Adenoma Implants Can Reverse Thymic Aging. *Proc Nat Acad Sci* 1986;83:5663.

13. Vahl N, et al. Growth Hormone (GH) Status is an Independent Determinant of Serum Levels of Cholesterol and Triglycerides in Healthy Adults. *Clin Endocrinol (Oxf)* 1999;51:309.

14. Vahl N, et al. The Favourable Effects of Growth Hormone (GH) Substitution on Hypercholesterolaemia in GH-Deficient Adults are Not Associated with Concomitant Reductions in Adiposity. A 12 Month Placebo-Controlled Study. *Int J Obes Relat Metab Disord* 1998;22:529.

15. O'Connor KG, et al. Interrelationships of Spontaneous Growth Hormone Axis Activity, Body Fat, and Serum Lipids in Healthy Elderly Women and Men. *Metabolism* 1999;48:1424.

16. Pfeifer M, et al. Growth Hormone (GH) Treatment Reverses Early Atherosclerotic Changes in GH-Deficient Adults. *J Clin Endocrinol Metab* 1999;84:453.

17. Russell-Aulet M, et al. In Vivo Semiquantification of Hypothalamic Growth Hormone-Releasing Hormone (GHRH) Output in Humans: Evidence for Relative GHRH Deficiency in Aging. *J Clin Endocrinol Metab* 1999;84:3490.

18. Bando H, et al. Impaired Secretion of Growth Hormone-Releasing Hormone, Growth Hormone and IGF-I in Elderly Men. *Acta Endocrinol (Copenh)* 1991;124:31.

19. Martin FC, Yeo AL, Sonksen PH. Growth Hormone Secretion in the Elderly: Ageing and the Somatopause. *Baillieres Clin Endocrinol Metab* 1997;11:223.

20. Sonntag WE, et al. Decreased Pulsatile Release of Growth Hormone in Old Male Rats. *Endocrinology* 1980;107:1875.

21. Rudman D, et al. Effects of Human Growth Hormone in Men over 60 Years Old. *N Engl J Med* 1990;323:1.

22. Rudman D. Growth Hormone, Body Composition, and Aging. *J Am Geriat Soc* 1985;33:800.

23. See, supra, note 21.

24. Id.

25. Rudman D, et al. Effects of Human Growth Hormone on Body Composition in Elderly Men. *Horm Res* 1991;36(Suppl):73S.

26. Rattan SI, Derventzi A, Clark BF. Protein Synthesis, Posttranslational Modifications, and Aging. *Ann N Y Acad Sci* 1992;663:48.

27. Parrado J, et al. Effects of Aging on the Various Steps of Protein Synthesis: Fragmentation of Elongation Factor 2. *Free Radic Biol Med* 1999;26:362.

28. Blazejowski CA, Webster GC. Decreased Rates of Protein Synthesis by Cell-Free Preparations from Different Organs of Aging Mice. *Mech Ageing Dev* 1983;21:345.

29. Klatz R. *Grow Young with HGH*. NY: Harper Collins 1997, p. 103-104.

30. See, supra, note 21.

31. Binnerts A, et al. The Effect of Growth Hormone Administration in Growth Hormone Deficient Adults on Bone, Protein, Carbohydrate and Lipid Homeostasis, as Well as on Body Composition. *Clin Endocrinol (Oxf)* 1992;37:79.

32. Baum HB, et al. Effects of Physiologic Growth Hormone Therapy on Bone Density and Body Composition in Patients with Adult-Onset Growth Hormone Deficiency. A Randomized, Placebo-Controlled Trial. *Ann Intern Med* 1996;125:883.

33. Cuttica CM, et al. Effects of Six-Month Administration of Recombinant Human Growth Hormone to Healthy Elderly Subjects. *Aging (Milano)* 1997;9:193.

34. Colgan M. *Hormonal Health*. BC Canada: Apple Publishing 1996, p. 194.

35. Yarasheski KE, Zachwieja JJ. Growth Hormone Therapy for the Elderly: The Fountain of Youth Proves Toxic. *JAMA* 1993;270:1694

36. Bengtsson BA, et al. GH Replacement in 1034 Growth Hormone Deficient Hypopituitary Adults: Demographic and Clinical Characteristics, Dosing and Safety. *Clin Endocrinol (Oxf)* 1999;50:703.

37. Malozowski S, et al. Acute Pancreatitis Associated with Growth Hormone Therapy for Short Stature. *N Engl J Med* 1995;332:401.

38. Shalet SM, Brennan BM, Reddingius RE. Growth Hormone Therapy and Malignancy. *Horm Res* 1997;48 (Suppl):29.

39. Hasegawa T, et al. Malignant Thymoma in a Patient with Growth Hormone Deficiency during Growth Hormone Therapy. *Eur J Pediatr* 1993;152:802.

40. Mills JL, et al. Status Report on the US Human Growth Hormone Recipient Follow-Up Study. *Horm Res* 1990;33:116.

41. Lehmann S, Cerra FB. Growth Hormone and Nutritional Support: Adverse Metabolic Effects. *Nutr Clin Pract* 1992;7:27.

42. Stahnke N, Zeisel HJ. Growth Hormone Therapy and Leukaemia. *Eur J Pediatr* 1989;148:591.

43. Boose AR, et al. [Growth Hormone Therapy and Leukemia]. *Tijdschr Kindergeneeskd* 1992;60:1. Dutch.

44. Demling RH. Comparison of the Anabolic Effects and Complications of Human Growth Hormone and the Testosterone Analog, Oxandrolone, after Severe Burn Injury. *Burns* 1999;25:215.

Chapter 3 - Growth Hormone and the Hormonal Revolution

Chapter 4

Putting Your Hormonal Army to Work for You

Every great advance in science has issued from a new audacity of imagination.
John Dewey

When we were young, you made me blush, go hot and cold, and turn to mush.
I still feel these things it's true, but is it menopause, or is it you?
Susan D. Anderson

They say aging is a one-way street. If that's true,
this is the one instance in which I don't mind waiting at stop lights.
Unknown

Hormonal Synergy

Growth hormone declines with advancing age in every animal species tested to date. The rate of decline varies with the individual, and is dictated by genetic and environmental/lifestyle factors. The steeper the drop-off in growth hormone, the more rapidly and visibly you age. Not only does growth hormone decline directly promote aging, but because all hormones are interconnected (a phenomenon called *hormonal synergy*) the fall in growth hormone has a ripple effect throughout the entire endocrine system. Conversely, enhancing growth hormone has a revitalizing effect on other hormones.

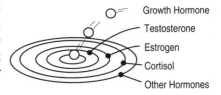

Growth Hormone
Testosterone
Estrogen
Cortisol
Other Hormones

Growth Hormone and Testosterone

A positive relationship exists between growth hormone and testosterone in men. Enhancing testosterone levels directly increases growth hormone levels.[1,2,3,4,5,6] Conversely, enhancing growth hormone exerts a more subtle positive effect on testosterone levels by bolstering *gonadotropins*, hormones that direct the testes to produce testosterone and sperm;[7,8,9] and by suppressing cortisol,[10] a hormone antagonistic to testosterone (see Chapter 22). Functionally, growth hormone and testosterone work together to build muscle[11] and bone,[12] and to facilitate fat burning.[13]

To illustrate the functional cooperation between growth hormone and testosterone, in studies of growth retardation testosterone fails to promote growth absent growth hormone.[14] In addition to being dependent on growth hormone for potentiation of its anabolic properties, testosterone's *androgenic* (sexual) action is impaired where growth hormone is deficient.[15] Hence, it is accurate to say that growth hormone and testosterone are "friendly" or complementary hormones. You will see shortly how this fact comes into play in the Natural Hormonal Enhancement strategy.

Growth Hormone and Estrogen

The relationship between growth hormone and estrogen is of great interest given widespread use of estrogen and growing popularity of growth hormone. Ostensibly, estrogen and growth hormone are complementary like testosterone and growth hormone. Estrogen and growth hormone levels are directly correlated (with both hormones higher in younger women than in older women), and administration of estrogen increases growth hormone.[16,17,18] Now for the confusing part: oral estrogen increases growth hormone via "negative feedback inhibition" by suppressing growth hormone's "sister hormone," IGF-1.[19,20] This probably accounts for conflicting studies showing estrogen assists[21] and opposes[22,23] the metabolic effects of growth hormone. The estrogen/growth hormone relationship is an example of the human body's penchant for throwing researchers curveballs and change-ups.

Chapter 11 explains that many of the beneficial effects of growth hormone are actually carried-out by IGF-1. This raises the dilemma of whether it's better to have higher growth hormone levels and lower IGF-1 levels, or lower growth hormone levels and higher IGF-1 levels. This inquiry is foreign to most practitioners, because higher growth hormone levels are associated with higher IGF-1 levels and vice versa. The question of the relative importance of growth hormone versus IGF-1 has long been a provocative one. But it has assumed a new dimension of practical significance insofar as it influences hormone replacement therapy dosages, especially where estrogen and growth hormone are administered together. (Specifically, if the objective is to raise IGF-1 levels in a woman taking oral estrogen, more growth hormone is necessary in order to counter the suppressive effect of oral estrogen.[24] If, however, the objective is to raise growth hormone levels, then a lower dose of growth hormone, or no dose at all, would be appropriate because estrogen raises growth hormone.)

To further muddy the waters, when progesterone is administered along with estrogen the effect on GH/IGF-1 changes. Progesterone offsets the suppressive effect of oral estrogen on IGF-1.[25,26] And to make matters even more complicated, transdermal and oral estrogen differ significantly in their effects on GH/IGF-1.[27,28] This difference is surely related to the fact that oral estrogen does a "first pass" through the liver, and the liver is the primary site of manufacture of IGF-1. The delivery-dependent difference in the effect of estrogen on GH/IGF-1 bears important implications for the long-term benefit of estrogen replacement therapy.

Hormone Replacement or Not?

Whether to correct an age-related hormonal deficiency by exogenous means is a difficult and controversial question; and it entails a weighing of risks (see "Exogenous Hormones vs. Endogenous Hormones," in Chapter 3). The argument in favor is stronger with respect to estrogen than testosterone or growth hormone for a couple of reasons. For one, testosterone in men and growth hormone can be naturally enhanced in older people whereas, after menopause, estrogen cannot. In addition, the "feedback problem" discussed in the last chapter, in which exogenous hormone administration causes the body to shut-down natural production, does not apply to estrogen because after menopause natural production shuts-down anyway. Nonetheless, there are always potential adverse side effects and long-term risks to be considered when hormones are taken into the body. A weighing of the risks of estrogen replacement against its benefits is beyond the scope of this book. But because of the magnitude of this decision in a woman's life, I will attempt to offer some helpful insight.

The Question Every Woman Faces: Estrogen Replacement or Not?

A properly formulated hormone replacement program can help ward-off two of the most prolific killers of postmenopausal women, cardiovascular disease and osteoporosis. Both of these diseases are relatively uncommon in premenopausal women. But after menopause, the risk of each jumps drastically. Hormonal changes, particularly the drop in estrogen, facilitate development of cardiovascular disease[29,30] and osteoporosis[31,32] in the postmenopausal period. Estrogen replacement has also been shown to improve cognitive function in older women,[33] and to reduce the risk of colorectal cancer (the second leading cause of cancer death in the United States[34]).[35,36]

While a "properly formulated" postmenopausal hormone replacement regimen can improve quality of life and combat degenerative disease, many hormone replacement regimens are not properly formulated. Errant replacement formulations can increase, rather than decrease, risk of disease. One problem involves dosage. As with testosterone and growth hormone, there are substantial inter-individual variations in estrogen levels. And just as many doctors miss this point when prescribing testosterone or growth hormone, they often commit the same oversight in relation to estrogen.

A woman's individual estrogen-replacement needs, determined by reference to her youthful levels, is often not taken into account or is crudely estimated by her doctor based on population-wide data. A particular dose of estrogen that is insufficient to offset menopausal decline in one woman may be excessive in another woman. In fact, there is evidence showing that, for many women, their doctor's prescription constitutes an "overdose." Too much estrogen relative to a woman's youthful physiological level can cause serious problems, and is responsible for many of the adverse side effects and long-term risks associated with estrogen replacement.

Youthful Level Baseline

At least three studies emerged in 1999 indicating that maximum hormone-replacement-generated protection against cardiovascular disease[37] and osteoporosis[38,39] can be achieved at very low doses. This view was publicly advanced by Dr. Michael Colgan in his 1996 book *Hormonal Health*,[40] in which he argued that optimal benefit from estrogen can be achieved at dosages ½ to ¼ as much as is commonly prescribed. Colgan also argues for the need to accompany exogenous estrogen with progesterone (natural not synthetic) and testosterone, both of which also decline after menopause.

I will defer to my esteemed colleague and his fine book for presentation of the specifics of this issue. On a conceptual level, I would refer to my repeated emphasis throughout this book that the hormonal system is an integrated and interconnected whole. Pursuant to this overriding principle, it is fundamentally unsound to replace exogenously one hormone while ignoring other hormones that are similarly no longer being naturally produced within the body. This has an unbalancing effect on your endocrine system. *Natural Hormonal Enhancement* contains numerous examples of how hormones operate in intricate patterns of cooperation and opposition. An example relevant to the present discussion is how progesterone works *with* estrogen favorably to preserve bone[41,42]; but works *against* estrogen unfavorably by blunting estrogen's beneficial effect on cholesterol levels,[43] and favorably by restraining estrogen's tendency to cause endometrial overgrowth and other hyperplasic changes associated with cancer.[44,45]

In summary, along with undue estrogen dosages, selective enhancement of estrogen to the exclusion of other menopausally diminished hormones is a source of much unnecessary suffering for women. Many doctors need to have their eyes pried open on this issue, and Dr. Colgan's research, presented in his book *Hormonal Health*, is a lever for doing that. I recommend *Hormonal Health* to each woman, and her doctor, confronted with the decision whether to undertake hormone replacement therapy.

13

Somatopause vs. Menopause

Like female menopause, age-related growth hormone decline in both sexes is predictable and its effects profound. For this reason, it has been given a similar name, "somatopause." Two differences between growth hormone decline and estrogen decline are *rate* and *reversibility*. Whereas estrogen drops like a stone, growth hormone descends slowly, taking other hormones and your youthfulness with it. And whereas the estrogen drop is unavoidable by natural means, growth hormone decline is now more a matter of choice than a fact of human destiny.

Actually, growth hormone production begins to fall-off long before we begin to "age" in the conventional sense of the word. Levels of this hormone are highest during the first and second years of life.[46] Growth hormone levels remain high during childhood and adolescence, powering the physical development that attends those life stages. The downward creep begins in early adulthood.

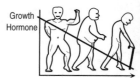

Absent hormonal enhancement measures, daily growth hormone production in men and women declines by about 14% per decade, so that by sixty years of age the average person's growth hormone output is less than 50% of what it was at twenty years of age.[47] By eighty years of age, the pituitary is squeezing-out about 25 micrograms per day, 5% as much as at age twenty - barely enough to grow a fingernail. The relentless decline of growth hormone and other hormones continues further, bridging the gap between old age and the grave.

Reversing Growth Hormone Decline

Many theories have been put forth to explain why growth hormone production drops-off with advancing age;[48] but as yet a consensus has not coalesced among researchers regarding the physiological mechanism responsible. What we do know is that growth hormone decline is not inevitable and can be reversed. Studies show that old pituitary somatotrophe cells (the cells that produce growth hormone) are capable of releasing as much growth hormone as young somatotrophe cells if adequately stimulated.[49,50,51] Dietary, exercise, lifestyle, and nutritional supplementation strategies are proven means of restoring growth hormone and other hormones to youthful levels.

Important as growth hormone is, it's only one in your hormonal ensemble. There are many others. If you're thinking it would require a ten-year course in endocrinology to learn how to get all these hormones working for you, remember "hormonal synergy," discussed earlier. "Good" hormones stimulate other "good" hormones; "bad" hormones stimulate other "bad" hormones. *This hormonal "ripple effect" enables you to get your entire hormonal army working for you in the battle against aging, disease, and excess bodyfat.*

14

You cannot permanently reduce bodyfat unless you alter the hormonal environment inside your body away from fat storage toward fat burning.

If, like the majority of Americans, you are currently losing the fight against fat it is probably because lipogenic hormones are dominant and they are sending the message: STORE FAT. As long as this message prevails, trying to lose fat will be like trying to walk up a downward-moving escalator. Because cells must obey hormonal directives, the only solution is to change these signals. This is not difficult task so long as you're willing to discard old beliefs and practices and embrace a new approach to fat loss. When you change the hormonal message from "store fat" to "burn fat," fat loss is natural and inevitable.

Principles of Natural Hormonal Enhancement: An Overview

♦ *Practically everything that goes on inside your body is regulated by hormones; they are the most powerful biological agents known to science.*

♦ *Hormones exert a dominant influence on body composition and aging.*

♦ *Many hormones that have a favorable effect on body composition, like growth hormone and testosterone/estrogen, also have other beneficial effects in connection with energy levels, aging, health, and sexual performance/reproductive function. Other hormones are "double-edged swords," like glucagon and insulin. With these two-faced hormones, the operative strategy is "optimization."*

♦ *Optimization is a key strategy of Natural Hormonal Enhancement. Optimization means maximizing the good while minimizing the bad. Optimization acknowledges and effectively addresses the fact that individual hormones perform several different functions and that some hormones can be either friend or foe, or a combination of both.*

♦ *The entire hormonal system is interconnected. Therefore, a change in one hormone equals a change in all hormones. This is the principle of hormonal synergy.*

♦ *Hormonal synergy works in such a way that "good" hormones tend to be mutually-reinforcing, and so do "bad" hormones. In effect, all hormonal effects are multiplied, either positively or negatively. This is why Natural Hormonal Enhancement is such a powerful force for good. It is also why your current dietary, exercise, and lifestyle practices may be a powerful force for bad.*

♦ *You have a great deal of control over hormonal status. In fact, every day of your life you influence your hormone levels, whether you realize it or not. By extension, you influence the composition and condition of your body. The problem is you are currently doing it haphazardly. If you have excess bodyfat, low energy levels, weak muscles, diminished sex drive, or look older than most people your age, chances are your uninformed shotgun method of hormonal manipulation is not working very well.*

Muscle Axis and Fat Axis: The Conceptual Foundation
MUSCLE AXIS
(Anabolic and Catabolic Hormones)

Anabolic Hormones   The word anabolic has gained notoriety as the word that usually precedes the word "steroids." This negative connotation is unwarranted. Anabolic hormones, like all hormones, are dangerous only when they enter the body from outside, thereby circumventing the body's system of checks and balances. Internally produced anabolic hormones favorably affect body composition, and they are central to the Natural Hormonal Enhancement anti-aging strategy.

Anabolism is a healthy process that goes on regularly inside your body, driven by naturally secreted anabolic hormones. Anabolism involves the growth, maintenance, and repair of cells and tissues by means of protein synthesis. Anabolic hormones maintain not only muscles, but also bones, connective tissues, and internal organs. As anabolic hormone production declines with advancing age, the strength, integrity, and functional capacity of the structures that comprise the human body diminish. It is the drop-off in anabolic hormone production (and the relative increase in catabolic hormones) that is responsible for the loss of the shapely, toned, firm look of youth, and the descent into the feeble frailty of old age.

The new, enlightened conception of aging views the debility and infirmity of old age as a result of an accumulation of damage at the cellular level. The cells' ability to function depends on the genetic material, DNA, which codes for all proteins, hormones, and enzymes essential to life. DNA is under continual assault from highly reactive oxygen atoms called free radicals. DNA has the ability to repair itself, but over time the damage accumulates. The basis for the proposition that antioxidants combat aging and help prevent disease is that they offset this cumulative damage process by neutralizing free radicals. While there is considerable merit to this theory, the latest research suggests that the anabolic hormones growth hormone and IGF-1 are far more powerful weapons in the battle against aging.

Whereas antioxidants can minimize damage to cells by countering free-radical-related oxidation, growth hormone and IGF-1 can "get under the hood" of the cells and repair damaged DNA. In this way, the aging process is directly counteracted. Conversely, if you allow growth hormone and IGF-1 to decline with age, cellular repair and renovation lags behind cellular damage and decay. The result is the degenerative process commonly referred to as "aging."

Natural Hormonal Enhancement aims naturally to enhance anabolic hormones as a means of building stronger, firmer, and more shapely muscles while combating aging and reducing bodyfat. Regarding building muscle, men can substantially increase muscle mass while women can only marginally, because of vastly differing testosterone/estrogen ratios between the sexes. Nonetheless, the three other anabolic hormones - growth hormone, insulin, and IGF-1 - are very important to women (and men) in their pursuit of a leaner, firmer, physiologically younger body.

16

Catabolic Hormones The opposite of anabolism, catabolism involves the breakdown of cells and tissues. Much of the muscle-wasting that attends disease and aging is attributable to catabolic hormones run amuck. While a certain level of catabolic activity is normal and healthy, misguided dietary, exercise, and lifestyle practices can elevate these hormones to a level at which they become detrimental to health and physique.

In addition to eating-away precious muscle tissue, high levels of catabolic hormones promote fat storage by reducing insulin sensitivity and can devastate the immune system. The pro-aging/anti-immunity effects of catabolic hormones, as well as the deleterious impact they can have on your physique, are graphically illustrated in patients with Cushing's syndrome, a disorder marked by abnormally high levels of cortisol, the chief catabolic hormone. Individuals with this disease experience premature aging, impaired wound healing, and abdominal obesity coupled with thin, wasted extremities.

Muscular development and health can be enhanced and aging can be meaningfully opposed by learning how naturally to keep catabolic hormones in check. And this is exactly what *Natural Hormonal Enhancement* teaches.

FAT AXIS
(Lipogenic and Lipolytic Hormones)

Lipogenic Hormones "Genesis" is Latin for "birth." Lipogenesis literally means "the birth of fat." These hormones make you fat and keep you fat. They *make* you fat by directing your body to store fat. They *keep* you fat by directing your body to burn sugar preferentially, as opposed to fat. Stated differently, lipogenic hormones make you a "sugar-burner" instead of a "fat-burner."

In the scope of human history, the widespread and ready availability of food is a very recent phenomenon, owed to mechanized agriculture and mass production of processed foodstuffs. In this milieu, in which people are more likely to eat themselves to death than starve to death, lipogenesis is more of a curse than a blessing. Insulin, the chief lipogenic hormone, is largely responsible for obesity and has been linked to other, more directly deadly diseases such as diabetes, heart disease, and cancer (see Chapter 8, 10, 11). In poorer countries, and the few remaining primitive societies in the world today, the incidence of degenerative diseases and obesity is far less than in industrialized societies. While there are many reasons for this disparity, sharply different dietary patterns and consequently differing hormonal responses to eating is a significant factor, and will be explored in subsequent chapters.

Insulin is not only lipogenic, but also anabolic. Therefore, the anti-insulin mentality advanced by the popular but relatively ineffective low-carbohydrate diet is misguided. Natural Hormonal Enhancement seeks to *optimize* insulin, which means exploiting its benefits while avoiding its detriments.

Unfortunately, out-of-control insulin levels, the true enemy of health and fitness has, for the most part, eluded attention while practically everyone has fixated, instead, on dietary fat. What is worse, the low-fat craze that has prevailed during the last twenty years has made matters worse by popularizing a form of eating that stimulates excessive insulin release. This is the principal reason why Americans have become fatter while cutting-back on dietary fat over the last two decades. It is also why well over 90% of people who go on a low-fat diet either fail to lose fat or regain every pound, and sometimes more, within six months of discontinuing the diet.

Lipolytic Hormones The opposite of lipogenesis, lipolysis involves the mobilization of fat for use as fuel. Fat is the human body's optimal fuel source for most daily activities and it yields higher energy levels than does glucose, the body's other fuel source. By naturally activating lipolytic hormones you can rid yourself of excess bodyfat, tap into unlimited energy, and prevent the accumulation of fat (triglyceride) in the blood thereby reducing a major coronary risk factor.

Taking a Turn for the Hearse, or Turning Back the Clock?

Hormonal changes for the worse are the main cause of the degenerative process we call "aging." Specifically, absent proper intervention, the following hormonal changes occur with advancing age.

- The ratio of catabolic hormones to anabolic hormones increases, causing people to shrink, wither, and deteriorate as they get older.

- The ratio of lipogenic hormones to lipolytic hormones increases, causing people to become fatter as they get older.

Change in Body Composition with Advancing Age

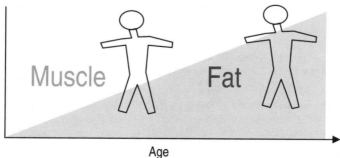

Muscle   Fat

Age

Change in Hormonal Status with Advancing Age

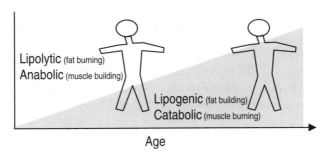

Lipolytic (fat burning)
Anabolic (muscle building)

Lipogenic (fat building)
Catabolic (muscle burning)

Age

In the words of Ronald Klatz, M.D.:

An aging body is like the creation of a Michelangelo sculpture, only in reverse - you move from the chiseled body of your youth back to a marble blob.[52]

It is widely believed that people gain weight as they get older. In fact, this is not completely true. People become fatter with advancing age,[53,54] but not necessarily heavier.* Concurrent with the age-related increase in bodyfat, men and women experience a loss of muscle, called *sarcopenia*.[55,56] From young adulthood to old age, human beings lose approximately 30% of their muscle mass.[57,58,59] Age-related muscle loss is the same for both sexes on a percentage basis. However, because women have less muscle mass, sarcopenia has a more severe physiological impact on them.

These two trends are interrelated insofar as the age-related decrease in metabolic rate, which promotes fat gain, is largely caused by loss of muscle.[60,61] As significant as are these body composition alterations, they are often not reflected, or are understated, by the scale. Because muscle weighs more than fat, many people remain about the same weight as they get older. Their bodyfat percentage increases, however, making them fatter, mushier, and weaker - more like a blob and less like a sculpture.

For those people who *do* gain weight as they get older, the weight gain generally indicates that they are growing fatter so rapidly that fat gain is outpacing the age-related loss of muscle, despite the fact that muscle weighs more than fat. These two trends, muscle loss and fat gain reflect the two hormonal trends discussed above: "fat axis" shifts toward lipogenic hormones away from lipolytic hormones, "muscle axis" shifts toward catabolic hormones away from anabolic hormones. *The key to combating aging successfully is to enhance anabolic and lipolytic hormones to counter the unfavorable shifting of the "muscle axis" and "fat axis," respectively.*

* Do people become heavier with age? Yes and no. Body weight tends to increase into the sixth decade and then decline.[61a,61b] This biphasic trend reflects the fact that from young adulthood to middle age the increase in fat outweighs the loss of muscle. This makes sense given that anabolic hormonal output remains relatively stable until middle age. After that, the self-perpetuating "downward spiral" that I described earlier begins to take hold, and muscle loss accelerates.[61c] Because muscle weighs more than fat, body weight is likely to fall when you are losing muscle – even if you are gaining fat at the same time.

Natural Hormonal Enhancement

The other important point here is that **weight is largely meaningless as an index of fitness, health, physical attractiveness, or practically anything else related to human beings**. Unless you are an athlete aiming to compete in a certain weight class, what matters is body composition, not weight. Bodyfat percentage is a measure of body composition. Unlike weight, bodyfat percentage addresses the all-important question of what your body is made-up of, and provides insight into the status of your "muscle axis" and "fat axis." You will be better able to appreciate and apply the materials in this book if you banish from your mind the concept of "weight," and replace it with "body composition."

Natural Hormonal Enhancement Strategy in a Nutshell

The five hormones listed below exert a profound influence on your health, body composition, and rate of aging. As previously noted, you influence each of these hormones every day. But with Natural Hormonal Enhancement, you will be strategically managing them for maximum benefit. Note the effect of each of these hormones on your "fat axis" and "muscle axis."

	Hormone Properties						Strategy			
	Anabolic +	Catabolic −	Lipogenic −	Lipolytic +	Pro-Immunity +	Anti-Aging +	Men		Women	
HORMONE							Enhance	Suppress	Enhance	Suppress
Growth Hormone (good)	■			■	■		■		■	
Testosterone (good)	■			■		■	■			
Insulin (double-edged sword)	■		■				* Optimize		* Optimize	
Glucagon (double-edged sword)		■		■			** Optimize		** Optimize	
Cortisol (bad)		■	Indirectly Lipogenic		Anti-Immunity	Pro-Aging		■		■

* Optimize (enhance muscle-enhancing properties, suppress fat-storage properties)
** Optimize (enhance fat-burning properties, suppress muscle-breakdown properties)

NOTE - This is a simplified, schematic model. It is not intended to depict the human endocrine system in all of its intricate splendor, nor would a comprehensive inventory of hormones be helpful from a practical standpoint. Because the endocrine system is an integrated network (see discussion of hormonal synergy, above), it is not necessary specifically to target every hormone, only the main ones. And by doing so, you can effect far-reaching positive changes in your health and physique.

References

1. Grinspoon S, et al. Effects of Androgen Administration on the Growth Hormone-Insulin-Like Growth Factor I Axis in Men with Acquired Immunodeficiency Syndrome Wasting. *J Clin Endocrinol Metab* 1998;83:4251.

2. Liu L, Merriam GR, Sherins RJ. Chronic Sex Steroid Exposure Increases Mean Plasma Growth Hormone Concentration and Pulse Amplitude in Men with Isolated Hypogonadotropic Hypogonadism. *J Clin Endocrinol Metab* 1987;64:651.

3. Martin LG, et al. Effect of Androgen on Growth Hormone Secretion and Growth in Boys with Short Stature. *Acta Endocrinol* (Copenh) 1979;91:201.

4. Hobbs CJ, et al. Testosterone Administration Increases Insulin-like Growth Factor-1 Levels in Normal Men. *J Clin Endocrinol Metab* 1993;77:776.

5. Silva ME, et al. Effects of Testosterone on Growth Hormone Secretion and Somatomedin-C Generation in Prepubertal Growth Hormone Deficient Male Patients. *Braz J Med Biol Res* 1992;25:1117.

6. Ulloa-Aguirre A, et al. Testosterone and Oxandrolone, a Nonaromatizable Androgen, Specifically Amplify the Mass and Rate of Growth Hormone (GH) Secreted Per Burst without Altering GH Secretory Burst Duration or Frequency or the GH Half-Life. *J Clin Endocrinol Metab* 1990;71:846.

7. Ohyama K, et al. Effects of Growth Hormone and Insulin-Like Growth Factor I on Testosterone Secretion in Premature Male Rats. *Endocr J* 1995;42:817.

8. Balducci R, et al. The Effect of Growth Hormone Administration on Testicular Response during Gonadotropin Therapy in Subjects with Combined Gonadotropin and Growth Hormone Deficiencies. *Acta Endocrinol* (Copenh) 1993;128:19.

9. Shoham Z, et al. Cotreatment with Growth Hormone for Induction of Spermatogenesis in Patients with Hypogonadotropic Hypogonadism. *Fertil Steril* 1992;57:1044.

10. Vierhapper H, Nowotny P, Waldhausl W. Treatment with Growth Hormone Suppresses Cortisol Production in Man. *Metabolism* 1998;47:1376.

11. Klindt J, Ford JJ, Macdonald GJ. Synergism of Testosterone Propionate with Growth Hormone in Promoting Growth of Hypophysectomized Rats: Effect of Sexual Differentiation. *J Endocrinol* 1990;127:249.

12. Prakasam G, et al. Effects of Growth Hormone and Testosterone on Cortical Bone Formation and Bone Density in Aged Orchiectomized Rats. *Bone* 1999;24:491.

13. Yang S, et al. Additive Effects of Growth Hormone and Testosterone on Lipolysis in Adipocytes of Hypophysectomized Rats. *J Endocrinol* 1995;147:147.

14. Zachmann M, Prader A. Anabolic and Androgenic Effect of Testosterone in Sexually Immature Boys and its Dependency on Growth Hormone. *J Clin Endocrinol* 1970;30:85.

15. Blok GJ, et al. Growth Hormone Substitution in Adult Growth Hormone-Deficient Men Augments Androgen Effects on the Skin. *Clin Endocrinol (Oxf)* 1997;47:29.

16. Dawson-Hughes B, et al. Regulation of Growth Hormone and Somatomedin-C Secretion in Postmenopausal Women: Effect of Physiological Estrogen Replacement. *J Clin Endocrinol Metab* 1986;63:424.

17. Marin G, et al. The Effects of Estrogen Priming and Puberty on the Growth Hormone Response to Standardized Treadmill Exercise and Arginine-Insulin in Normal Girls and Boys. *J Clin Endocrinol Metab* 1994;79:537.

18. Moe KE, et al. Growth Hormone in Postmenopausal Women after Long-Term Oral Estrogen Replacement Therapy. *J Gerontol A Biol Sci Med Sci* 1998;53:B117.

19. Shah N, Evans WS, Veldhuis JD. Actions of Estrogen on Pulsatile, Nyctohemeral, and Entropic Modes of Growth Hormone Secretion. *Am J Physiol* 1999;276:R1351.

20. Bermann M, et al. Negative Feedback Regulation of Pulsatile Growth Hormone Secretion by Insulin-Like Growth Factor I. Involvement of Hypothalamic Somatostatin. *J Clin Invest* 1994;94:138.

21. Beckett PR, et al. Combination Growth Hormone and Estrogen Increase Bone Mineralization in Girls with Turner Syndrome. *Pediatr Res* 1999;45:709.

22. Josimovich JB, Mintz DH, Finster JL. Estrogenic Inhibition of Growth Hormone-Induced Tibial Epiphyseal Growth in Hypophysectomized Rats. *Endocrinology* 1967;81:1428.

23. Schwartz E, et al. Estrogenic Antagonism of Metabolic Effects of Administered Growth Hormone. *J Clin Endocrinol* 1969;29:1176.

24. Cook DM, Ludlam WH, Cook MB. Route of Estrogen Administration Helps to Determine Growth Hormone (GH) Replacement Dose in GH-Deficient Adults. *J Clin Endocrinol Metab* 1999;84:3956.

25. Campagnoli C, et al. Effect of Progestins on IGF-I Serum Level in Estrogen-Treated Postmenopausal Women. *Zentralbl Gynakol* 1997;119(Suppl)2:7S.

26. Malarkey WB, et al. Differential Effects of Estrogen and Medroxyprogesterone on Basal and Stress-Induced Growth Hormone Release, IGF-1 Levels, and Cellular Immunity in Postmenopausal Women. *Endocrine* 1997;7:227.

27. Weissberger AJ, Ho KK, Lazarus L. Contrasting Effects of Oral and Transdermal Routes of Estrogen Replacement Therapy on 24-Hour Growth Hormone (GH) Secretion, Insulin-Like Growth Factor I, and GH-Binding Protein in Postmenopausal Women. *J Clin Endocrinol Metab* 1991;72:374.

28. Ho KK, Weissberger AJ. Impact of Short-Term Estrogen Administration on Growth Hormone Secretion and Action: Distinct Route-Dependent Effects on Connective and Bone Tissue Metabolism. *J Bone Miner Res* 1992;7:821.

29. Stampfer MJ, Colditz GA, Willett WC. Menopause and Heart Disease. *Ann N Y Acad Sci* 1990;592:193.

30. Rosano GM, Panina G. Oestrogens and the Heart. *Therapie* 1999;54:381.

31. Richelson LS, et al. Relative Contributions of Aging and Estrogen Deficiency to Postmenopausal Bone Loss. *N Engl J Med* 1984;311:1273.

32. Sunyer T, et al. Estrogen's Bone-Protective Effects May Involve Differential IL-1 Receptor Regulation in Human Osteoclast-Like Cells. *J Clin Invest* 1999;103:1409.

33. Steffens DC, et al. Enhanced Cognitive Performance with Estrogen Use in Nondemented Community-Dwelling Older Women. *J Am Geriatr Soc* 1999;47:1171.

34. Grodstein F, Newcomb PA, Stampfer MJ. Postmenopausal Hormone Therapy and the Risk of Colorectal Cancer: A Review and Meta-Analysis. *Am J Med* 1999;106:574.

35. Paganini-Hill A. Estrogen Replacement Therapy and Colorectal Cancer Risk in Elderly Women. *Dis Colon Rectum* 1999;42:1300.

36. Troisi R, et al. A Prospective Study of Menopausal Hormones and Risk of Colorectal Cancer. *Cancer Causes Control* 1997;8:130.

37. Walsh BW, et al. Relationship between Serum Estradiol Levels and the Increases in High-Density Lipoprotein Levels in Postmenopausal Women Treated with Oral Estradiol. *J Clin Endocrinol Metab* 1999;84:985.

38. No authors listed. Are Lower Doses of Estrogen Effective against Osteoporosis? *Healthc Demand Dis Manag* 1999;5:125.

39. Recker RR, et al. The Effect of Low-Dose Continuous Estrogen and Progesterone Therapy with Calcium and Vitamin D on Bone in Elderly Women. A Randomized, Controlled Trial. *Ann Intern Med* 1999;130:897.

40. Colgan M. *Hormonal Health.* BC Canada: Apple Publishing 1996.

41. No authors listed. Effects of Hormone Therapy on Bone Mineral Density: Results from the Postmenopausal Estrogen/Progestin Interventions (PEPI) Trial. The Writing Group for the PEPI. *JAMA* 1996;276:1389.

42. Grey A, et al. Medroxyprogesterone Acetate Enhances the Spinal Bone Mineral Density Response to Oestrogen in Late Post-Menopausal Women. *Clin Endocrinol (Oxf)* 1996;44:293.

43. Chen FP, Lee N, Soong YK. Changes in the Lipoprotein Profile in Postmenopausal Women Receiving Hormone Replacement Therapy. Effects of Natural and Synthetic Progesterone. *J Reprod Med* 1998;43:568.

44. Ross D, et al. Randomized, Double-Blind, Dose-Ranging Study of the Endometrial Effects of a Vaginal Progesterone Gel in Estrogen-Treated Postmenopausal Women. *Am J Obstet Gynecol* 1997;177:937.

45. Gambrell RD Jr. Cancer and the Use of Estrogens. *Int J Fertil* 1986;31:112.

46. Franchimont P, Burger H. *Human Growth Hormone and Gonadotrophins in Health and Disease*. Amsterdam, Holland: North Holland Publishing Company 1975, p. 75-78.

47. Iranmanesh A, Lizarralde G, Veldhuis JD. Age and Relative Adiposity are Specific Negative Determinants of the Frequency and Amplitude of Growth Hormone (GH) Secretory Bursts and the Half-Life of Endogenous GH in Healthy Men. *J Clin Endocrinol Metab* 1991;73:1081.

48. Thorner MO, et al. Growth Hormone-Releasing Hormone and Growth Hormone-Releasing Peptide as Therapeutic Agents to Enhance Growth Hormone Secretion in Disease and Aging. *Recent Prog Horm Res* 1997;52:215.

49. Micic D, et al. Growth Hormone Secretion after the Administration of GHRP-6 or GHRH Combined with GHRP-6 Does Not Decline in Late Adulthood. *Clin Endocrinol (Oxf)* 1995;42:191.

50. Ghigo E, et al. Short-Term Administration of Intranasal or Oral Hexarelin, a Synthetic Hexapeptide, Does Not Desensitize the Growth Hormone Responsiveness in Human Aging. *Eur J Endocrinol* 1996;135:407.

51. Chapman IM, et al. Stimulation of the Growth Hormone (GH)-Insulin-Like Growth Factor I Axis by Daily Oral Administration of a GH Secretogogue (MK-677) in Healthy Elderly Subjects. *J Clin Endocrinol Metab* 1996;81:4249.

52. Klatz R. *Grow Young with HGH*. NY: Harper Collins Publishers 1997, p. 103.

53. Bemben MG, et al. Age-Related Patterns in Body Composition for Men Aged 20-79 Yr. *Med Sci Sports Exerc* 1995;27:264.

54. Pascot A, et al. Age-Related Increase in Visceral Adipose Tissue and Body Fat and the Metabolic Risk Profile of Premenopausal Women. *Diabetes Care* 1999;22:1471.

55. Baumgartner RN, et al. Cross-Sectional Age Differences in Body Composition in Persons 60+ Years of Age. *J Gerontol A Biol Sci Med Sci* 1995;50:M307.

56. Evans WJ, Campbell WW. Sarcopenia and Age-Related Changes in Body Composition and Functional Capacity. *J Nutr* 1993;(Suppl):465S.

57. Lexell J. Human Aging, Muscle Mass, and Fiber Type Composition. *J Gerontol A Biol Sci Med Sci* 1995;50:11.

58. Rogers MA, Evans WJ. Changes in Skeletal Muscle with Aging: Effects of Exercise Training. *Exerc Sport Sci Rev* 1993;21:65.

59. Faulkner JA, Brooks SV, Zerba E. Muscle Atrophy and Weakness with Aging: Contraction-Induced Injury as an Underlying Mechanism. *J Gerontol A Biol Sci Med Sci* 1995;50:124.

60. Poehlman ET, Horton ES. Regulation of Energy Expenditure in Aging Humans. *Annu Rev Nutr* 1990;10:255.

61. Harper EJ. Changing Perspectives on Aging and Energy Requirements: Aging, Body Weight and Body Composition in Humans, Dogs and Cats. *J Nutr* 1998;128(Suppl):2627S.

61a. Schemmel R, ed. *Nutrition, Physiology, and Obesity*. Boca Raton, FL: CRC Press 1980 (citing, Hathaway ML, Foard ED. Heights and Weights of Adults in the United States, Home Economics Research Report No. 10, U.S. Dept. of Agriculture, U.S. Government Printing Office, Washington D.C. 1960, 65; Anon., Skinfolds, Body Girths, Biacromial Diameter, and Selected Anthropometric Indices of Adults, United States, 1960-62, Public Health Service Publication No. 1000-Series 11-No. 35, Public Health Service, U.S. Department of Health, Education, and Welfare, Washington D.C., 1970, 35; Center for Disease Control, Ten-State Nutrition Survey 1968-1970, Clinical, Anthropometry, Dental, Vol. 3, DHEW Publication No. (HSM) 72-8131, Health Services and Mental Health Administration, U.S. Department of Health, Education, and Welfare, Atlanta, 1972).

61b. Losonczy KG, et al. Does Weight Loss from Middle Age to Old Age Explain the Inverse Weight Mortality Relation in Old Age? *Am J Epidemiol* 1995;141:312.

61c. Carmeli E, Reznick AZ. The Physiology and Biochemistry of Skeletal Muscle Atrophy as a Function of Age. *Proc Soc Exp Biol Med* 1994;206:103.

Chapter 5

You Can Learn a Lot from an Ancient Warrior:

Looking Back to Prehistory to Unlock Secrets to Super-Health

From a genetic standpoint, humans living today are Stone Age hunter-gatherers displaced through time to a world that differs from that for which our genetic constitution was selected.
Boyd S.B., Konner M., Shostak M. Stone Agers in the Fast Lane: Chronic Degenerative Diseases in Evolutionary Perspective. *American Journal of Medicine* 1988;84:739.

The deviation of man from the state in which he was originally placed by nature seems to have proved to him a prolific source of diseases.
Edward Jenner

The eating patterns of our ancient ancestors may seem to be a trivial fact of concern only to anthropologists or *Jeopardy* contestants. To the contrary, the inquiry into what humans ate for the overwhelming majority of our existence yields critical insight into how to eat for optimal health, fitness, and well-being. The Natural Hormonal Enhancement Eating Plan is patterned after the diets of early man and woman, a category of people who, according to anthropologists and paleontologists, were characterized by lean, well-built physiques and an almost complete absence of the degenerative diseases that afflict modern Western civilization.

Although we have a tendency to think otherwise, the fact is that modern man and woman have occupied this planet for a tiny fraction of human existence. By definition, "history" does not include "prehistory." But prehistory is where all the action took place in terms of the metabolic and hormonal adaptations that now hold the keys to our physical destiny.

Anatomically modern human beings, *Homo sapiens*, originated in Africa approximately 150,000 years ago.[1,2,3] Though it seems a colossal duration, 150,000 years is like a snap of a finger when you consider that a similar, earlier version of human beings, *Homo erectus,* existed for about two million years before that.[4,5] Going back another two million years, protohumans like *Homo hablis* and australopithecus, who had a larger jaw and a smaller brain[6,7] but walked upright *and had the same hormonal system as we do*, inhabited the earth. Therefore, based on the latest DNA and fossil research, bipedal (upright-walking) hominids have populated our planet for at least four million years.[8,9] For 99.8% of that time, human beings and their genetic forebears consumed a diet profoundly different from that which has been adopted in the most recent .2% - and herein lies a major cause of the rampant health problems that plague modern man and woman.

You may be surprised to learn that our uncivilized predecessors from bygone eras possessed the same hormonal system as we do today. In fact, the insulin/glucagon axis, which governs metabolism in an astonishingly wide array of animals, was in place millions of years before the first mammal stood upright. So by the time human-like creatures evolved, the hormones that regulate energy use/storage were already up and running. Since the emergence of mammals approximately 60 million years ago,[10] our hormonal and metabolic systems have been shaped by the eating habits of early man.

The modern day onslaught of obesity and degenerative disease is readily explained as resulting, in large part, from the hormonal effects of the modern Western diet. Not only were our *Homo sapien* ancestors free of most of the health problems we experience today, but such is the case with regard to members of technologically primitive cultures in more modern times, as well.[11,12] * Even more telling is the fact that when primitive populations embrace a Western diet and lifestyle, either by migrating or by adopting it on their home soil, the prevalence of cardiovascular disease, obesity, diabetes, and many types of cancer increases sharply and invariably.[13,14,15,16,17,18]

To say that evolutionary adaptation is a slow process is dramatic understatement, similar to saying the universe is spacious. With individual human experience ranging up to 100 years or so, and the entire evolutionary process that contributed to the human genome (a species' total genetic makeup) lasting more than a billion years,[19] the same difficulties of comprehension arise when contemplating the duration of evolution as when pondering the expansiveness of the universe. To give you an idea of how incredibly protracted is the evolutionary process, consider that the genome of humans and chimpanzees differs by 1.6 percent,[20] even though researchers believe five million years have past since the two species diverged.[21,22]

Given the millions of years required for genetic adaptation to occur, any changes in the human diet that took place within the last few thousand years are immaterial from an evolutionary standpoint – they have not altered our genetic blueprint. Therefore, to understand the kind of diet for which humans are genetically programmed, we must refer to the eating patterns that prevailed over the many millions of years during which adaptations were gradually occurring. As you will see, during the last .002 of humanoid existence dietary patterns have radically diverged from those which dominated the other 998/100ths, such that we now consume a diet that we were not evolutionarily designed to handle. The resulting mismatch between physiology and food corrodes the underpinnings of human wellness.

---

* It is tempting to suppose that the longer life expectancy of people in industrialized societies is the only reason why degenerative disease has become such a dynamic force. In other words, phrased as a question: do primitive folk avoid degenerative disease merely because they die before these diseases have a chance to take hold? The answer is no; although, obviously, a person who dies of tuberculosis or dysentery early in life never gets much of an opportunity to develop cardiovascular disease, adult-onset diabetes, cancer, or any other disease that results from cumulative damage and degeneration.
   Among technologically primitive cultures, it is more difficult to attain middle age due to the poverty of medical treatment and the consequently greater likelihood of dying from conditions that would pose no great threat of death in a technologically advanced society. However, those individuals who survive to the age of 60 years or more remain relatively free of the degenerative diseases that afflict their civilized counterparts.[22a,22b] Furthermore, young people in industrialized societies often have early-stage asymptomatic forms of these conditions, but youthful members of primitive societies do not.[22c,22d,22e,22f]

25

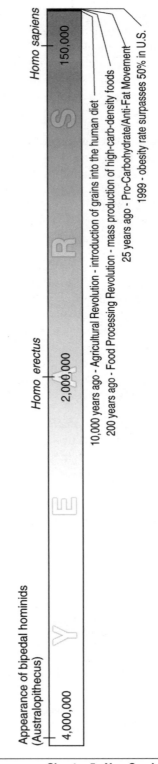

Appearance of bipedal hominids
(Australopithecus)

4,000,000

Homo erectus

2,000,000

Homo sapiens

150,000

10,000 years ago - Agricultural Revolution - introduction of grains into the human diet
200 years ago - Food Processing Revolution - mass production of high-carb-density foods
25 years ago - Pro-Carbohydrate/Anti-Fat Movement
1999 - obesity rate surpasses 50% in U.S.

A Departure from the Ancient Warrior Diet: Throwing Your Hormones a Curve

In a nutshell, there have been three developments, along the same line, that have transformed the human diet. In effect, these dietary alterations have changed for the worse the hormonal effects of eating. The three developments occurred, respectively, 10,000 years ago, 200 years ago, and 25 years ago. Each one has taken us further from our natural diet. In so doing, these developments have created disharmony between the foods we eat and our biological constitution.

Agricultural Revolution

10,000 years ago, the agricultural revolution occurred and grains became a dietary staple, displacing the traditional diet of the hunter-gatherers: meat, supplemented by a wide range of uncultivated plant foods such as berries, seeds, nuts, and roots.[23,24] The wide variety of natural foods eaten by the hunter-gatherers supplied them with vitamins and minerals in much higher quantities than the woefully inadequate, but much revered, RDA.[25,26] * The high-meat diet of the hunter-gatherers is estimated to have contained two to five times as much protein as the average American diet, and to have contained cholesterol in excess of the U.S. Senate Select Committee's recommended cholesterol intake level.[27] As nomads, the hunter-gatherers' unreliable foraging and hunting pursuits compelled them to eat on an availability, not a preference, basis. Therefore, protein and carbohydrate were "cycled" (in a manner similar to the NHE Eating Plan) as geographic and seasonal variations made different types of foods available at different times.[28,29]

The cereal grains introduced by the agricultural revolution were the human metabolism's first exposure to regular feedings of high-density carbohydrate food. In effect, our metabolic hormones (insulin and glucagon) were "thrown a curve," having never been exposed to such foods over the millions of years during which evolution transpired. Moreover, these new grain products dislocated protein from its position of centrality, and meat became a less significant dietary constituent.[30]

In addition, the agricultural revolution made a consistent food surplus possible for the first time. This was the turning point that gave rise to civilization, as energy could be devoted to cultural endeavors rather being allocated predominately to food procurement; and stable population centers could be formed as people no longer had to travel around hunting and gathering their food.[31] From a different perspective, the unprecedented food surplus introduced the potential of bodyfat excess. This potential would, thousands of years later in the 20th and 21st centuries, come to widespread fruition.

* On the subject of the "woefully inadequate" RDA, which will be attacked more fully later, it is interesting to note that the diet of monkeys in zoos is supplemented with 23 times the RDA for vitamins and minerals.[31a] Even in animals less closely related to humans, the practice of nutritional supplementation is widely employed by breeders. In Chapter 7, I note how intriguing it is to ponder a health-care system in which financial interest is aligned with health rather than sickness. This is the case in the animal breeding industry, where the breeders' bottom line is directly harmed by the occurrence of sickness and death among their animals. Breeders have found that the relatively cheap cost of nutritional supplementation pays for itself many times over in healthier and longer-living animals. Spurred by business considerations, breeders have come to understand that there is a wide gulf between adequate nutrition and optimal nutrition. The notion that this precept applies to animals but not to humans defies common sense, especially when one considers that animal studies are a leading avenue of research into human nutrition.

27

Interestingly, although food availability increased after the advent of farming, the average height of human beings *decreased* by six inches - down from an average of five feet, ten inches for men and five feet, six inches for women in the Paleolithic Era.[32] In addition to a reduction in stature, postagricultural man and woman exhibited a decrepit skeletal frame in place of the strong and healthy bone structure that characterized the hunter-gatherers.[33] The decrease in protein intake is likely a cause of these adverse morphological changes.

Ancient Warrior

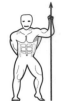

Since the Industrial Revolution, food in general and protein in particular has become more abundant, and we have recaptured the lost inches of height.[34] We are now about as tall as were the first anatomically modern human beings, but we are unequal to them in all other physical respects. They had the chiseled physique of a world class athlete whereas the average American has an unfit, somewhat rotund body, with the muscular definition of a jelly donut.

Modern Warrior

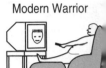

The next major development was the Industrial Revolution, which began approximately 200 years ago. One of the prominent technical developments of this period was machinery for mass-producing white flour, which marked the advent of modern food processing. While food processing made food cheaper to produce and more widely available, it also heralded the virtual disappearance of dietary fiber (which acts as a brake on insulin by slowing the rate at which ingested carbohydrate is converted to blood sugar[35,36,37,38]) from the human diet. Food processing produced a denatured, devitalized form of food that has a longer shelf-life but is relatively devoid, not only of fiber, but of vitamins and minerals too.[39] Food processing led to such dietary innovations as the Twinkie, the Fruit Loop, the potato chip, and the rice cake, all of which generate a highly fattening insulin spike (except when properly cycled into your diet, as with the NHE Eating Plan).

Food Processing Revolution

The food processing revolution - which enabled widespread availability of nutrient-deplete white flour and sugar, and made refined-carbohydrate-based products the centerpiece of the human diet in the Western world - correlates with the emergence of most of the degenerative diseases that afflict modern Western civilization (see Chapter 8). Refined foods were formerly the exclusive privilege of "refined" people: noblemen and aristocrats. But thanks to the technology of food processing, even common folk can experience these foods - and the degenerative conditions they bring in their wake.

Then 25 years ago, the hormonal imbalance between insulin and glucagon was exacerbated by the pro-carbohydrate, anti-fat movement. This spawned a renewed burst of production of highly processed, high-density carbohydrate foods - but this time without the fat. These foods send insulin levels skyrocketing. And compounding their hyperinsulinemic effect is the fact that people feel they have license to consume these foods with unrestrained abandon since they are "lowfat" or "nonfat." Furthermore, food processors typically endeavor to offset the "taste-deficit" caused by the removal of fat, by adding more sugar. This has resulted

Anti-Fat Movement

in production of foods of unprecedented carbohydrate density. Additionally, the anti-fat movement has encouraged people to shun protein foods (because they often contain fat), thereby further aggravating the imbalance between insulin and glucagon. Perversely, the pro-carbohydrate/anti-fat movement has induced people to substitute foods alien to human metabolism for foods that have been a central source of human sustenance for more than 100,000 years.

In April of 1992 A.D., the trend which began 10,000 years ago, and gathered explosive momentum through the food processing revolution and later the pro-carbohydrate movement, was institutionalized when the United States government, which is watched and followed on matters of nutrition by other governments around the world, put its official stamp of approval on the hormonally unbalanced, high-carbohydrate diet by adopting the Food Pyramid in lieu of the traditional Four Food Groups. The Food Pyramid recommends that carbohydrate foods - particularly bread, cereal, rice, and pasta - be the foremost source of calories in one's diet, places protein foods higher on the pyramid, signifying that one should eat less of them relative to carbohydrate, and positions fats along with sweets at the apex of the pyramid.

Carbs Institutionalized

The Modern Day Ancient Warrior

Akin to the diet consumed by the ancient warrior men and women who populated the earth long before the advance of civilization radically altered the human diet, the NHE Eating Plan promotes hormonal balance between insulin and glucagon. Hence, the Eating Plan turns back the clock (or rather the timeline) to an era in which hormonal balance was the norm and obesity was non-existent. But unlike the ancient warrior men and women, you will not have to club your dinner to death, rather you can easily capture it at your local grocery store or at restaurants.

Like your lean and terrifically well-built *Homo sapien* counterparts from the Paleolithic Era, you will be eating a variety of nutrient-dense, carbohydrate-sparse, protein-rich foods, along with high-quality fats. These foods are eaten within a dietary framework that maximizes fat burning, energy levels, and physical and mental performance. And like the ancient folks, who enjoyed superb health at least until such time as they got run-down by a saber-toothed tiger or some other highly untame fanged creature, you will be cycling your food intake. But whereas they cycled out of necessity, you will be cycling to achieve hormonal benefits that were beyond their reach, and to allow you to indulge intelligently and advantageously in the carbohydrate-dense foods that have become a part of American culture.

Modern Day Ancient Warrior

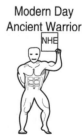

References

1. Seielstad M, et al. A View of Modern Human Origins from Y Chromosome Microsatellite Variation. *Genome Res* 1999;9:558.

2. Ayala FJ, Escalante AA. The Evolution of Human Populations: A Molecular Perspective. *Mol Phylogenet Evol* 1996;5:188.

3. Horai S. Evolution and the Origins of Man: Clues from Complete Sequences of Hominoid Mitochondrial DNA. *Southeast Asian J Trop Med Public Health* 1995;26(Suppl):146.

4. Franciscus RG, Trinkaus E. Nasal Morphology and the Emergence of Homo Erectus. *Am J Phys Anthropol* 1988;75:517.

5. Wood B, Collard M. The Human Genus. *Science* 1999;284:65.

6. McHenry HM. Tempo and Mode in Human Evolution. *Proc Natl Acad Sci U S A* 1994;91:6780.

7. Ruff CB, Trinkaus E, Holliday TW. Body Mass and Encephalization in Pleistocene Homo. *Nature* 1997;387:173.

8. Leakey MG, et al. New Specimens and Confirmation of an Early Age for Australopithecus Anamensis. *Nature* 1998;393:62.

9. Leakey M, Walker A. Early Hominid Fossils from Africa. *Sci Am* 1997;276:74.

10. Benton MJ. Early Origins of Modern Birds and Mammals: Molecules vs. Morphology. *Bioessays* 1999;21:1043.

11. Truswell AS. Diet and Nutrition of Hunter-Gatherers. *Ciba Found Symp* 1977;:213.

12. O'Dea K. Cardiovascular Disease Risk Factors in Australian Aborigines. *Clin Exp Pharmacol Physiol* 1991;18:85.

13. O'Dea K, Spargo RM, Nestle PJ. Impact of Westernization on Carbohydrate and Lipid Metabolism in Australian Aborigines. *Diabetologia* 1982;22:148.

14. Cohen AM, et al. Diabetes, Blood Lipids, Lipoproteins and Change of Environment; Restudy of the 'New Immigrant Yemenites' in Israel. *Metabolism* 1979;28:716.

15. O'Dea. Westernisation, Insulin Resistance and Diabetes in Australian Aborigines. *Med J Aust* 1991;155:258.

16. Hildes JA, Schaefer O. The Changing Picture of Neoplastic Disease in the Western and Central Canadian Arctic (1950-1980). *Can Med Assoc J* 1984;130:25.

17. Ostwald R, Gerbe-Medhin M. Westernization of Diet and Serum Lipids in Ethiopians. *Am J Clin Nutr* 1978;31:1028.

18. Trostler N. Health Risks of Immigration: The Yemenite and Ethiopian Cases in Israel. *Biomed Pharmacother* 1997;51:352.

19. Eaton SB, Konner M, Shostak M. Stone Agers in the Fast Lane: Chronic Degenerative Diseases in Evolutionary Perspective. *Am J Med* 1988;84:739.

20. Id.

21. Horai S, et al. Recent African Origin of Modern Humans Revealed by Complete Sequences of Hominoid Mitochondrial DNAs. *Proc Natl Acad Sci U S A* 1995;92:532.

22. Adachi J, Hasegawa M. Improved Dating of the Human/Chimpanzee Separation in the Mitochondrial DNA Tree: Heterogeneity among Amino Acid Sites. *J Mol Evol* 1995;40:622.

22a. Eaton SB, Konner M. Paleolithic Nutrition. *N Engl J Med* 1985;312:283.

22b. Truswell AS. Diet and Nutrition of Hunter-Gatherers. *Ciba Found Symp* 1977;:213.

22c. Bergstrom E, et al. Insulin Resistance Syndrome in Adolescents. *Metabolism* 1996;45:908.

22d. Anding JD, et al. Blood Lipids, Cardiovascular Fitness, Obesity, and Blood Pressure: The Presence of Potential Coronary Heart Disease Risk Factors in Adolescents. *J Am Diet Assoc* 1996;96:238.

22e. Ronnemaa T, et al. Serum Insulin and other Cardiovascular Risk Indicators in Children, Adolescents and Young Adults. *Ann Med* 1991;23:67.

22f. McGill HC Jr, et al. Determinants of Atherosclerosis in the Young. Pathobiological Determinants of Atherosclerosis in Youth (PDAY) Research Group. *Am J Cardiol* 1998;82:30T.

23.   Swanson C. *The Natural History of Man.* NJ: Prentice Hall 1973.

24.   O'Dea K. Traditional Diet and Food Preferences of Australian Aboriginal Hunter-Gatherers. *Philos Trans R Soc Lond B Biol Sci* 1991;334:233.

25.   See, supra, note 19.

26.   See, supra, note 22a.

27.   See, supra, notes 19 and 22a.

28.   Harding RDS, Teleki G, eds. *Omnivorous Primates: Gathering and Hunting in Human Evolution.* NY: Columbia University Press 1981.

29.   Speth JD, Spielmann KA. Energy Source, Protein Metabolism, and Hunter-Gatherer Subsistence Strategies. *J Anthropol Archaeol* 1983;2:1.

30.   See, supra, note 22a.

31.   Swanson C. *The Natural History of Man.* NJ: Prentice Hall 1973.

31a. Colgan M. *Optimum Sports Nutrition.* NY: Advanced Research Press 1993, p. 229 (citing, Kallman B. Micronutrient Intakes in Laboratory Animals and Humans. *J Appl Nutr* 1989;41:23).

32.   See, supra, note 22a.

33.   Id.

34.   Id.

35.   Ullrich IH, Albrink MJ. The Effect of Dietary Fiber and other Factors on Insulin Response: Role in Obesity. *J Environ Pathol Toxicol Oncol* 1985;5:137.

36.   Potter JG, et al. Effect of Test Meals of Varying Dietary Fiber Content on Plasma Insulin and Glucose Response. *Am J Clin Nutr* 1981;34:328.

37.   Anderson JW, et al. Postprandial Serum Glucose, Insulin, and Lipoprotein Responses to High- and Low-Fiber Diets. *Metabolism* 1995;44:848.

38.   Jenkins DJ, Jenkins AL. Dietary Fiber and the Glycemic Response. *Proc Soc Exp Biol Med* 1985;180:422.

39.   Mount JL. *The Food and Health of Western Man.* London, England: Butterworth and Co. 1971.

Chapter 6

The Misinformation Age

Information (or misinformation) has trickled down to us through the grapevine as rumors, hearsay, advertising copy, popular articles by reporters . . . doctors untrained in nutrition, and industry "experts."
Dr. Udo Erasmus, *Fats that Heal Fats that Kill*

I am told that we have a health-care crisis in this country, but I don't think so. I think we have a sick-care crisis. And if we took better care to prevent the healthy from becoming sick, we wouldn't have a crisis.
Rob Faigin

Most physicians and surgeons received little instruction in [nutrition] in medical school and have picked up much misinformation since their graduation.
Dr. Linus Pauling, *How to Live Longer and Feel Better*

The health and fitness industry has become a circus sideshow. But instead of the one-armed midget and the two-headed woman, we've got tummy tucks, cellulite creams, magic pills, and belly vibrators.
Rob Faigin

Go into any bookstore in the U.S. and you will find that the bookshelves are overflowing with diet books. Surf the channels of your television set and you will see a dizzying array of fitness devices being sold. It seems like there is a health club at every street corner in America and more are opening all the time. In view of these facts, as well as the fact that more people are dieting now than ever and fat consumption is at an all-time low, you might logically assume that the fitness renaissance is producing a trimmer, healthier America.

This assumption, however, while reasonable to make, is contradicted by the facts. The shocking reality is that obesity has risen steadily over the last twenty years, concurrently with the low-fat craze, and is approaching epidemic proportions (see below). Similarly, although Americans have diligently heeded admonitions from health authorities to reduce dietary fat and cholesterol, the high incidence of cardiovascular disease, cancer, and diabetes has not abated.

Highly publicized pronouncements to the effect that these diseases are on the decline obscure the fact that the *incidence* (not to be confused with the death rate) of degenerative diseases is holding fast, or increasing, in the U.S.[1,2,3,4,5,6,7,8] In other words, medical science is making progress at treating, and sometimes curing, diseased people; but is making zero progress (zippo, nil) at preventing people from becoming afflicted with degenerative diseases. Consequently, the death rate from these diseases may be declining as sick people are cured or kept alive longer. But the rates of affliction of cancer, cardiovascular disease, osteoporosis, obesity, and diabetes in the United States are the highest in the world. The fact that the U.S. is the world's leader in medical technology AND Americans are the fattest and sickest people on the planet is an incongruity that demands an explanation.

This book is devoted to resolving the problem, not investigating its sources. However, the glaring and alarming discrepancy highlighted above cries out so loudly for an explanation that it simply must be addressed. I feel that you will benefit from understanding how this grievous state of affairs, which I call the "health misinformation age," has come into being. *Because if you don't understand what drives it, you will continue to be victimized by it.*

In part, it has been a case of decent, well-intentioned scientists and medical professionals simply being wrong: mistaking *correlational* connections for *causal* connections (a tricky distinction for even the most disciplined and well-schooled minds), and the related mistake of treating the *symptom* rather than the *cause*. For instance, fat consumption is correlated with obesity in the United States; but so is sugar consumption, which is higher in the United States than in any other country. Which of these is the cause or are they both causes? (I'll address this question in Chapter 8.) As to the symptom/cause distinction, you will learn in this book that excess bodyfat is, in many cases, a symptom of hormonal imbalance. Because practically everyone is focused on the symptom not the cause, it's no wonder most fat loss efforts fail - it is like trying to correct illiteracy by enlarging the print in books.

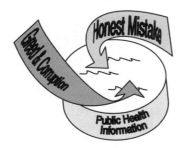

Another explanation for how so many people have been led astray relates to the greed and unscrupulousness of people in the fitness industry whose sole objective is to extract money from decent people earnestly searching for answers to how to lose fat and get in shape. Unfortunately, "honest misinformation" and "dishonest misinformation" are mutually reinforcing: the more mistaken the "experts" are, the more misled the public becomes; the more misled the public becomes, the more people fail in their efforts to lose fat; the more people fail in their efforts to lose fat, the more desperate they become; the more desperate they become, the more receptive they become to the come-ons, scams, frauds, and farces that pervade the fitness industry; and finally, the dishonest misinformation disseminated in order to make a sale leaks into the general pool of information and is adopted as truth by decent, honest people who repeat it as truth; thus, the line is blurred between dishonest misinformation and honest misinformation.

The result of all this is that Americans are becoming fatter, sicker, and are getting pick-pocketed at every turn by snake-oil scamsters promising to have the answer to the fat loss question. Unfortunately, not much help can be obtained from the abundance of well-intentioned medical doctors in this country (many of whom are sporting a spare tire of their own) because nutritional training is not a significant part of the medical school curriculum due to the inertia of tradition and the influence of pharmaceutical

33

companies on both the course content of medical schools and on the politics of medical associations.

While being ripped-off is certainly no fun, the failure of the medical community to make even the slightest inroad into the obesity epidemic has spurred the development of treatments that pose new health risks, sometimes worse than the health risks associated with being fat. The 1997 recall of the diet pills Redux and Fen-phen exemplifies this paradox in which the treatment is more harmful than the disorder it is intended to treat. When considering how many millions of people have taken these drugs, one can only speculate how much as-yet-undetected damage has been caused by these ill-fated, but highly profitable, "magic pills."

What is even more troubling is the fact that the full extent of the danger of these pills could have been easily discovered had the rush to cash-in been less hasty. The FDA, which regularly interferes with the availability of nutritional supplements based on scant or nonexistent evidence of their harmful potential, managed to overlook numerous scientific articles that reported the harmful effects of Redux, including studies showing that Redux causes brain damage in laboratory animals. The dangerousness of Fen-phen was even more apparent to those who cared to look. I don't suppose that the fact that Redux and Fen-phen were supported by the immensely powerful pharmaceutical lobby, which profited grandly from this health disaster, had anything to do with the approval of these drugs, do you?*

Similarly, fat loss failure has given rise to a motley assortment of ghastly medical procedures which, in many cases, would not have been necessary had fat loss recommendations been more accurate. These include: liposuction, stomach stapling, removal of part of the intestine, jaw-wiring, and insertion of a balloon into the stomach to lessen stomach capacity. All of these procedures are fraught with adverse side effects, and none addresses the underlying metabolic and hormonal conditions that caused the fat gain in the first place.

In summary, the "health misinformation age" is a product of greed and corruption combined with honest mistake. But there is another, more insidious, force at work. You see, greed and corruption can be detected and frequently backfire; and honest mistake strives to correct itself. However, intellectual arrogance/conformism among the people to whom we look for guidance in matters of health is the most potent enemy of truth. It may not be clear to you, right now, what I mean by "intellectual arrogance/conformism" or why it is such a monster; but it will be clear in a moment when I lay-out the graphic details. I think you will find the next chapter to be both enlightening and shocking. But first, let's look at one offspring of the misinformation crisis - conventional dieting - and its consequences.

* Incidentally, remember L-tryptophan, the amino acid supplement that, despite a 50-year track record of safe and beneficial human use, was banned by the FDA after several people died from taking L-tryptophan pills that were later conclusively linked to a contaminated batch from oversees? Well, L-tryptophan, still banned, has been quietly approved as a prescription drug for insomnia and depression. This leaves us with the bizarre situation in which the same substance that is safe when purchased from a pharmacy is deadly when bought at a health food store.

34

Conventional Dieting is One of the Largest and Most Costly Failures in the History of Humanity

-- The *Journal of the American Medical Association*[9] (Oct. 1999) estimates that approximately 300,000 deaths per year in the U.S. are attributable to obesity, *placing excess bodyfat second only to smoking as a preventable cause of death.*

-- The United States spends more money on weight-reduction research than on cancer research. But, because of hormonally unsound approaches to the problem, the cure rate for obesity is lower than for cancer. The general success rate for curing cancer is 40%,[10] whereas a much lower percentage of people are successful at losing fat and keeping it off for one year[11,12,13] (losing fat temporarily does not amount to a cure - it's a remission).

-- The direct cost of obesity in the U.S. is approximately 60 billion dollars,[14,15] a 50% increase from 1986.[16]

Fact #1 - Americans spend billions of dollars per year on weight loss.

> **Result #1** - Americans are fatter than ever. More than half of all adult Americans are "significantly overweight" (translation: FAT).[17]

Fact #2 - Fat consumption in the U.S has been steadily declining over the last decade.[18]

> **Result #2** - See Result #1; and the prevalence of obesity has increased sharply during the last decade.[19]

Fact #3 - More Americans are dieting than ever before.

> **Result #3** - See Result #1. See Result #2. And, over 90% of people who diet either fail to lose fat or regain the lost fat within six months. At the one-year mark, the statistic becomes even more pathetic; by then, 95% of those who lost fat initially have regained it all. In view of this statistic, conventional dieting is practically a sure-fire way *not* to lose fat.

References

1. Burke JP, et al. Rapid Rise in the Incidence of Type 2 Diabetes from 1987 to 1996: Results from the San Antonio Heart Study. *Arch Intern Med* 1999;159:1450.

2. Blot WJ, McLaughlin JK. The Changing Epidemiology of Esophageal Cancer. *Semin Oncol* 1999;26(Suppl):2.

3. Miller BA, Feuer EJ, Hankey BF. Recent Incidence Trends for Breast Cancer in Women and the Relevance of Early Detection: An Update. *CA Cancer J Clin* 1993;43:27.

4. Rosamond WD, et al. Trends in the Incidence of Myocardial Infarction and in Mortality Due to Coronary Heart Disease, 1987 to 1994. *N Engl J Med* 1998;339:861.

5. Iqbal MM. Osteoporosis: Epidemiology, Diagnosis, and Treatment. *South Med J* 2000;93:2.

6. Davis DL, Dinse GE, Hoel DG. Decreasing Cardiovascular Disease and Increasing Cancer among Whites in the United States from 1973 through 1987. Good News and Bad News. *JAMA* 1994;271:431.

7. No authors listed. Trends in the Prevalence and Incidence of Self-Reported Diabetes Mellitus -- United States, 1980-1994. *MMWR Morb Mortal Wkly Rep* 1997;46:1014.

8. Harris MI. Diabetes in America: Epidemiology and Scope of the Problem. *Diabetes Care* 1998;21(Suppl):C11.

9. Allison DB, et al. Annual Deaths Attributable to Obesity in the United States. *JAMA* 1999;282:1530.

10. American Cancer Society. *Cancer Facts and Figures* 1997, p. 2.

11. Skender ML, et al. Comparison of 2-Year Weight Loss Trends in Behavioral Treatments of Obesity: Diet, Exercise, and Combination Interventions. *J Am Diet Assoc* 1996;96:342.

12. Yost TJ, Jensen DR, Eckel RH. Weight Regain Following Sustained Weight Reduction is Predicted by Relative Insulin Sensitivity. *Obes Res* 1995;3:583.

13. Kramer FM, et al. Long-Term Follow-Up of Behavioral Treatment for Obesity: Patterns of Weight Regain among Men and Women. *Int J Obes* 1989;13:123.

14. Colditz GA. Economic Costs of Obesity and Inactivity. *Med Sci Sports Exerc* 1999;31(Suppl):S663.

15. Wolf AM, Colditz GA. Current Estimates of the Economic Cost of Obesity in the United States. *Obes Res* 1998;6:97.

16. Colditz GA. Economic Costs of Obesity. *Am J Clin Nutr* 1992;55(Suppl):503S.

17. Must A, et al. The Disease Burden Associated with Overweight and Obesity. *JAMA* 1999;282:1523.

18. Lichtenstein AH, et al. Dietary Fat Consumption and Health. *Nutr Rev* 1998;56:3S.

19. Mokdad AH, et al. The Spread of the Obesity Epidemic in The United States, 1991-1998. *JAMA* 1999;282:1519.

Chapter 7

The Truth Can Hurt,
But the Absence of Truth Can Kill

In the fitness industry today there is a traffic jam on the road to riches,
while the road to truth languishes in quiet desolation.
Rob Faigin

It is easier to believe a falsehood that has been repeated a thousand times,
than a truth that is said for the first time.
Unknown

Because all scientific evidence must be filtered through the interpretive process before meaning can be extracted, it can be used to prove anything, even the truth - and it can, like an expert witness, be called upon to testify for either side. For this reason, blind faith in everything that is represented to you as science makes you as vulnerable to being misled as placing your trust in everyone claiming to possess psychic powers.
Rob Faigin

According to the Journal of the American Medical Association (April 1998),[1] 106,000 Americans die each year from properly prescribed medicine taken in prescribed doses. This makes doctor-prescribed drugs the sixth most common cause of death in the United States!

A miracle drug is a drug that actually remedies the problem
it is supposed to, without causing other more serious problems.
Rob Faigin

All truth passes through three stages. First, it is ridiculed.
Second, it is violently opposed. Third, it is accepted as self-evident.
Arthur Schopenhauer

Orthodox medicine has not found an answer to your complaint.
However, luckily for you, I happen to be a quack.
Charles Richter cartoon caption

The American Medical Association, operating from a platform of negative vigilance, presents
no solutions but busily fights each change and then loudly supports it against the next proposal.
John H. Knowles

In general, orthodox beliefs die slow, painful deaths. At the same time, the presumption of being mistaken automatically attaches to those who dissent from widely accepted principles. Compounding the inertia of conventional thought is the fact that "experts" often have more difficulty than others admitting their mistakes because being wrong on a major issue would be viewed, by some, as invalidating their status as expert.

Now factor-in the inordinate pressure to conform that dominates the conservative fields of science and medicine. In these circles, dissenting from the consensus places the dissenter's hard-earned reputation and status in jeopardy. In fact, a doctor or scientist who departs from the confines of the intellectual community by disavowing the official dogma risks being branded a quack - a devastating stigma for someone who has spent tremendous amounts of time, energy, and dollars in an effort to establish the opposite status.

While the rewards for renouncing the status quo and advancing a new and different view can be great, intellectual revolutions rarely happen overnight. More commonly, the status quo staggers on for quite some time before falling. For the doctor or scientist who divorces himself from the intellectual community, being branded a quack is likely to be a severe career hindrance until such time as his quackish views become accepted, which could take years or may not happen in his lifetime. Until then, where will the scientist find grant money, and where will the doctor find patients? Except when desperate, people are justifiably disinclined to invest their money or entrust their health in someone who is at odds with the weight of authority in his field.

There are innumerable examples, throughout history, of visionaries being spurned and ostracized. When Galileo announced his finding that the Earth revolves around the sun, he was rewarded with a trip to jail. He made his telescope and his mathematical proofs available to the ecclesiastical and scientific authorities, but they refused to look. Subsequently, Galileo was put on trial and the outcome of the proceeding was as follows: recant or die. He recanted and thus was exiled rather than executed. When the average person hears the story of Galileo, he/she is sympathetic but finds it irrelevant to modern times. To the contrary, this drama has been repeated throughout the centuries - with different actors but the same tragic storyline.

One such contemporary instance involves Dr. Linus Pauling. Pauling, the great humanitarian and scientist, whose work was inspired by his passionate desire, in his words, to "minimize human suffering" was forced to endure some suffering of his own when, despite having extraordinary credentials which included two Nobel Prizes, Dr. Pauling was ridiculed and essentially dumped by the scientific community when in the early 1970's he argued that vitamin C helps prevent sickness and disease and recommended multi-gram doses. Years later, Pauling, the only living recipient of two Nobel Prizes (for Chemistry in 1954 and for Peace in 1962), found himself unable to get his exceedingly important and enlightening article "Solution to the Puzzle of Human Cardiovascular Disease" published. Instead, this article, concerning the leading cause of death in the civilized world, written by one of the great scientists of the twentieth century, was published in an obscure journal with a tiny circulation of about 500.[2]

Dr. Pauling's arguments in favor of vitamin C were eventually confirmed by hundreds of studies showing the myriad benefits of vitamin C at levels substantially greater than the paltry RDA. Pauling, though, was unable to do much gloating, even if he had wanted to, because all of his major critics were dead by the time he was vindicated, while he continued swimming, lecturing, writing books, and taking multi-gram doses of vitamin C well into his tenth decade, when his brilliant career, and life, finally ended.

Pauling, thanks to his own stubborn longevity, lived to enjoy a large measure of vindication (although even today you can find doctors who cling to the idea that nutritional intake above minimal levels affords no benefits whatsoever). Other visionaries, however, have been less fortunate than Linus Pauling. In 1847, Ignaz Philipp Semmelweis argued that doctors should wash their hands after delivering one infant before going to the next one. In his clinic in Vienna and then in Budapest, Semmelweis, by implementing this procedure, reduced the childbirth infant mortality rate from 16 percent to 1 percent. Nonetheless, his idea brought him personal abuse and was rejected for years. He became embittered and dejected and went insane before he died in 1865.

This type of thing has happened over and over throughout recent history, and society has paid a horrific price for the close-minded fixation on preferred theories and treatments. The most recent instance relates to the homocysteine theory of heart disease. The homocysteine theory holds that heart disease is caused, in large part, by sub-optimal intake of vitamins B6, B12, and folic acid. Homocysteine is an intermediate by-product routinely created when the body metabolizes the amino acid methionine.[3] When adequate amounts of B6, B12, and folic acid are present, homocysteine is promptly converted to other, harmless, substances.[4] But when these vitamins, which are cofactors in protein metabolism, are lacking, homocysteine accumulates to toxic levels.

What is today regarded as a breakthrough in heart disease has in fact been around since the early 1970's, when Dr. Kilmer McCulley first advanced the theory. By the 1980's, studies had been published in the Netherlands, the United States, Japan, and other countries, validating the homocysteine theory to an extent that would pique the interest of anyone with any degree of intellectual curiosity in the areas of disease prevention and health. By the turn of the century, the scientific journals were so filled with studies (hundreds) indicating the cardio-pathogenic influence of elevated homocysteine levels that to deny the association between homocysteine and cardiovascular disease was to deny the stars in the sky.[5,6,7,8,9,10,11,12,13,14,15,16,17,18,19,20,21,22]

Why then is the public only getting wind of the homocysteine theory now, more than a quarter-century later, after countless millions of people have died of heart disease? Why didn't investigation of the homocysteine/heart disease connection commence upon Dr. McCulley's publishing his findings more than two decades ago? As is too often the case, Dr. McCulley, then a young Harvard pathologist, was rewarded with disdain, rather than acclaim, for his monumental discovery.

Dr. McCulley's findings were met with, in his words, "stony silence" from the medical community and "a refusal to acknowledge the significance of this work."[23] Dr. McCulley was exiled from Harvard, denied money for research, and blackballed from the medical community. By upsetting the applecart of conventional thought and offending the egos and interests of those who jealously guard it, McCulley had, in effect, committed professional suicide. Subsequently, Dr. McCulley found work at the Veterans' Administration Medical Center in Providence, Rhode Island where he continued his research in obscurity for close to thirty years.

The homocysteine theory does not negate the importance of LDL cholesterol and serum triglyceride as cardiovascular risk factors. Rather, all of these factors interrelate. Because the homocysteine theory does not entirely overturn conventional medical wisdom, there is a possibility that it will someday be embraced by the medical establishment. But at the moment, even as Dr. McCulley's views have captured the attention of the media and the more progressive elements of the scientific community, the medical establishment maintains an askance view of the homocysteine theory and refuses to accept its therapeutic implications. And people continue dying, by the hundreds of thousands per year, of heart disease.

This is not to diminish the amazing and wonderful treatments that have been developed by the pharmaceutical/medical establishment. And, in a free market system, it is not at all objectionable that virtually every amazing and wonderful innovation has carried the potential to enrich doctors and drug companies. But what *is* objectionable, and inexcusable, is the way in which potentially lifesaving information about treatments and preventative measures that offer no profit potential to the establishment have been suppressed or ignored (like Dr. Pauling's message, and Dr. McCulley's message, and Dr. Semmelweis's message, and so many others like them). *How many people have been cut-open, radiated, poisoned by chemotherapeutic drugs, or subjected to other hazardous cash-ectomy procedures because compelling preventative theories have gone unexplored?* Too many, I would argue.

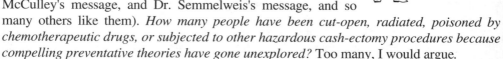

Am I overstating my case? Am I exaggerating the extent to which money, politics, and self-interest cripple the delivery of crucial health information to the public? Consider that vitamin therapy has been shown to promptly and reliably lower homocysteine levels. Folic acid and vitamin B6, in particular, are typically deficient in individuals with elevated homocysteine levels, and supplementing these vitamins has been shown to reduce this coronary risk factor. [24,25,26,27,28,29]

Equally persuasive evidence exists for other nutrients in connection with other diseases. But, alas, patents are not available on natural substances. Absent the exclusivity that a patent confers, competition forces the price of a product down to an equitable level. But armed with a patent and aided by a complicit medical establishment that shares in the bounty, drug companies are able to charge outrageous sums for marginal products. Consequently, the public hears all about the latest grossly overpriced "miracle drug," while information concerning inexpensive natural substances that can make many of these drugs unnecessary languishes in deadening silence.

My opponents will argue that "long-term, controlled studies do not exist proving conclusively that vitamins and antioxidants reduce mortality or morbidity." To this pathetic argument I have two responses. First, reduction of a major disease risk factor (homocysteine, for instance) is a sufficient basis for recommending an inexpensive substance bearing no adverse side effects when hundreds of thousands of people per year are dying from the disease for which this risk factor is a predictive indicator. Second, is "long-term, controlled studies proving conclusively reduced mortality or morbidity" the invariable standard for getting a drug approved for sale to the pubic? No. Rather, a double standard exists, predicated on considerations other than the reasoned assessment of a substance's potential for beneficial human use. When a plane crashes and a hundred people die, it is a heartbreaking tragedy and garners worldwide attention. But where is the outrage and grief at the millions of people who have suffered and died because of the institutional indifference toward, and denial of, alternative health care approaches?

Part of the problem is that nowhere in the world can one earn an advanced degree denoting expertise in *health promotion* and *disease prevention*. Instead, we have a world full of doctors who, although they provide an indispensable service to society, are trained to cure and treat diseases, many of which arise from the failure to take appropriate *health-promoting, disease-preventative* measures. What's wrong with this picture?

Medical students are typically imbued with an admirable work ethic, and often they are motivated by the best of intentions. But upon beginning medical school, they are indoctrinated into a view of "health care" devoid of any concept of the meaning of health or how to promote it. Brilliant independent thinkers rarely emerge from an educational system that fosters and rewards intellectual conformity. Instead, time-honored misconceptions and prejudices are perpetuated, and ignorance and arrogance act to sustain each other while forming an insuperable barrier to the acceptance of new ideas. It is largely for this reason that doctors more readily prescribe expensive drugs of questionable efficacy bearing adverse side effects than recommend cheap, harmless nutrients proven to reduce risk factors for deadly diseases.

A health-care system should be concerned solely with caring for peoples' health; this leaves no room for politics and vested interest. Caring for health entails *promoting* health, a concept alien to our current system in which crisis intervention, symptom control, and disease treatment predominate. The objectives of true health care could be best served by replacing the current malady-management system with a system in which doctors are paid to keep people healthy and fined when sickness occurs. The fine could then be used by the patient to pay for treatment.

This system is not likely ever to be instituted, but it is interesting to ponder a regime in which financial interest is aligned with health rather than illness. I suspect that the incidence of sickness and disease would decrease drastically in this scenario, as doctors would be compelled to stay on the cutting-edge of the fast-paced developments occurring in the fields of nutrition and other natural approaches to health. Every doctor would have subscriptions to every major scientific journal and would study them with the same inspired diligence with which a Wall Street trader reads the business section. Doctors would be driven constantly to develop and refine their knowledge of how best to keep people healthy, and the fight against disease would be waged by means of preemptive attack rather than retaliatory response. In this way, society could more constructively harness the enormous intellectual resource that the medical community represents.

What makes matters worse is that the defenders of the status quo always have ammunition. The average lay person views science as being black and white: clinical experiments yield clear, unequivocal results, right? Wrong. All data are subject to interpretation; and researchers will often reach different conclusions from the same data, *especially if they have preconceived ideas about what is the correct answer.*

Natural Hormonal Enhancement

Even in those relatively rare instances in which the data point in only one direction, there remains a question as to the validity of the experiment that generated the data. No matter how carefully a study is designed, it is practically impossible to control all the variables that could taint the results (especially in human studies). Experimental design and protocol is a science in itself, replete with its own lexicon of confusing terms, such as: "randomized," "crossover," "double-blind," and "placebo-controlled."

Just as an astute lawyer can find loopholes, exceptions, and hair-splitting technicalities in any legal issue, so an astute scientist can do so with any scientific issue. This is why there will always be scientific evidence that can be cited in support of almost any theory, and the "fat makes you fat" theory, which we will examine in the next chapter, is no exception. When considering the bias issue in this connection, take note of the fact that sugar- and starch-based foods are, by far, the cheapest foods to produce and that a tremendously profitable lowfat/nonfat industry has grown-up around the anti-fat movement. Therefore, the "low-fat cats" have a lot to gain by perpetuating the notion that fat makes you fat; and there is no doubt that hundreds of millions of dollars can buy a lot of ostensible legitimacy. But does the low-fat theory have merit? We will now address that question.

References

1. Lazarou J, Pomeranz BH, Corey PN. Incidence of Adverse Drug Reactions in Hospitalized Patients: A Meta-Analysis of Prospective Studies. *JAMA* 1998;279:1200.

2. Rath M, Pauling L. Solution to the Puzzle of Human Cardiovascular Disease: Its Primary Cause is Ascorbate Deficiency Leading to the Deposition of Lipoprotein (a) and Fibrogen/Fibrin in the Vascular Wall. *J Orthomol Med* 1991;6:125.

3. Braverman ER. *The Healing Nutrients Within*. Conn:Keats Publishing 1997, 199-200.

4. Id.

5. Andreotti F, et al. Homocysteine and Risk of Cardiovascular Disease. *J Thromb Thrombolysis* 2000;9:13.

6. Saw SM. Homocysteine and Atherosclerotic Disease: The Epidemiologic Evidence. *Ann Acad Med Singapore* 1999;28:565.

7. Pasceri V, Willerson JT. Homocysteine and Coronary Heart Disease: A Review of the Current Evidence. *Semin Interv Cardiol* 1999;4:121.

8. Whincup PH, et al. Serum Total Homocysteine and Coronary Heart Disease: Prospective Study in Middle Aged Men. *Heart* 1999;82:448.

9. Bostom AG, et al. Nonfasting Plasma Total Homocysteine Levels and Stroke Incidence in Elderly Persons: The Framingham Study. *Ann Intern Med* 1999;131:352.

10. Guthikonda S, Haynes WG. Homocysteine as a Novel Risk Factor for Atherosclerosis. *Curr Opin Cardiol* 1999;14:283.

11. Hyanek J, et al. [Diagnostic Significance of Mild Hyperhomocysteinemia in a Population of Children with Parents or Grandparents who have Peripheral or Coronary Artery Disease]. *Cas Lek Cesk* 1999;138:333. Czech.

12. Ridker PM, et al. Homocysteine and Risk of Cardiovascular Disease among Postmenopausal Women. *JAMA* 1999;281:1817.

13. Bostom AG, et al. Nonfasting Plasma Total Homocysteine Levels and All-Cause and Cardiovascular Disease Mortality in Elderly Framingham Men and Women. *Arch Intern Med* 1999;159:1077.

14. Joubran R, et al. Homocysteine Levels and Coronary Heart Disease in Syria. *J Cardiovasc Risk* 1998;5:257.

15. Stehouwer CD, et al. Serum Homocysteine and Risk of Coronary Heart Disease and Cerebrovascular Disease in Elderly Men: A 10-Year Follow-Up. *Arterioscler Thromb Vasc Biol* 1998;18:1895.

16. Aronow WS, Ahn C. Association between Plasma Homocysteine and Coronary Artery Disease in Older Persons. *Am J Cardiol* 1997;80:1216.

17. Nygard O, et al. Plasma Homocysteine Levels and Mortality in Patients with Coronary Artery Disease. *N Engl J Med* 1997;337:230.

18. Montalescot G, et al. Plasma Homocysteine and the Extent of Atherosclerosis in Patients with Coronary Artery Disease. *Int J Cardiol* 1997;60:295.

19. Ubbink JB, et al. Plasma Homocysteine Concentrations in a Population with a Low Coronary Heart Disease Prevalence. *J Nutr* 1996;126(Suppl):1254S.

20. van den Berg M, et al. Plasma Homocysteine and Severity of Atherosclerosis in Young Patients with Lower-Limb Atherosclerotic Disease. *Arterioscler Thromb Vasc Biol* 1996;16:165.

21. Clarke R, et al. Hyperhomocysteinemia: An Independent Risk Factor for Vascular Disease. *N Engl J Med* 1991;324:1149.

22. Robinson K, et al. Hyperhomocysteinemia and Low Pyridoxal Phosphate. Common and Independent Reversible Risk Factors for Coronary Artery Disease. *Circulation* 1995;92:2825.

23. Mitchell T. Life Extension Magazine (interview with Dr. Kilmer McCully) Nov. 1997, p. 27.

24. Lobo A, et al. Reduction of Homocysteine Levels in Coronary Artery Disease by Low-Dose Folic Acid Combined with Vitamins B6 and B12. *Am J Cardiol* 1999;83:821.

25. Pietrzik K, Bronstrup A. The Role of Homocysteine, Folate and other B-Vitamins in the Development of Atherosclerosis. *Arch Latinoam Nutr* 1997;47(Suppl):9S.

26. Gallagher PM, et al. Homocysteine and Risk of Premature Coronary Heart Disease. Evidence for a Common Gene Mutation. *Circulation* 1996;94:2154.

27. Verhoef P, et al. Homocysteine Metabolism and Risk of Myocardial Infarction: Relation with Vitamins B6, B12, and Folate. *Am J Epidemiol* 1996;143:845.

28. Robinson K, et al. Low Circulating Folate and Vitamin B6 Concentrations: Risk Factors for Stroke, Peripheral Vascular Disease, and Coronary Artery Disease. European COMAC Group. *Circulation* 1998;97:437.

29. Boushey CJ, et al. A Quantitative Assessment of Plasma Homocysteine as a Risk Factor for Vascular Disease. Probable Benefits of Increasing Folic Acid Intakes. *JAMA* 1995;274:1049.

You Broil, Never Fry,
But You've Been Living a Lie

While the Natural Hormonal Enhancement Eating Plan is not a high-fat diet, and you may find yourself eating less fat on the Eating Plan than you are currently, fat-phobia must be expunged so that you will not balk at the notion of "Using Dietary Fat to Burn Bodyfat" (Chapter 18). Moreover, the low-fat craze presents an insightful window into the forces operating to perpetuate the misinformation crisis that has riddled the fat loss efforts and undermined the health and confidence of so many Americans. This chapter also explores the actual causes of cardiovascular disease, the leading killer in the civilized world, and clarifies the relationship between dietary fat and bodyfat. As you will see, popular belief and scientific evidence have diverged to an alarming extent.

A physician who is a lover of wisdom is the equal to a god.
Hippocrates

The superior doctor prevents sickness;
The mediocre doctor attends to impending sickness;
The inferior doctor treats actual sickness.
Chinese Proverb

The medical problems that confound us today will probably amaze scientists in the twenty-first century as they puzzle over why we medical pioneers of today were unable to reach out and grab the obvious, why we were so advanced in certain areas of medical treatment yet so abysmally deficient in others. Why, they may ask, could our surgeons perform open-heart surgery so skillfully as to make it a routine operation while at the same time our nutritional experts couldn't determine the optimal diet for preventing most of the problems necessitating that procedure? Why spend so much time and effort developing complex surgical techniques and other wondrous medical procedures that prolong the life of the diseased body for a few months or, at best, a few years instead of focusing on nutritional changes capable of prolonging healthy life for decades? Why can't we see the big picture? (emphasis mine)
Michael Eades M.D. and Mary Dan Eades M.D., authors of *Protein Power*

For more than 20 years, the "experts" have told us to avoid fat: fat makes you fat, fat causes disease, reduce fat intake or suffer the consequences. And so you do. You pay homage to the Lords of Lowfat every day by separating the eggs yolks from the whites, surgically removing all visible fat from any piece of meat that you eat, and always buying reduced-fat foods, no matter how much like sawdust they may taste.

As a good, fat-fearing person, you accept the sacrifice and deprivation visited upon you by the Lords of Lowfat as the price you must pay to have a healthy, attractive body. When you do not lose bodyfat like you are supposed to, you humbly accept the blame - the fault is obviously yours. You renew your fight against fat by reaffirming your goal to eliminate dietary fat and redoubling your efforts toward that end. And so goes the plight of the average American. Occasionally, you hear a statistic about how Americans are getting fatter, and it gives you pause - how strange that in twenty years the lowfat movement has not registered even the slightest evidence of success. But your skepticism quickly passes - all those "experts" can't possibly be wrong. But they are . . . you've been living a big, *fat,* lie.

Actually, for the most part, health authorities have not been lying any more than a jury is lying that wrongly convicts an innocent person. And like the justice system (which, once judgment is rendered, it is difficult to overturn the conviction even when new, exculpatory evidence surfaces), judgments in the medical and scientific community are not easily overturned. We would like to believe otherwise: that the medical/scientific community is constantly and open-mindedly reexamining current theories, ready at all moments to proclaim loudly, "we were wrong." But as you learned in the last chapter, that is simply not the case.

Appealingly Simple and Intuitively Inviting

The "fat makes you fat" theory is wonderfully appealing in its simplicity. Eat less fat and you'll become less fat (also known as the "less in, less on" theory). The low-fat diet has the same seductive simplicity and seeming obviousness as the flat-Earth theory did - and both are equally mistaken.

Fat has both an incriminating name and an incriminating appearance. The word "fat" is one of the most hated words in the English language, and it is so easy to look at the fat encircling a slab of beef and envision it encircling your waist. Because the fat you eat and the fat hanging off your body are essentially the same in appearance, composition, and consistency, the association between dietary fat and bodyfat is intuitively inviting. Add the fact that, gram for gram, fat has more than twice the calories of protein or carbohydrate and there seems to be a strong scientific basis for the low-fat dietary prescription. Then look at the fact that high fat consumption is correlated with high rates of obesity in the United States (but be sure to ignore the fact that lower fat consumption, the trend in recent years, is correlated with an even higher rate of obesity[1]) and the "fat makes you fat" theory appears bulletproof.

It seems to make perfect sense that, since fat has nine calories per gram and carbohydrate has four calories per gram, if you replace fat with carbohydrate you will consume fewer calories and lose bodyfat. This simplistic reasoning lies at the heart of the low-fat dietary paradigm. However, while the logic is sound, both of the underlying assumptions are flawed. (This situation is similar to adding five plus eight and getting thirteen, and then looking more closely and discovering that the five is really a six - the arithmetic is correct but the result is nonetheless inaccurate.)

For one, reducing calories is generally not an effective way to reduce bodyfat because your metabolism up-regulates or down-regulates to match caloric intake (see Chapter 9). In other words, calorie restriction induces a metabolic slowdown that offsets the calorie deficit. The other assumption, that you will consume fewer calories when carbohydrate is substituted for fat, is also incorrect. Fat tends to reduce cravings (see Chapter 18) while carbohydrate tends to stimulate cravings,[2,3] by generating *hormonal hunger* (see Chapter 11). In fact, although fat contains more than twice the calories per gram of carbohydrate, fat keeps away hunger for about three times as long.[4] So guess what happens when you replace fat with carbohydrate. You wind-up eating at least as many calories as you had before you reduced your fat intake. But now your diet is less pleasurable, and you are not getting the fat-burning effects of fat described in Chapter 18.

45

When you consider how many people have been following the "experts'" instruction to cut fat and increase carbohydrate intake, while becoming fatter and enduring the misery of cravings as a result, you realize what a colossal mistake this has been. The high-carb/low-fat blunder recalls a similar error from years ago that still holds sway over many people today: we were given dire warnings by health authorities to cut cholesterol. Like the "fat makes you fat" theory, the anti-cholesterol theory makes sense on the surface. But, also like the "fat makes you fat" theory, the missing piece of the puzzle is hormones.

Hormones Regulate Cholesterol and Triglyceride Levels

After putting the cholesterol scare into everyone, a realization dawned upon the medical community: the amount of cholesterol you consume has minimal bearing upon the amount of cholesterol in your blood. In fact, most of the cholesterol in the body is produced by the body itself, and a feedback mechanism exists such that the less cholesterol one eats the more one makes, and vice versa.[5,6,7,8]

The disconnect between dietary cholesterol and blood cholesterol was demonstrated in 1970 by the multi-million dollar Framingham study, and has been repeatedly confirmed since that time.[9,10,11,12,13,14,15,16] For example, a study published in the *American Journal of Clinical Nutrition* reports that although the mean cholesterol intake among South African egg farm workers is 1,240 mg per day, their serum cholesterol levels average 181.4 mg/dl.[17] The distinct unimportance of dietary cholesterol for the average person was further dramatized in an article published in the *New England Journal of Medicine*,[18] which reported on an 88-year-old man who ate 25 eggs a day for thirty years. Despite his consistent intake of 5,000 mg. of cholesterol per day (approximately

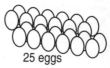

25 eggs

sixteen times the normal recommended amount) this eccentric fellow had normal cholesterol levels and sported a svelte 6'2'', 185-pound physique. (When asked why he ate so many eggs, he blandly replied that he never really thought about it.) These studies, combined with the fact that cholesterol consumption has remained roughly the same during the last 100 years while cardiovascular disease has skyrocketed,[19] exonerates dietary cholesterol as an independently significant cause of cardiovascular disease.

Furthermore, just as dietary cholesterol has minimal bearing upon total serum cholesterol, total serum cholesterol has minimal bearing upon the risk of developing cardiovascular disease. Rather, coronary risk is correlated with the ratio of low-density lipoprotein (LDL) cholesterol to high-density lipoprotein (HDL) cholesterol and with serum triglyceride. Apolipoproteins, as well, are emerging as significant modifiers of coronary risk.[20,21,22,23,24] Additionally, oxidation of cholesterol within the body, which is influenced by dietary intake of antioxidants, is an important (and perhaps the paramount) mechanism by which the artherogenic potential of LDL is actuated.[25,26,27,28,29,30,31,32,33] This kaleidoscope of factors, rather than merely how much cholesterol you have in your blood, determines coronary risk. Thus, it is not surprising that on the island of Crete, where the incidence of cardiovascular disease is the lowest in the world,[34] the average serum cholesterol level of the islanders is over 200.[35]

Nevertheless, drug companies have made, and continue to make, a fortune selling cholesterol-lowering drugs (statins) that lower heart-protective HDL cholesterol along with LDL, produce adverse side effects in many individuals, and have been linked to cancer.[36,37,38,39] As Dr. Udo Erasmus points-out, "it makes no sense to be saved from a heart attack only to be fed to cancer."[40] I would add that it makes even less sense *not* to be saved from a heart attack and fed to cancer. Moreover, as discussed in Chapter 22, cholesterol is the raw material that the body uses to produce the prohormones dehydroepiandrosterone (DHEA) and pregnenolone. These hormones are precursors to testosterone and estrogen, may have important health properties of their own, and decline with advancing age. If you consume less cholesterol, your body makes more of it via the feedback mechanism described above. But if you cripple your body's ability to make cholesterol by taking cholesterol-lowering drugs, you could short-circuit production of anti-aging hormones.

So the resounding question is: what regulates production of cholesterol, and, more importantly, what regulates the ratio of HDL to LDL cholesterol and the production of triglyceride? The answer is hormones. Specifically, insulin and glucagon, which also govern whether you store fat or burn it. When insulin becomes dominant over glucagon, fat storage, total cholesterol, LDL cholesterol, and serum triglyceride levels increase, and vice versa.[41,42,43,44,45,46,47,48,49,50,51,52,53,54] Moreover, new research indicates that a high insulin/glucagon ratio goes even further in promoting cardiovascular disease, by increasing susceptibility of LDL to oxidation.[55,56] All of this research is soundly reinforced by statistical data showing that even slight elevations in baseline insulin levels correspond with increased coronary risk; and consistently high baseline insulin is a powerful discriminator of who develops heart disease and who does not.[57,58,59,60,61,62,63]

In recent years, health authorities have revised their recommendation for preventing heart disease. Recognizing belatedly that dietary cholesterol is all but irrelevant for most people, they instead advise against saturated fat, or *all* fat, which is where the generic "fat promotes heart disease" myth came from. I doubt that any health authority actually believes that dietary fat in general causes cardiovascular disease. Rather, "fat causes heart disease" is a lazy generalization substituted for the fact that certain kinds of fat (saturated and trans fat) can contribute to heart disease while other kinds of fat (monounsaturated and omega 3) can help prevent heart disease. Thus, "dietary fat causes heart disease" is not a simplification, but rather a distortion, of the truth. It is equally accurate to say, "dietary fat prevents heart disease." Nonetheless, sweeping and indiscriminate indictments of dietary fat as a health hazard are common in our fat-phobic society.

The more narrowly tailored "*saturated* fat causes heart disease" is a marked improvement on its anti-cholesterol predecessor. The recommendation to avoid saturated fat at least has the virtue of having some basis in scientific fact given that saturated fat tends to raise both HDL and LDL cholesterol.[64,65,66] But as discussed a moment ago, the insulin/glucagon axis regulates the HDL/LDL ratio and triglyceride levels. Hence, while saturated fat consumption influences serum cholesterol levels, its net health effect is dictated by hormonal status. Trans fatty acids, though far less condemned by health authorities than saturated fat, have a more detrimental impact on health – and their pernicious effect does not depend on hormonal status (see Chapter 18).

47

In light of the fact that insulin predominance raises both LDL and triglyceride levels while lowering HDL, is it any surprise that the high-carbohydrate/low-fat dietary recommendation has proven ineffective, not only as a means of reducing bodyfat, but also as a means of improving blood lipid profile? A strict high-carb/low-fat diet often does result in a modest lowering of total serum cholesterol, depending on the pre-intervention diet,* but the LDL/HDL ratio is usually unaffected. The reason why cholesterol status rarely improves on a high-carbohydrate/low-fat diet is because, in addition to lowering LDL cholesterol, this diet also lowers HDL cholesterol. High-density lipoprotein cholesterol is an established negative risk factor for cardiovascular disease – meaning that high HDL is protective and low HDL is conducive, to heart disease.[67,68,69,70,71,72,73,74] A high-carbohydrate/low-fat diet has repeatedly been shown to suppress HDL cholesterol.[75,76,77,78,79,80,81,82] But let us not forget, cholesterol is only one factor determining who clutches his/her chest and falls over dead.

Like high LDL cholesterol, high serum triglyceride levels foretell cardiac doom. And dietary carbohydrate is strongly correlated with serum triglyceride levels. To put it more precisely: a high-carbohydrate diet raises serum triglyceride levels relative to a lower-carbohydrate diet.[83,84,85,86,87,88,89,90,91] The underlying factor linking high carbohydrate intake with high serum triglyceride is insulin.[92,93,94,95,96,97,98,99] Insulin converts excess blood sugar (derived from ingested carbohydrate) into triglyceride and blocks the burning of triglyceride for energy. The latter effect is the more potent of the two in terms of raising serum triglyceride levels: by inhibiting uptake and utilization of triglyceride by the muscles, these fats remain, and accumulate, in the blood.[100,101,102,103]

Carbohydrate Consumption   Serum Triglyceride

The triglyceride-raising effect of a high-carbohydrate diet is particularly disturbing in light of growing evidence showing that elevated serum triglyceride is a more forceful cardiovascular risk factor than previously believed,[104,105,106,107,108,109,110] and may synergistically interact with low HDL cholesterol to heighten dramatically cardiovascular risk in individuals whose blood lipid profile reflects both of these features.[111,112,113,114] For example, a research report presented at the 1995 American Heart Association meeting concluded that an elevated triglyceride to HDL cholesterol ratio can make a heart attack *seventeen times* more likely.[115] No wonder that several human studies of high-carbohydrate diets in recent years have been aborted due to ethical concerns about adverse coronary-risk-profile changes.

Serum Triglyceride   Heart Disease Rate

---

* Naturally, the net effect of a high-carb/low-fat diet depends on what one's blood lipid profile was before beginning such a diet. If one is switching from the typical unhealthy American diet (high in both carbohydrate *and* fat), to a high-carbohydrate/low-fat diet, blood lipid levels may undergo a relative improvement. Keep this "worse to bad" scenario in mind next time you hear one of the "experts" cite a study purportedly proving the heart-healthy effects of a high-carb/low-fat diet.

(This illustrates a major advantage of animal studies: experiments can be undertaken that maim, torment, or destroy the subjects. Of course, the animals aren't nearly as enthusiastic as the researchers about these experiments.) The high-carbohydrate/low-fat diet, with its powerful capability of raising triglyceride levels and its suppressive effect on HDL cholesterol, appears to be an even graver miscalculation than previously thought.

With painful slowness, the medical community is beginning to take notice. For example, widely respected cardiologist K. Lance Gould wrote in a letter published in the *Journal of the American Medical Association*: "Frequently, triglyceride levels increase and HDL cholesterol levels decrease for individuals on vegetarian, high-carbohydrate diets. Since low HDL cholesterol, particularly with high triglycerides, incurs substantial risk of coronary events, I do not recommend a high-carbohydrate strict vegetarian diet."[116] Despite these remarks and the compelling scientific evidence underlying them, most members of the medical community are still held captive by their entrenched pro-carbohydrate, anti-fat, bias.

The following provides an example of the destructive impact of institutionalized low-fat bias. A high-carbohydrate/low-fat diet continues to be widely prescribed to Type II diabetics (a group at exceptionally high risk for developing cardiovascular disease[117,118,119]), even though the vast weight of the scientific evidence shows that such a diet will worsen their condition and further elevate their risk of cardiovascular disease. For instance, a study published in the *Journal of the American Medical Association*,[120] comparing a higher-carbohydrate/lower-fat diet with a lower-carbohydrate/higher-fat diet in Type II diabetic patients found, in the words of the authors of the study, that the higher-carbohydrate diet "caused persistent deterioration of glycemic control and accentuation of hyperinsulinemia, as well as increased plasma triglyceride and very-low-density lipoprotein cholesterol levels." It went on to conclude that these effects "may not be desirable" - what? A bad haircut may not be desirable; exacerbation of the diabetic condition and raising of coronary risk factors in an already high-risk group is *definitely, highly* undesirable.

In contrast to, and in spite of, the vast majority of the medical community, enlightened physicians like Michael and Mary Dan Eades, authors of *Protein Power,* and Robert Atkins have compiled impressive records of success at treating their patients with a dietary plan that is relatively high in overall fat, allows for unlimited saturated fat consumption, and aims at the internal (hormonal) controls that govern cholesterol and triglyceride formation. The low-carbohydrate approach espoused by these doctors is certainly not new. In fact, the first popular diet book in the United States, *Bantings Letter on Corpulence* written by William Banting in the mid-1800s, advocated low-carbohydrate eating. Since then, the low-carbohydrate diet has periodically faded away and reemerged. About once every twenty years it is trotted-out by an enterprising person who is clever enough to market it as a breakthrough (or "new revolution" in the case of the bestselling *Dr. Atkins' New Diet Revolution*).

49

While the low-carbohydrate diet is neither new nor revolutionary, it has assumed new relevance in recent years as a counterpoint to the high-carbohydrate/low-fat dietary paradigm. Dr. Atkins and Dr.s Michael and Mary Dan Eades, and others like them, have been raising the hackles of the medical establishment while lowering the LDL cholesterol levels of their patients with their heretical dietary approach of low carbohydrate and unlimited fat. While I believe that the low-carbohydrate diet has serious flaws (see p. 139) and thus I do not endorse it, the Atkins/Eades approach lends crucial insight into the impact of dietary fat upon health.

Dr. Atkins, in particular, a cardiologist by trade who expanded into the lucrative diet industry with his reinvented version of the low-carbohydrate diet, has successfully treated thousands of *cardiac patients* with a high-fat/low-carbohydrate diet during the last twenty-five years at the Atkins Center in New York. According to conventional wisdom, this is tantamount to advising lung cancer patients to take-up cigarette smoking. But the consistently positive, often dramatic, results achieved with this dietary prescription invalidate any comparison between Dr. Atkins and Dr. Kevorkian.

Despite the problematic nature of the low-carbohydrate/high-fat diet as a vehicle for body composition improvement and permanent fat loss, the rebellious physicians who promote it deserve credit for proving (regardless of whether the medical establishment chooses to acknowledge the proof) that neither fat in general, nor saturated fat in particular, is the principal causative agent in cardiovascular disease. Why won't the medical establishment acknowledge the superiority of the low-carbohydrate diet over the low-fat diet for improving blood lipid profile? In the words of Dr. Atkins, "American medicine is more responsive to the dogmatic pronouncements of academicians appointed to consensus panels than it is to scientific research."[121] Notwithstanding our differences, I couldn't agree more with the good doctor on this point.

The impressive success of the low-carbohydrate diet as a means of improving blood lipid profile contrasts sharply with its abysmal record as a means of effecting positive and lasting body composition changes. The point here is that, while a large percentage of people who go on a low-carbohydrate/high-fat diet regain all the lost fat within six months of quitting the diet, fat gain *while on the diet* virtually never happens. Think about this for a moment: a high-fat diet, when employed in the context of carbohydrate restriction, virtually never results in fat gain! What does this tell you about the dominant dietary belief of the last twenty years - that fat makes you fat?

The experience of doctors like Atkins and Eades, successfully treating cardiac patients with what often amounts to a high-fat diet, is not an anomaly.[122] Nor is the dismal track record of the low-fat diet difficult to explain. In fact, the scientific journals are filled with studies showing that fat is not necessarily fattening, and indicating that hormonal state is the decisive factor in this connection. Many, but certainly not all, such studies are referenced in this book. I encourage you to review the scientific evidence for yourself.

Examining History and Other Cultures

As you can see, both the weight of scientific evidence and the teachings of practical experience indicate that the low-fat approach to fat loss and health is a dietary debacle. After hearing the chorus of anti-fat sentiment over the last twenty years, most people are shocked to learn that they have had all their egg whites in the wrong basket for all this time. By contrast, students of history and those who have studied other cultures of the world have been quizzically scratching their heads over the Great Fat Scare of the late 20th century ever since its inception.

The Eskimos of Greenland, Canada, and Alaska have subsisted for most of their existence on a very high-fat/-cholesterol, very low-carbohydrate diet consisting largely of fish, marine mammals, and reindeer - and yet they traditionally survive to a ripe-old age with exceedingly low rates of heart disease and diabetes.[123,124,125,126,127,128] Dietary fat was so highly valued by the Greenlandic Eskimos that rent on land in some places was paid with butter.[129] And yet, as Dr. Mauro Di Pasquale observes, "no one keeled over on their way to the landlord."[130] Obesity, too, is historically rare among the Eskimos (despite the cartoons),[131,132] refuting the "fat makes you fat" myth.

Recently, though, the incidence of heart disease, diabetes, and obesity have increased sharply among many Eskimo populations. The anti-fat crowd would have you believe that the Eskimos' centuries of uncanny good luck had finally run-out. But no, the Eskimos who have begun succumbing to heart disease in American-like fashion are the ones who have undergone the dietary changes attendant with the advance of Western civilization upon their culture in recent decades.[133] As I explain throughout this book, the modern Western diet – characterized by refined carbohydrates, trans fatty acids, processed vegetable oil, and a relative absence of fiber - unfavorably alters hormone levels, thereby promoting obesity and disease.

In Iceland, heart disease and diabetes were very rare since time immemorial, despite the predominance of a high-fat diet. Enter refined carbohydrates into the Icelandic diet in the early part of the twentieth century, and enter both of these afflictions about twenty years later. Similarly, the Masai, a cattle-raising pastoral tribe of East Africa, suffer virtually zero incidence of heart disease despite high consumption of animal fat.[134] However, as the Western dietary influence encroaches upon the African continent, more and more black African populations are experiencing cardiovascular disease for the first time.[135,136,137] A study of Yemenite Jews performed by Dr A. M. Cohen is in accord with these findings. Cohen observed that after moving from Yemen where the typical diet was high in animal fat and low in sugar, to Israel, and adopting the high-sugar westernized diet of that country, coronary disease

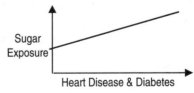

and diabetes increased commensurately with length of time in Israel.[138] When Ethiopians emigrated to Israel many years later, in 1987, the same pattern was observed. Five years after their arrival in Israel, the incidence of diabetes was up 1500% among Ethiopian immigrants.[139]

The point often missed is that fat consumption is correlated with cardiovascular disease and obesity, but so is sugar consumption. The tricky part is that refined carbohydrate consumption and fat consumption *are highly correlated with each other* - both are defining dietary characteristics of affluent, westernized societies.[140,141] With urbanization and industrialization comes the mass production of inexpensive, processed foodstuffs - and that means sugar and other forms of refined carbohydrate. This is *in addition to* higher intake of fat resulting from 1) partially hydrogenated fat (trans fat) added to processed foods to extend shelf life, 2) greater supply of meat and dairy products owing to advanced methods of animal husbandry that increase yield but reduce nutritive content and adversely alter fatty acid composition, and 3) widespread availability of mass-marketed, heavily processed vegetable oil. **It is this combination of high consumption of refined carbohydrates and low-quality fat, more so than either of these factors individually, which is the health scourge of the industrialized world**.

You don't have to be a logic whiz to realize that in industrialized nations, *association* cannot be equated with *causation* of degenerative disease or obesity because we do not know which of these two co-existent dietary factors – refined carbohydrate, or fat, or a combination

association
≠
causation

of both - is at fault. In order to tease-out the causal agent, we have to examine the exceptions - those cultures in which these two eating patterns do not converge. In the industrialized world, such exceptions are not to be found. The United States, however, represents an instructive case study. As discussed in Chapter 6, fat consumption in the U.S. has decreased in recent years due to the low-fat craze, and carbohydrate consumption has increased for the same reason. Result: obesity afflicts a greater percentage of people in the U.S. now than ever, and the big three killers - heart disease, cancer, and diabetes - continue their devastating rampage through American society.

According to the low-fat gospel, the late twentieth century was a time of soaring fat consumption in the United States and, consequently, soaring incidence of heart disease. But only the second part of that statement is true. In response to the implication that fat consumption was much lower back in the good old days, an obvious question arises: since the food processing revolution, which introduced refined flour, high fructose corn syrup, and cola into the American diet and made sugar-based products cheaply and widely available, did not occur until the latter part of the Industrial Revolution, in the 1890's, what did people eat in the U.S. before that time? Certainly they did not eat cookies, white bread, breakfast cereal, or potato chips - these foods did not exist. Answer: meat, eggs, butter, and lard, along with fruits and vegetables and some high-fiber, unprocessed starchy foods - a typical preindustrial diet. Not coincidentally, heart disease was an insignificant factor before the 1900's.[142] So insignificant in fact, that although research was being done and medical journals were being published, the first study of heart disease did not appear until 1912.[143]

It is true that life expectancy today is considerably higher in the United States than it was in the early 1900's. But is this because of the dietary changes that have occurred since then, or in spite of them? It is often overlooked that infant mortality and the death rate among citizens under sixteen years of age have fallen dramatically during the twentieth century, due to a national program of vaccinations and medical advances in pediatric and prenatal care. When you factor these figures in with the elimination of hazardous working conditions, improved housing and sanitation, and the tremendous medical advances that have enabled sick and diseased persons to either be cured or kept alive longer, the question becomes: why aren't we living longer?* The answer to that question is simple: because Americans are being mowed-down by degenerative diseases like heart disease, cancer, diabetes, and osteoporosis at a rate unparalleled in human history. In view of this, I doubt that we owe a debt of gratitude to the modern American diet.

Another culture that contradicts the prevailing bias against dietary fat held in the United States is the French. The "French Paradox," as it is called, has attracted a great deal of attention in recent years, including being featured on *Sixty Minutes*. The French take pride in their gourmet cooking which centers upon butter, cheese, ham, sausage, and other rich, high-fat foods. Their diet is higher in fat than the typical American diet, but substantially lower in sugar and other refined carbohydrates. The low-fat devotees in this country would predict that such a diet would have the French people dropping like flies from clogged arteries. In fact, the French experience flies in the face of such a prediction. To the puzzlement of American experts steeped in lowfat lore, heart disease in France is not nearly the force it is in the United States, and neither is obesity.[144,145,146]

More recently, a 1995 article was published entitled, "The Spanish Paradox."[147] The Spanish, like the French, consume a high-fat/low-refined-carbohydrate diet and enjoy a low incidence of cardiovascular disease.[148] Even more "paradoxical" is the fact that fat consumption has been rising steadily in the last few decades in Spain, while cardiovascular disease has been declining.[149] Nevertheless, in a study published in the *European Journal of Clinical Nutrition* the authors state, "the rise in fat intake in Spain urges dietary interventions."[150] Why? Is cardiovascular disease too low in Spain?

---

* In fact, back in the old days, if you could make it through your infant and teenage years, you had a pretty good shot at living a long life. Benjamin Franklin lived to 84, President Van Buren lived to 80, President Adams lived to 91, President Jefferson lived to 83, President Madison lived to 85, and President Quincy Adams lived to 81. All of these men were born in the 1700's when medical science was relatively primitive (no lasers, no organ transplants, no angioplasty – today we've got the artificial heart, back then they had the wooden leg). Even so, plenty of people in that era, presidents and average citizens alike, lived beyond today's life expectancy, and they tended to be more vigorous and active in their later years than are today's elderly. (Benjamin Franklin negotiated the Treaty of Paris, in which Britain formally acknowledged American independence, at the age of 77.)

Unfortunately, the turn of the twentieth century has not proven auspicious for U.S. presidents, even though it has witnessed the development of cures and treatments for diseases that were untreatable in prior centuries. Among the twentieth century presidents, Wilson died at 68, Harding died at 58, Coolidge died 61, FDR died at 63, and Johnson died at 65; only Hoover, Nixon, Truman, and Reagan made it into their 80's. It's true that there are more centenarians now than ever in the U.S.; but it is also true that there are many more people overall in the U.S. now than ever. The fact is that only 1 in 10,000 Americans reach 100 years of age.[150a] And among centenarians, about half are disabled, most are institutionalized, and only 30% have full command of their faculties.[150b] Self-congratulatory hype and false cheer to the contrary notwithstanding, the truth is that the highly-celebrated increase in life expectancy in the twentieth century is no great shakes when you consider the exponential advances in medical science that have occurred during this period.

And let's not forget about the Eskimo Paradox, and the Masai Paradox, and the Cretans. Inhabitants of the Mediterranean island of Crete consume a high-fat diet (40%-45% of total calories).[151] Incidence of heart disease in Crete: lowest in the world.[152] Why did I not refer to this as a paradox? Because according to an article published in a prestigious journal, the Cretan experience is not a paradox, but rather a "miracle."[153] The use of a word reserved for divine acts of the Almighty to describe the incidence of heart disease on the island of Crete illustrates the enormous difficulty the scientific community is having in coming to grips with the fact that dietary fat does not cause heart disease. We should all pray to have arteries as pristine as the Cretans. And perhaps by increasing our intake of the right kind of fats, our cardiovascular systems, too, can be immaculate exceptions to the low-fat gospel.

As incredible as it may seem, few researchers consider carbohydrate consumption when performing studies of diet/disease. Instead, either assuming that carbs can't possibly be the culprit or unwilling to challenge conventional thought at the risk of their professional reputation, researchers simply "round-up the usual suspects": total fat and saturated fat. This is why there is a voluminous body of epidemiological research showing that fat intake is *correlated* with cardiovascular disease, but scant published studies of this kind connecting refined carbohydrates to cardiovascular disease – *even though* in most populations where fat consumption is high so is consumption of soft drinks, white flour, and sugar. A recent study that did take carbohydrate consumption into account, and which examined dietary links to heart disease in 32 countries, found a stronger association for sugar than for fat. And guess which food was most strongly correlated with heart disease. Answer: non-fat milk.[154] Who are the people most likely to drink non-fat milk? Answer: people on a low-fat, high-carbohydrate diet. Rather than being itself a contributor to coronary disease, might non-fat-milk consumption be a statistical marker of a low-fat, high-carb eating pattern?

Epidemiological studies like these, which trace the incidence of diseases among various populations, are downplayed by most scientists, and rightfully so. It is impossible to track-down all the variable cultural factors that could influence the findings. For instance, it has been suggested that red wine consumption is responsible for the French Paradox, and that the high omega 3 fat content of the fish eaten by Eskimos exerts a cardioprotective effect. Nobody knows for sure exactly what mix of factors accounts for these findings. What is clear, though, from 1) the worldwide epidemiological evidence, 2) the experience of doctors in the U.S. who have departed from the low-fat party line in treating their patients, 3) the clinical studies, 4) the twenty-year low-fat misadventure in the U.S. is that: the proposition that fat makes you fat and promotes heart disease is inaccurate on both counts.

Ignore-ance Defeats Truth and Causes Death

All of this evidence, however, is ignored by health authorities who would rather enjoy the comfort and prestige of parroting mainstream views than critically to probe the basis of such views. Sadly, I suspect that health authorities who have staked their reputation on the low-fat theory will continue for quite some time to avert their eyes from the clear and convincing evidence refuting their doctrine. And where willful blindness fails, they will continue to conjure-up ever-more-tortured reasoning to justify their anti-fat prejudices.

Because the hormonal root of obesity and heart disease has been lost on most health authorities, we have been led astray as heart disease, the leading cause of death and disability in the United States, continues to exact a terrible toll.[155,156] In the case of the saturated fat bogeyman, we have been pointed away from butter and other naturally saturated fats that people in our society and others thrived on long before heart disease was even a footnote in medical textbooks, and toward margarine and other sources of trans fatty acids, polyunsaturated processed vegetable oil, and low-fat products loaded with refined carbohydrates. Trans fat and refined carbs are each a greater menace to health than saturated fat, and many types of vegetable oil raise serious health concerns as well (see Chapter 18).

Together, trans fatty acids and refined carbohydrates are a potent pathogenic combo, and they are likely responsible for much of the mischief blamed on fat in general and saturated fat in particular. In contrast to saturated fat which has been consumed in significant quantities since the days when "fast food" referred to animals fleet-a-foot and hard to catch, refined carbohydrates and trans fatty acids are relatively recent additions to the human diet. And both refined carbs and trans fat correlate much more closely, in both historical and cross-population analyses, with the degenerative diseases that afflict modern man and woman than does cholesterol or saturated fat.

Ironically, the instruction to lower saturated fat often *does* lead to improvements in serum cholesterol, but for the wrong reason. Most Americans are in a fat-storing cholesterol-producing state due insulin/glucagon imbalance, promoted by the Standard American Diet (S.A.D. - a fitting acronym). *In this hormonal environment*, with the insulin/glucagon axis out-of-kilter in favor of insulin, saturated fat is, indeed, as unhealthy as health authorities make it out to be. This is why I stated on p. 52 that the combination of refined carbohydrates (which raise insulin levels) and fat, more so than either factor individually, is the health scourge of the industrialized world. But when you improve your hormonal state, saturated fat becomes a toothless tiger. In any event, doesn't it make more sense to attack the underlying problem, hormonal imbalance, especially since it causes other health problems, including obesity?

This chapter has been critical, and maybe even a bit caustic, in outlining a series of errors pertaining to dietary fat in general, cholesterol, and saturated fat. It is not the errors that are reprehensible, but the persistence of the errors in the face of the available scientific evidence. We laugh at the obtuse ivory tower complacency of Galileo's contemporaries who refused to open their minds to the concept that the Earth moves around the sun. But I am not so inclined to laugh at similar close-mindedness in this advanced age, especially when the issue relates not to the relationship between heavenly bodies, but to the health of human bodies.

Propaganda to the contrary aside, *more than 50% of Americans* are now either overweight or obese[157] in spite of, and probably in part because of, the low-fat/high-carbohydrate diet that has been foisted on them by the so-called health experts. The low-fat authorities have egg on their face (whole egg that is, yolk and all) – and Americans are fatter and sicker than ever. Mortality (death rate) may be falling as doctors become ever more proficient at treating the sick and dying, but the incidence of cancer, diabetes, osteoporosis, cardiovascular disease, and especially obesity (which contributes to the four other diseases) is *much* higher today than it was one-hundred years ago.

The "experts" had better begin to acknowledge the handwriting on the wall, or rather on the death certificates - according to the *Journal of the American Medical Association* (October 1999) at least 300,000 deaths per year in the U.S. could be linked to being overweight, placing excess bodyfat second only to smoking as a preventable cause of death.[158] The economic cost is similarly staggering with obesity-related medical problems now costing approximately 60 billion dollars in the U.S., up approximately 50% from 1986 (see p. 35). Clearly, the problem is getting worse, and our health-care system is being crushed under the weight of obesity.

Smoking #1
Obesity #2

The "experts" often blame it on the public, casting the American people as lazy, weak-willed gluttons. I strongly disagree. I have found that most people are willing to commit themselves to improving their appearance and their health. It is not a failure of execution but a flawed plan of action that is the problem. The statistics support my observations. When the "experts" said cut cholesterol, egg sales dropped like a lead anchor. When the "experts" said that we should cut fat, that is exactly what people did - fat consumption decreased sharply. When the "experts" said replace butter with margarine, margarine consumption skyrocketed and butter joined eggs on the blacklist. When the "experts" said carbohydrate is the key to being lean and healthy, Americans made carbohydrate the centerpiece of their diet and bought all the tasteless lowfat products that the fat-loss industry manufactured to exploit this misbegotten dietary trend.

Where has all this obedience gotten us? As I mentioned a moment ago, Americans are fatter now than ever and the U.S. is at or near the top of the list in all categories of degenerative disease. In view of these statistics, I believe that it is unconscionable for the same "experts" who have misled us on matters of health and fat loss, albeit unintentionally, to continue to espouse the same tired, old recommendations that helped put us in our current sorry state of health in the first place, while dismissing new approaches supported by overwhelming evidence simply because the medical establishment has yet to remove the blinders that keep them wedded to the tried and untrue, factually discredited views of old.

Having said all of this, it is important to recognize the segment of health professionals who do not fall into this category, who are constantly reexamining their views and open-mindedly searching for new solutions. An example of this progressive spirit can be seen in the quotation at the beginning of this chapter from Dr.s Michael and Mary Dan Eades. It is that mindset which holds the promise of a reversal of the current awful health record of the United States, toward a brighter future of health, fitness, and longevity.

Furthermore, to their credit, many health professionals are beginning to acknowledge that the low-fat movement has been a movement backwards (or if we're talking about waistlines - outwards). Evidence that some members of the medical community are willing to admit they were wrong and embark on an open-minded search for truth can be found in *Hippocrates* (May 1997):

"Study after study from around the world shows that fat isn't the bad guy we've made it out to be."

In a Nutshell, Here's What You Need to Know about Dietary Fat:

♦ **Just as you do not need redwood to build a red house, your body does not need dietary fat to make bodyfat**. Your body can convert carbohydrate and even protein to bodyfat, and when lipogenic (fat-storage) hormones are active, that's exactly what happens.

♦ **Ultimately, it does not matter how much fat you eat, it matters how much fat you store**. The fat you eat and the fat on your body are the same for energy purposes. When your body is efficient at using fat for energy (i.e., you are a "fat-burner") your body uses-up bodyfat as well as dietary fat at a high rate. On the other hand, if your hormonal state makes you a "sugar-burner," eating fat is like pumping kerosene into your car instead of gasoline: your body is not efficient at using fat for fuel, so when you consume fat you wind-up wearing it instead of burning it.

Sugar-Burner or Fat-Burner?

As you can see, the truth concerning dietary fat is at variance with what the twenty-year-old anti-fat hysteria has led you to believe. Now make sure you are sitting down for this shocking bit of information: dietary fat is not only helpful but is *necessary* for shedding bodyfat and improving your body composition. Accordingly, I have devoted Chapter 18 to teaching you how to use dietary fat to burn bodyfat.

The American public's misguided aversion to dietary fat is one of the reasons why Americans have grown fatter over the years, while fat consumption has decreased. However, the fact that you need dietary fat in order to burn fat, DOES NOT mean that increasing fat consumption in the context of your current dietary habits will cause you to lose fat. It will not necessarily, and it will probably make you fatter. If this seems confusing or contradictory, recall that hormones regulate fat storage and fat burning. Accordingly, whether or not dietary fat is fattening depends on your hormonal state. When you are in a

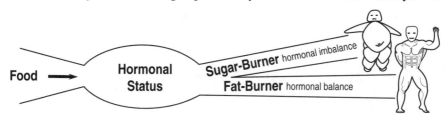

fat-storing state (i.e., you are a sugar-burner) everything you put in your mouth - fat, carbohydrate, even protein - has a greater likelihood of being turned into bodyfat. Conversely, when your hormonal state makes you a fat-burner, everything you eat is less likely to be stored as fat.

As a fat-burner, it is unnatural for your body to store dietary fat in quantity sufficient to produce excess bodyfat. Your body's energy needs are tremendous. Innumerable processes are going on right now as you read this book: respiration, circulation, digestion, protein synthesis, immune system activity, etc.; and this is while you are reading a book - imagine when you are moving around or exercising! Every cell of your body (trillions) are constantly demanding their share of energy: more, more, more, now, now, now. As a fat-burner, fat from food and from adipose tissue will be used to fulfill your energy needs, twenty-four hours a day, seven days a week. The aim of the NHE Eating Plan is to activate a metabolic shift from being a sugar-burner, which you have probably been for most or all of your life, to being a fat-burner. The fat-burning state is the natural one, and there are many other benefits to being a fat-burner besides maintaining low bodyfat. These include: better health, better athletic performance, and higher energy levels.

References

1. Lichtenstein AH, et al. Dietary Fat Consumption and Health. *Nutr Rev* 1998;56:S3.

2. Holt S, et al. Relationship of Satiety to Postprandial Glycemic, Insulin, and Cholecystokinin Responses. *Appetite* 1992;18:129.

3. Holt SH, Miller JB. Increased Insulin Responses to Ingested Foods are Associated with Lessened Satiety. *Appetite* 1995;24:43.

4. Erasmus U. *Fats that Heal Fats that Kill*. BC, Canada: Alive Books 1993, p. 196

5. Maranhao RC, Quintao EC. Long Term Steroid Metabolism Balance Studies in Subjects on Cholesterol-Free and Cholesterol-Rich Diets: Comparison between Normal and Hypercholesterolemic Individuals. *J Lipid Res* 1983;24:167.

6. Nestel PJ, Poyser A. Changes in Cholesterol Synthesis and Excretion when Cholesterol Intake is Increased. *Metabolism* 1976;25:1591.

7. Jones PJ, et al. Dietary Cholesterol Feeding Suppresses Human Cholesterol Synthesis Measured by Deuterium Incorporation and Urinary Mevalonic Acid Levels. *Arterioscler Thromb Vasc Biol* 1996;16:1222.

8. Rudel L, et al. Dietary Cholesterol and Downregulation of Cholesterol 7 Alpha-Hydroxylase and Cholesterol Absorption in African Green Monkeys. *J Clin Invest* 1994;93:2463.

9. McNamara DJ. Dietary Cholesterol and the Optimal Diet for Reducing Risk of Atherosclerosis. *Can J Cardiol* 1995;(Suppl):123G.

10. Namara DJ. Cholesterol Intake and Plasma Cholesterol: An Update. *J Am Coll Nutr* 1997;16:530.

11. Flaim E, et al. Plasma Lipid and Lipoprotein Cholesterol Concentrations in Adult Males Consuming Normal and High Cholesterol Diets under Controlled Conditions. *Am J Clin Nutr* 1981;34:1103.

12. Glick M, et al. Dietary Cardiovascular Risk Factors and Serum Cholesterol in an Old Order Mennonite Community. *Am J Public Health* 1998;88:1202.

13. Bowman MP, et al. Effect of Dietary Fat and Cholesterol on Plasma Lipids and Lipoprotein Fractions in Normolipidemic Men. *J Nutr* 1988;118:555.

14. McNamara DJ, et al. Heterogeneity of Cholesterol Homeostasis in Man. Response to Changes in Dietary Fat Quality and Cholesterol Quantity. *J Clin Invest* 1987;79:1729.

15. Edington J, et al. Effect of Dietary Cholesterol on Plasma Cholesterol Concentration in Subjects following Reduced Fat, High Fibre Diet. *Br Med J (Clin Res Ed)* 1987;294:333.

16. Flynn MA, et al. Effect of Dietary Egg on Human Serum Cholesterol and Triglycerides. *Am J Clin Nutr* 1979;32:1051.

17. Vorster HH, et al. Serum Cholesterol, Lipoproteins, and Plasma Coagulation Factors in South African Blacks on a High-Egg but Low-Fat Intake. *Am J Clin Nutr* 1987;46:52.

18. No authors listed. Normal Plasma Cholesterol in a Man Who Eats 25 Eggs a Day. *N Engl J Med* 1991;325:584.

19. Erasmus U. *Fats that Heal Fats that Kill.* BC, Canada: Alive Books 1993, p. 326.

20. Breckenridge WC. The Role of Lipoproteins and Apolipoproteins in Prediction of Coronary Heart Disease Risk. *Clin Invest Med* 1990;13:196.

21. Kottke BA, Apolipoproteins and Coronary Artery Disease. *Mayo Clin Proc* 1986;61:313.

22. Maciejko JJ, et al. Apolipoprotein A-I as a Marker of Angiographically Assessed Coronary-Artery Disease. *N Engl J Med* 1983;309:385.

23. Puchois P, et al. Apolipoprotein A-I Containing Lipoproteins in Coronary Artery Disease. *Atherosclerosis* 1987;68:35.

24. Barbir M, et al. High Prevalence of Hypertriglyceridaemia and Apolipoprotein Abnormalities in Coronary Artery Disease. *Br Heart J* 1988;60:397.

25. Rong JX, et al. Arterial Injury by Cholesterol Oxidation Products Causes Endothelial Dysfunction and Arterial Wall Cholesterol Accumulation. *Arterioscler Thromb Vasc Biol* 1998;18:1885.

26. Gey KF. The Antioxidant Hypothesis of Cardiovascular Disease: Epidemiology and Mechanisms. *Biochem Soc Trans* 1990;18:1041.

27. Linseisen J, et al. Effect of a Single Oral Dose of Antioxidant Mixture (Vitamin E, Carotenoids) on the Formation of Cholesterol Oxidation Products after Ex Vivo LDL Oxidation in Humans. *Eur J Med Res* 1998;3:5.

28. Sparrow CP, et al. Low Density Lipoprotein is Protected from Oxidation and the Progression of Atherosclerosis is Slowed in Cholesterol-Fed Rabbits by the Antioxidant N,N'-Diphenyl-Phenylenediamine. *J Clin Invest* 1992;89:1885.

29. Jialal I, Devaraj S. Low-Density Lipoprotein Oxidation, Antioxidants, and Atherosclerosis: A Clinical Biochemistry Perspective. *Clin Chem* 1996;42:498.

30. Bjorkhem I, et al. The Antioxidant Butylated Hydroxytoluene Protects against Atherosclerosis. *Arterioscler Thromb* 1991;11:15.

31. Steinberg D. Clinical Trials of Antioxidants in Atherosclerosis: Are We Doing the Right Thing? *Lancet* 1995;346:36.

32. Frei B. Cardiovascular Disease and Nutrient Antioxidants: Role of Low-Density Lipoprotein Oxidation. *Crit Rev Food Sci Nutr* 1995;35:83.

33. Jialal I, Devaraj S. The Role of Oxidized Low Density Lipoprotein in Atherogenesis. *J Nutr* 1996;126:1053S.

34. Menotti A, et al. Food Intake Patterns and 25-Year Mortality from Coronary Heart Disease: Cross-Cultural Correlations in the Seven Countries Study. The Seven Countries Study Research Group. *Eur J Epidemiol* 1999;15:507.

35. Lindholm LH, et al. Risk Factors for Ischaemic Heart Disease in a Greek Population. A Cross-Sectional Study of Men and Women Living in the Village of Spili in Crete. *Eur Heart J* 1992;13:291.

36. Zureik M, Courbon D, Ducimetiere P. Decline in Serum Total Cholesterol and the Risk of Death from Cancer. *Epidemiology* 1997;8:137.

37. Geurian KL. The Cholesterol Controversy. *Ann Pharmacother* 1996;30:495.

38. Davidson KW, et al. Increases in Depression after Cholesterol-Lowering Drug Treatment. *Behav Med* 1996;22:82.

39. Chang AK, Barrett-Connor E, Edelstein S. Low Plasma Cholesterol Predicts an Increased Risk of Lung Cancer in Elderly Women. *Prev Med* 1995;24:557.

40. Erasmus U. *Fats that Heal Fats that Kill*. BC, Canada: Alive Books 1993, p. 73.

41. Lindberg O, et al. Inverse Association of Serum Cholesterol with Plasma Insulin in the Elderly. Cross-Sectional and Prospective Analyses. *Aging (Milano)* 1998;10:137.

42. Jeppesen J, Facchini FS, Reaven GM. Individuals with High Total Cholesterol/HDL Cholesterol Ratios are Insulin Resistant. *J Intern Med* 1998;243:293.

43. Laws A, et al. Relation of Fasting Plasma Insulin Concentration to High-Density Lipoprotein Cholesterol and Triglyceride Concentrations in Men. *Arterioscler Thromb* 1991;11:1636.

44. Hubbard R, et al. Effect of Dietary Protein on Serum Insulin and Glucagon Levels in Hyper- and Normocholesterolemic Men. *Atherosclerosis* 1989;76:55.

45. Laws A, Reaven GM. Evidence for an Independent Relationship between Insulin Resistance and Fasting Plasma HDL-Cholesterol, Triglyceride and Insulin Concentrations. *J Intern Med* 1992;231:25.

46. Godsland IF, et al. Influence of Insulin Resistance, Secretion, and Clearance on Serum Cholesterol, Triglycerides, Lipoprotein Cholesterol, and Blood Pressure in Healthy Men. *Arterioscler Thromb* 1992;12:1030.

47. Stalder M, Pometta D, Suenram A. Relationship between Plasma Insulin Levels and High Density Lipoprotein Cholesterol Levels in Healthy Men. *Diabetologia* 1981;21:544.

48. Winocour PH, et al. Relation between Insulinemia, Body Mass Index, and Lipoprotein Composition in Healthy, Nondiabetic Men and Women. *Arterioscler Thromb* 1992;12:393.

49. Ghiselli G, et al. Regulatory Function of Glucose and Insulin on High-Density Lipoprotein Cholesterol in Normolipidemic Subjects. *Metabolism* 1994;43:1332.

50. Capaldo B, et al. Relationship between Insulin Response to Intravenous Glucose and Plasma Lipoproteins in Healthy Men. *Artery* 1985;13:108.

51. Karhapaa P, Malkki M, Laakso M. Isolated Low HDL Cholesterol. An Insulin-Resistant State. *Diabetes* 1994;43:411.

52. Abbasi F, et al. Fasting Remnant Lipoprotein Cholesterol and Triglyceride Concentrations Are Elevated in Nondiabetic, Insulin-Resistant, Female Volunteers. *J Clin Endocrinol Metab* 1999;84:3903.

53. Bruce R, et al. Associations between Insulin Sensitivity, and Free Fatty Acid and Triglyceride Metabolism Independent of Uncomplicated Obesity. *Metabolism* 1994;43:1275.

54. Bazelmans J, Nestel PJ, Nolan C. Insulin-Induced Glucose Utilization Influences Triglyceride Metabolism. *Clin Sci* 1983;64:511.

55. Rifici VA, Schneider SH, Khachadurian AK. Stimulation of Low-Density Lipoprotein Oxidation by Insulin and Insulin Like Growth Factor I. *Atherosclerosis* 1994;107:99.

56. Quinones-Galvan A, et al. Evidence that Acute Insulin Administration Enhances LDL Cholesterol Susceptibility to Oxidation in Healthy Humans. *Arterioscler Thromb Vasc Biol* 1999;19:2928.

57. Despres JP, et al. Hyperinsulinemia as an Independent Risk Factor for Ischemic Heart Disease. *N Engl J Med* 1996;334:952.

58. Job FP, et al. Hyperinsulinism in Patients with Coronary Artery Disease. *Coron Artery Dis* 1994;5:487.

59. Mykkanen L, et al. Low Insulin Sensitivity is Associated with Clustering of Cardiovascular Disease Risk Factors. *Am J Epidemiol* 1997;146:315.

60. Lamarche B, et al. Fasting Insulin and Apolipoprotein B Levels and Low-Density Lipoprotein Particle Size as Risk Factors for Ischemic Heart Disease. *JAMA* 1998;279:1955.

61. Bao W, Srinivasan SR, Berenson GS. Persistent Elevation of Plasma Insulin Levels is Associated with Increased Cardiovascular Risk in Children and Adults. *Circulation* 1996;93:54-59.

62. Burchfiel CM, et al. Hyperinsulinemia and Cardiovascular Disease in Elderly Men: The Honolulu Heart Program. *Arterioscler Thromb Vasc Biol* 1998;18:450.

63. Burchfiel CM, et al. Distribution and Correlates of Insulin in Elderly Men. The Honolulu Heart Program. *Arterioscler Thromb Vasc Biol* 1995;15:2213.

64. Hayes KC, et al. Saturated Fatty Acids and LDL Receptor Modulation in Humans and Monkeys. *Prostaglandins Leukot Essent Fatty Acids* 1997;57:411.

65. Dietschy JM. Dietary Fatty Acids and the Regulation of Plasma Low Density Lipoprotein Cholesterol Concentrations. *J Nutr* 1998;128:444S.

66. Hayek T, et al. Dietary Fat Increases High Density Lipoprotein (HDL) Levels both by Increasing the Transport Rates and Decreasing the Fractional Catabolic Rates of HDL Cholesterol Ester and Apolipoprotein (Apo) A-I. Presentation of a New Animal Model and Mechanistic Studies in Human Apo A-I Transgenic and Control Mice. *J Clin Invest* 1993;91:1665.

67. Salonen JT, et al. HDL, HDL2, and HDL3 Subfractions, and the Risk of Acute Myocardial Infarction. A Prospective Population Study in Eastern Finnish Men. *Circulation* 1991;84:129.

68. Toikka JO, et al. Constantly Low HDL-Cholesterol Concentration Relates to Endothelial Dysfunction and Increased In Vivo LDL-Oxidation in Healthy Young Men. *Atherosclerosis* 1999;147:133.

69. Stampfer MJ, et al. A Prospective Study of Cholesterol, Apolipoproteins, and the Risk of Myocardial Infarction. *N Engl J Med* 1991;325:373.

70. Uhl GS, et al. Relation between High Density Lipoprotein Cholesterol and Coronary Artery Disease in Asymptomatic Men. *Am J Cardiol* 1981;48:903.

71. Frick MH, et al. HDL-Cholesterol as a Risk Factor in Coronary Heart Disease. An Update of the Helsinki Heart Study. *Drugs* 1990;40 (Suppl):7S.

72. Drexel H, et al. Relation of the Level of High-Density Lipoprotein Subfractions to the Presence and Extent of Coronary Artery Disease. *Am J Cardiol* 1992;70:436.

73. Wilson PW, Abbott RD, Castelli WP. High Density Lipoprotein Cholesterol and Mortality. The Framingham Heart Study. *Arteriosclerosis* 1988;8:737.

74. Abbott RD, et al. High Density Lipoprotein Cholesterol, Total Cholesterol Screening, and Myocardial Infarction. The Framingham Study. *Arteriosclerosis* 1988;8:207.

75. Oster P, et al. Diet and High Density Lipoproteins. *Lipids* 1981;16:93.

76. Starc TJ, et al. Greater Dietary Intake of Simple Carbohydrate is Associated with Lower Concentrations of High-Density-Lipoprotein Cholesterol in Hypercholesterolemic Children. *Am J Clin Nutr* 1998;67:1147.

77. Ingram DD, et al. U.S.S.R. and U.S. Nutrient Intake, Plasma Lipids, and Lipoproteins in Men Ages 40-59 Sampled from Lipid Research Clinics Populations. *Prev Med* 1985;14:264.

78. Liu G, et al. The Effect of Sucrose Content in High and Low Carbohydrate Diets on Plasma Glucose, Insulin, and Lipid Responses in Hypertriglyceridemic Humans. *J Clin Endocrinol Metab* 1984;59:636.

79. Coulston AM, Liu GC, Reaven GM. Plasma Glucose, Insulin and Lipid Responses to High-Carbohydrate Low-Fat Diets in Normal Humans. *Metabolism* 1983;32:52.

80. Zimmerman J, et al. Effect of Moderate Isocaloric Modification of Dietary Carbohydrate on High-Density Lipoprotein Composition and Apolipoprotein A-1 Turnover in Humans. *Isr J Med Sci* 1986;22:95.

81. Coulston AM, et al. Deleterious Metabolic Effects of High-Carbohydrate, Sucrose-Containing Diets in Patients with Non-Insulin-Dependent Diabetes Mellitus. *Am J Med* 1987;82:213.

82. Wolf RN, Grundy SM. Influence of Exchanging Carbohydrate for Saturated Fatty Acids on Plasma Lipids and Lipoproteins in Men. *J Nutr* 1983;113:1521.

83. Nelson GJ, Schmidt PC, Kelley DS. Low-Fat Diets Do Not Lower Plasma Cholesterol Levels in Healthy Men Compared to High-Fat Diets with Similar Fatty Acid Composition at Constant Caloric Intake. *Lipids* 1995;30:969.

84. Wolfe BM, Piche LA. Replacement of Carbohydrate by Protein in a Conventional-Fat Diet Reduces Cholesterol and Triglyceride Concentrations in Healthy Normolipidemic Subjects. *Clin Invest Med* 1999;22:140.

85. Liu GC, Coulston AM, Reaven GM. Effect of High-Carbohydrate-Low-Fat Diets on Plasma Glucose, Insulin and Lipid Responses in Hypertriglyceridemic Humans. *Metabolism* 1983;32:750.

86. Fuh MM, et al. Effect of Low Fat-High Carbohydrate Diets in Hypertensive Patients with Non-Insulin-Dependent Diabetes Mellitus. *Am J Hypertens* 1990;3:527.

87. Liu B, et al. [Effect of High Carbohydrate and High Fat Diets on Plasma Glucose, Insulin and Lipids in Normal and Hypertriglyceridemic Subjects]. *Hua Hsi I Ko Ta Hsueh Hsueh Pao* 1990;21:145. Chinese.

88. Reaven GM. Effects of Differences in Amount and Kind of Dietary Carbohydrate on Plasma Glucose and Insulin Responses in Man. *Am J Clin Nutr* 1979;32:2568.

89. Coulston AM, et al. Persistence of Hypertriglyceridemic Effect of Low-Fat High-Carbohydrate Diets in NIDDM Patients. *Diabetes Care* 1989;12:94.

90. Lithell H, et al. Decrease of Lipoprotein Lipase Activity in Skeletal Muscle in Man during a Short-Term Carbohydrate-Rich Dietary Regime. With Special Reference to HDL-Cholesterol, Apolipoprotein and Insulin Concentrations. *Metabolism* 1982;31:994.

91. See, supra, notes 78-82.

92. Laws A, Reaven GM. Evidence for an Independent Relationship between Insulin Resistance and Fasting Plasma HDL-Cholesterol, Triglyceride and Insulin Concentrations. *J Intern Med* 1992;231:25.

93. Bruce R, et al. Associations between Insulin Sensitivity, and Free Fatty Acid and Triglyceride Metabolism Independent of Uncomplicated Obesity. *Metabolism* 1994;43:1275.

94. Burchfiel CM, et al. Association of Insulin Levels with Lipids and Lipoproteins in Elderly Japanese-American Men. *Ann Epidemiol* 1998;8:92.

95. Laws A, et al. Relation of Fasting Plasma Insulin Concentration to High Density Lipoprotein Cholesterol and Triglyceride Concentrations in Men. *Arterioscler Thromb* 1991;11:1636.

96. Zavaroni I, et al. Evidence for an Independent Relationship between Plasma Insulin and Concentration of High Density Lipoprotein Cholesterol and Triglyceride. *Atherosclerosis* 1985;55:259.

97. Bazelmans J, Nestel PJ, Nolan C. Insulin-Induced Glucose Utilization Influences Triglyceride Metabolism. *Clin Sci* 1983;64:511.

98. Cambien F, et al. Body Mass, Blood Pressure, Glucose, and Lipids. Does Plasma Insulin Explain their Relationships? *Arteriosclerosis* 1987;7:197.

99. Chaiken RL, et al. Metabolic Effects of Darglitazone, an Insulin Sensitizer, in NIDDM Subjects. *Diabetologia* 1995;38:1307.

100. See, supra, note 90.

101. Lithell H, et al. Is Muscle Lipoprotein Lipase Inactivated by Ordinary Amounts of Dietary Carbohydrates? *Hum Nutr Clin Nutr* 1985;39:289.

102. See, supra, note 90.

103. Julius U, et al. Insulin Resistance in Diabetics and Non-Diabetics with Impaired Triglyceride Removal. *Exp Clin Endocrinol* 1984;83:225.

104. Sprecher DL. Triglycerides as a Risk Factor for Coronary Artery Disease. *Am J Cardiol* 1998;82:49U.

105. Austin MA. Plasma Triglyceride as a Risk Factor for Cardiovascular Disease. *Can J Cardiol* 1998;14 (Suppl):14B.

106. Assmann G, et al. The Emergence of Triglycerides as a Significant Independent Risk Factor in Coronary Artery Disease. *Eur Heart J* 1998;19(Suppl):M8.

107. Stampfer MJ, et al. A Prospective Study of Triglyceride Level, Low-Density Lipoprotein Particle Diameter, and Risk of Myocardial Infarction. *JAMA* 1996;276:882.

Chapter 8 - You Broil, Never Fry, But You've Been Living a Lie

108. Hokanson JE, Austin MA. Plasma Triglyceride Level is a Risk Factor for Cardiovascular Disease Independent of High-Density Lipoprotein Cholesterol Level: A Meta-Analysis of Population-Based Prospective Studies. *J Cardiovasc Risk* 1996;3:213.

109. Patsch JR, et al. Relation of Triglyceride Metabolism and Coronary Artery Disease. Studies in the Postprandial State. *Arterioscler Thromb* 1992;12:1336.

110. Durrington PN. Triglycerides are More Important in Atherosclerosis than Epidemiology has Suggested. *Atherosclerosis* 1998;141 (Suppl):S57.

111. Tenkanen L, et al. The Triglyceride Issue Revisited. Findings from the Helsinki Heart Study. *Arch Intern Med* 1994;154:2714.

112. Kaukola S, Manninen V, Halonen PI. Serum Lipids with Special Reference to HDL Cholesterol and Triglycerides in Young Male Survivors of Acute Myocardial Infarction. *Acta Med Scand* 1980;208:41.

113. Brinton EA, Eisenberg S, Breslow JL. Increased Apo A-I and Apo A-II Fractional Catabolic Rate in Patients with Low High Density Lipoprotein-Cholesterol Levels With or Without Hypertriglyceridemia. *J Clin Invest* 1991;87:536.

114. Assmann G, Schulte H. Role of Triglycerides in Coronary Artery Disease: Lessons from the Prospective Cardiovascular Munster Study. *Am J Cardiol* 1992;70:10H.

115. American Heart Association. "Heart Disease and Strokes Deaths Rising." Jan. 24, 1996, press release.

116. Gould KL. Very Low-fat Diets for Coronary Heart Disease: Perhaps But Which One? *JAMA* 1996;275:1402.

117. Howard BV. Risk Factors for Cardiovascular Disease in Individuals with Diabetes. The Strong Heart Study. *Acta Diabetol* 1996;33:180.

118. Kannel WB, McGee DL. Diabetes and Cardiovascular Disease. The Framingham Study. *JAMA* 1979;241:2035.

119. Uusitupa M, et al. The Relationship of Cardiovascular Risk Factors to the Prevalence of Coronary Heart Disease in Newly Diagnosed Type 2 (Non-Insulin-Dependent) Diabetes. *Diabetologia* 1985;28:653.

120. Garg A, et al. Effects of Varying Carbohydrate Content of Diet In Patients with Non-Insulin-Dependent Diabetes Mellitus. *JAMA* 1994;271:1421.

121. Atkins R. *Dr. Atkins' New Diet Revolution*. NY: M. Evans and Company 1992, p. 138.

122. Newbold HL. Reducing Serum Cholesterol Level with a Diet High in Animal Fats. *S Med J* 1988;81:61.

123. Dyerberg J. Coronary Heart Disease in Greenland Inuit: A Paradox. Implications for Western Diet Patterns. *Arctic Med Res* 1989;48:47.

124. Young TK, Moffatt ME, O'Neil JD. Cardiovascular Diseases in a Canadian Arctic Population. *Am J Public Health* 1993;83:881.

125. Bjerregaard P, Mulvad G, Pedersen HS. Cardiovascular Risk Factors in Inuit of Greenland. *Int J Epidemiol* 1997;26:1182.

126. Davidson M, Bulkow LR, Gellin BG. Cardiac Mortality in Alaska's Indigenous and Non-Native Residents. *Int J Epidemiol* 1993;22:62.

127. Schraer CD, et al. Prevalence of Diabetes Mellitus in Alaskan Eskimos, Indians, and Aleuts. *Diabetes Care* 1988;11:693.

128. Young TK, et al. Prevalence of Diagnosed Diabetes in Circumpolar Indigenous Populations. *Int J Epidemiol* 1992;21:730.

129. Di Pasquale M. *The Anabolic Diet*. Optimum Training Systems 1995, p. 19.

130. Id.

131. Thouez JP, et al. Obesity, Hypertension, Hyperuricemia and Diabetes Mellitus among the Cree and Inuit of Northern Quebec. *Arctic Med Res* 1990;49:180.

132. Young TK. Obesity, Central Fat Patterning, and their Metabolic Correlates among the Inuit of the Central Canadian Arctic. *Hum Biol* 1996;68:245.

133. Murphy NJ, et al. Hypertension in Alaska Natives: Association with Overweight. Glucose Intolerance, Diet and Mechanized Activity. *Ethn Health* 1997;2:267.

134. Mann GV, et al. Atherosclerosis in the Masai. *Am J Epidemiol* 1972;95:26.

135. Walker AR, Sareli P. Coronary Heart Disease: Outlook for Africa. *J R Soc Med* 1997;90:23.

136. Watkins LO. Coronary Heart Disease and Coronary Disease Risk Factors in Black Populations in Underdeveloped Countries: The Case for Primordial Prevention. *Am Heart J* 1984;108:850.

137. Seftel HC. The Rarity of Coronary Heart Disease in South African Blacks. *S Afr Med J* 1978;54:99.

138. Cohen AM, Marom L. Diabetes and Accompanying Obesity, Hypertension And ECG Abnormalities in Yemenite Jews 40 Years after Immigration to Israel. *Diabetes Res* 1993;23:65.

139. Trostler N. Health Risks of Immigration: The Yemenite and Ethiopian Cases in Israel. *Biomed Pharmacother* 1997;51:352.

140. Cleave TL. *The Saccharine Disease*. New Canaan, CN: Keats 1978.

141. Temple NJ. Coronary Heart Disease--Dietary Lipids or Refined Carbohydrates? *Med Hypotheses* 1983;10:425.

142. Perry TM. The New and Old Diseases: A Study of Mortality Trends in the United States, 1900-1969. *Am J Clin Pathol* 1975;63:453.

143. Herrick JB. Clinical Features of Sudden Obstruction of Coronary Arteries. *JAMA* 1912;LIX:2105.

144. Dolnick E. "Le Paradoxe Francais." *Hippocrates,* May/June, 1990 p. 37.

145. Drewnowski A, et al. Diet Quality and Dietary Diversity in France: Implications For the French Paradox. *J Am Diet Assoc* 1996;96:663.

146. Burr ML. Explaining the French Paradox. *J R Soc Health* 1995;115:217.

147. Serra-Majem L, et al. How Could Changes in Diet Explain Changes in Coronary Heart Disease Mortality in Spain? The Spanish Paradox. *Am J Clin Nutr* 1995;61(Suppl):1351S.

148. Id.

148a. Rimer S. "Reaching 100 - Not What It Used to Be," *Sun-Sentinel,* June 22, 1998 3A.

148b. Id.

149. Serra-Majem L, et al. Changing Patterns of Fat Consumption in Spain. *Eur J Clin Nutr* 1993;47 (Suppl)1:13S.

150. Id.

151. Kafatos A, et al. Nutrition Status of the Elderly in Anogia, Crete, Greece. *J Am Coll Nutr* 1993;12:685.

152. Menotti A, et al. Food Intake Patterns and 25-Year Mortality from Coronary Heart Disease: Cross-Cultural Correlations in the Seven Countries Study. The Seven Countries Study Research Group. *Eur J Epidemiol* 1999;15:507.

153. Simini B. Serge Renaud: From French Paradox to Cretan Miracle. *Lancet* 2000;355:48 .

154. Grant WB. Milk and other Dietary Influences on Coronary Heart Disease. *Altern Med Rev* 1998;3:281.

155. Hahn RA, Heath GW, Chang MH. Cardiovascular Disease Risk Factors and Preventive Practices among Adults-- United States, 1994: A Behavioral Risk Factor Atlas. Behavioral Risk Factor Surveillance System State Coordinators. *Mor Mortal Wkly Rep CDC Surveill Summ* 1998;47:35.

156. Oberman A, Kuller LH, Carleton RA. Prevention of Cardiovascular Disease--Opportunities for Progress. *Prev Med* 1994;23:727.

157. Must A, et al. The Disease Burden Associated with Overweight and Obesity. *JAMA* 1999;282:1523.

158. Allison DB, et al. Annual Deaths Attributable to Obesity in the United States. *JAMA* 1999;282:1530.

The Key to Permanent Fat Loss: Working with Your Body, Not Against It.

Don't count calories, make calories count by eating the right foods.
Unknown

The only worthwhile fat loss is permanent fat loss.
Unknown

It is natural to be healthy because health is our natural state.
Dr. Udo Erasmus

Millions of years of evolution have made the human body a brilliant adaptive organism. Within its genetic constraints, the body will alter its functioning to accommodate external conditions with a remarkable degree of precision and efficiency. There are several dietary implications of this phenomenon, which are capitalized upon by the NHE Eating Plan.

Calorie Restriction - A No-Win Proposition

The human body is much more sophisticated than many dieters realize. In order to survive over hundreds-of-thousands of years through food shortages, extreme weather conditions, the continual onslaught of predatory enemies, the constant attack of viruses and bacteria, and other threats to human existence, *Homo sapiens* and their genetic predecessors developed an intricate array of checks and balances. Among these survival mechanisms is regulation of metabolic rate in response to caloric intake.

When caloric intake is restricted, the body compensates by reducing metabolic rate.[1,2,3,4] Consequently, fewer calories and less fat is burned.[5,6,7] Much obesity research has been directed at defining the physiological mechanisms involved in fat regain subsequent to fat loss, because researchers believe that this avenue of investigation may yield treatments or a cure for obesity. In this vein, the discovery of the hormone-like substance *leptin*, produced by fat cells under the direction the "ob" gene,[8,9] created a sensation in the research community a few years ago. Since then, a profusion of studies have been performed, which have generated more questions than answers about this enigmatic substance. Leptin levels are higher in obese individuals and are altered by weight loss.[10,11,12,13,14] However, while it is highly probable that leptin plays an important role in bodyfat regulation generally, *lipoprotein lipase* and thyroid hormones appear to be more instrumental in regulating metabolism in response to short-term changes in caloric intake.

Lipoprotein lipase, a lipogenic (fat-storing) enzyme, increases markedly when calories are restricted.[15,16,17] At the same time, production of the thyroid hormone *triiodothyronine* (T3) decreases.[18,19,20] The downregulation of T3 slows metabolism, resulting in retention of muscle mass but also bodyfat.[21,22,23,24,25] The metabolic adjustments to reduced caloric intake make sense from the standpoint of survival: the slower one's metabolism, the more "mileage" one gets out of a given quantity of stored energy (fat), and the longer one remains alive during a famine (and the longer one remains alive during a famine, the greater the likelihood that conditions will change, food will be found, and death will be averted). But for those individuals more likely to perish from gluttony than from starvation, these energy-conserving adaptations are curses not blessings.

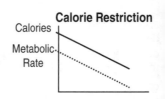

When the restrictive dieter resumes normal eating, lipoprotein lipase activity remains elevated and metabolic rate remains depressed, causing him/her to quickly regain the lost fat, and maybe even a little extra fat as insurance against the next "famine."[26,27,28] Stated differently, the rate of fat storage is increased after a period of calorie restriction, and it stays that way until the pre-diet level of bodyfat is re-established. *This demonstrates the futility of trying to achieve permanent fat loss solely by means of calorie restriction.*

In addition, the restrictive dieter invariably loses precious muscle tissue. This further retards metabolism and adversely affects the shape, tone, and functional ability of the body. Muscle loss resulting from restrictive dieting ranges from 20% - 40% of total weight loss.[29,30,31,32,33,34] With this muscle loss to fat loss ratio, body composition may only improve marginally while on the diet. And when the diet ends, and the fat returns but the muscle does not, body composition worsens. In this vicious cycle, you go from being fat and flabby, to being less fat but more flabby, to ultimately becoming fatter and flabbier than ever.

"Wasting" Calories

Whereas restricting calories causes a metabolic slowdown, consuming extra calories causes your body to step-up metabolic rate in order to "waste" calories.[35,36,37,38] Thyroid activity,[39,40,41] thermogenesis,[42,43,44,45] and leptin levels[46,47] each increase during overfeeding. The relative contribution of each of these mechanisms to counteracting caloric excess is a subject of debate among researchers.

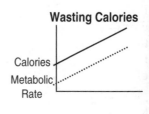

Although questions exist concerning the mechanisms responsible for dissipating extra calories, there is no doubt that it happens. Consider this: whatever your current daily calorie consumption average is, let's say that you increased it by an average of 400 calories per day for a year, without deliberately changing your activity level. Then let's say you increased your average calorie consumption by another 600 calories per day for the following year. If you do the math, with a pound of fat equaling 3500 calories, this would mean that in those two years you should gain over 100 pounds, right? Not likely.

Chapter 9 - Working With Your Body, Not Against It

You would likely gain *some* weight in the scenario depicted above, but, time and again, studies have shown that a consistent linear positive relationship between calorie consumption and weight gain simply does not exist.[48,49,50,51] Furthermore, when weight is gained as a result of overfeeding, there is a strong tendency to gravitate back to the pre-overfeeding weight following resumption of normal eating.[52,53,54] Incidentally, the hypothetical presented in the foregoing paragraph describes an actual study carried-out by a German scientist. At the end of the second year he weighed almost the same as he did before the study began![55] Where did the extra 365,000 calories go? Not to his waist, or his hips, or his arms or legs. Answer: they were "wasted" by the body as part of a million-year-old metabolic adaptation.

Overriding Your Fat Setpoint

Similarly, if there existed an airtight mathematical relationship between caloric intake and weight loss, cutting daily caloric intake from 3000 to 1000 calories would result in a 60,000 calorie deficit and, correspondingly, a 17-pound weight loss in the first month - that's possible (although much of it would be water and glycogen loss, not fat loss) - and would result in a *200-pound weight loss* after a year. What if the person began the diet weighing 200 pounds, would he disappear?

Clearly, there exists a weight-regulating mechanism, mediated by genetic and hormonal factors, which determines how much, if any, extra calories will be stored, and how much will be burned-up or "wasted." The genetic influence accounts for wide inter-individual differences; a 1999 study published in *Science* found ten-fold variation in fat storage among subjects in response to overfeeding.[56] Insulin and glucagon are the principal hormones involved in weight regulation,[57,58] and we will examine them more closely in the next chapter.

The effort to explain weight regulation has led to the elaboration of a "fat setpoint" theory.[59,60,61] The setpoint theory holds that bodyfat is maintained in each individual according to a predetermined, "preferred" level. The test of a good scientific theory is whether it provides a rational, unifying explanation for established clinical observations. The setpoint theory meets this standard by plausibly explaining why bodyfat tends to hover around a certain level, which varies with the individual, in defiance of mathematical predictions of the outcome of caloric restriction or excess.

% Bodyfat

While there is considerable merit to the setpoint theory, it is important to bear in mind that it describes only a genetically ordained advantage or disadvantage in relation to losing fat. Ultimately, though, as with anything else, disadvantage does not mean defeat, nor does advantage mean victory. This is especially so with respect to fat loss as studies show that neither the number of fat cells one possesses, nor the size of fat cells, is genetically fixed.[62,63,64,65,66,67,68] Likewise, the fat setpoint is not unalterably dictated by genetics.

The Natural Hormonal Enhancement program aims at tweaking two factors that can lower your fat setpoint: 1) insulin/glucagon 2) quantity of metabolically active tissue (i.e., muscle mass). Hence, it is both possible and practically feasible to change your fat setpoint, but it requires sustained effort and a sound plan. Fad diets and quick fixes won't do the trick. *To override your fat setpoint and build the body you want regardless of genetic advantage or disadvantage you must change your metabolism and your internal hormonal environment.*

The Calorie Theory Refuted

The problems with the calorie theory go even deeper. At the most fundamental level, the concept of calories as human energy units is questionable. The calorie counts you see on food labels and charts were determined without reference to human biochemistry. Rather, calorie counts for foods are obtained by burning food in a calorimeter and measuring the heat produced. To assume that the 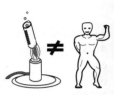 same rules that govern combustion in a calorimeter govern human metabolism is like assuming that because life exists on Earth, life must also exist on Pluto. Nonetheless, the values of four calories per gram for carbohydrate and protein, and nine calories per gram for fat, which are approximations conceived almost a hundred years ago, have become a central fixture of dietary mythology.

Fat metabolism provides one example of how the intricacies of human metabolism defy calorimeter-derived generalizations. The textbook rule, which is one of the many faulty rationales underlying the "fat makes you fat" myth, is that fat contains 2¼ times as many calories as carbohydrate (9 and 4, respectively). The practical reality of the matter, though, is that the caloric value of fat varies depending on hormonal state and type of ingested fat.

When the insulin/glucagon ratio is low for several days as result of a diet low in carbohydrate and high in fat, fat molecules are burned incompletely, yielding less energy and producing fat fragments called *ketones* which are excreted via the breath, stool, and urine.[69,70,71] Under these metabolic conditions, more fat must be burned to provide a given amount of energy. Similarly, the chemical structure of fats, particularly the degree of unsaturation, influences their fate within the body. Specifically, unsaturated fats are less likely to be stored as fat because they burn at a higher rate.[72,73,74,75,76,77]

There is an even more basic reason why the calorie theory should be discarded. Even if the popularly accepted caloric values were correct, ultimately what matters is not how many calories you ingest but how many calories you absorb. Fiber, by binding with fat, and by speeding the transit of digested food through the intestines, reduces the bioavailability of ingested fat.[78,79,80,81,82,83] The upshot is that butter is less fattening when eaten with broccoli than with white bread, because less of the butter is absorbed. In the final analysis, whether a gram of fat has 9 calories or 900 is immaterial if it is not absorbed. Although the difference in fat absorption rates for fat plus fiber versus fat by itself is marginal when viewed on a per meal basis, it can add-up - and my point is that the calorie theory ignores fat absorption rate differences.

Along the same lines, protein and essential fatty acids, in contrast to carbohydrate, serve vital functions in the body aside from their role as an energy source. Essential fatty acids and protein form the structures of the body, all the way down to the cellular level. Fats and proteins that are used for building purposes are not available for use as energy or for energy storage in the form of bodyfat. The calorie theory does not take this basic fact into consideration, and instead it incorrectly assumes that all calories are equally available for use as energy.

There are two practical consequences of all this:

1) Calorie restriction, while it may be logical on paper, is not effective in practice. As millions of star-crossed dieters can attest, upon quitting a restrictive diet the missing fat comes bounding back like a golden retriever playing fetch. The setpoint theory, described above, explains why fat returns so doggedly after a period of reduced caloric intake. In order to lose fat, you must change your approach to the problem, addressing it from the inside, out - by altering your metabolism and the hormones that influence it, rather than using a simplistic ploy like calorie restriction to try to outsmart your body.

2) Because your metabolism will speed up or slow down in response to how many calories you consume, you have a certain amount of "wiggle room" in regard to calorie consumption. In other words, more calories does not necessarily translate to more fat storage. Within a certain range, greater or fewer calories does not make a difference because your body will up-regulate or down-regulate metabolism to match caloric intake.

But what if you go outside that range on the upside - will consuming excess calories make you fat? It may, but that virtually never happens to people on the NHE Eating Plan even though calorie counting is strictly prohibited. The reason for this relates back to the human body as a "brilliant adaptive organism."

Counting Calories is Strictly Prohibited

Liberation from calorie counting is one of the many benefits of the NHE Eating Plan. As noted above, excessive caloric intake can make you fat. But consuming an excessive amount of calories is not natural. Think about it: the human body possesses highly efficient self-protective mechanisms. Your body is constantly striving to protect itself from disease and sickness and keep itself in a state of health and wellness - this is your body's foremost and overriding priority. In view of this, why on earth would your body tell you to consume an excessive amount of calories so you become fat and unhealthy?

Nowadays, we have come to accept being fat, overeating, and constantly struggling against cravings as normal - but it's not. Looked at in the scope of human history, widespread obesity is an aberration specific to industrialized nations in the modern era. And contrary to what you might suppose, food cravings and overeating are caused neither by the abundance of tantalizing foods available nor by the mouth-watering TV

69

commercials that promote them. Rather, the reason why people engage in the unnatural practice of consuming too many calories is *hormonal hunger* (discussed in Chapter 11).

At high levels, insulin not only causes fat storage but it also causes intense food cravings, especially for carbohydrates which, in turn, causes you to overeat carbohydrates, which stimulates more insulin, which generates more cravings! Constantly stimulating high levels of the hormone that tells your body to store fat AND generates irresistible cravings guarantees failure for anyone trying to lose fat. Conversely, when you break this vicious cycle, cravings disappear like magic.

If you are currently consuming a diet high in carbohydrate, **your particular food desires and your sense of hunger are warped**.

When you eliminate the corrupting influence of hormonal hunger, you eat less and calorie consumption, governed by a part of the brain called the hypothalamus,[84,85,86] becomes self-regulating for the great majority of people. With lower insulin levels, and no more overeating, your fat setpoint will undergo a gradual downward readjustment. You will then instinctively eat the right amount of food to maintain your new, lower level of bodyfat.

In summary, without hormonal hunger throwing a monkey wrench into your calorie thermostat, you will no longer experience the cravings that lead people to consume too many calories. This is why calorie counting is unnecessary, and potentially counterproductive, on the NHE Eating Plan.

Fat Consumption and Hormonal Hunger: A Disastrous Combination

Absent excess carbohydrate, fat consumption, like calorie consumption, is self-regulating. If you are doubtful, answer this question: when was the last time you saw someone eat a tub of plain butter, or munch a block of cream cheese like it was a candy bar, or drink a tall cool glass of vegetable oil? Not only have you never seen it, but the mere thought probably turns your stomach. This illustrates that, in fact, people generally have a low tolerance for dietary fat.

So why does it seem like so many people have an insatiable appetite for fat? Because the whole equation changes when fat is eaten along with carbohydrate. For one, when fat is diluted with carbohydrate, it does not register the same way with your hypothalamic appetite control center.[87,88,89] This is the case with potato chips, doughnuts, cakes, ice cream, etc. You can easily consume sixty or seventy grams of fat when the fat is part of french fries or cookies, but try eating it in a *much less caloric form* (i.e., alone) and you probably would not be able to, or would not want to. By contrast, carbohydrates can palatably be eaten alone in high quantities; consider all the nonfat foods that people are stuffing themselves with these days.

Moreover, when too much carbohydrate (which stimulates an excessive amount of insulin) is consumed at one sitting, the archenemy of fat loss - hormonal hunger - rears its ugly head. Once hormonal hunger enters the ballgame, all bets are off. Not only will fat coupled with carbs eaten in the presence of hormonal hunger taste delicious, but the fat will be more likely to be converted to bodyfat.

High Dietary Fat   +   High Insulin   =   Bad Combination
(both in terms of health and fat loss)

Accordingly, with the NHE Eating Plan your meals are cycled such that when fat intake is higher, insulin is low; and when insulin is higher (during and after the carb-load) fat intake is low.

References

1. Vansant G, et al. Short and Long Term Effects of a Very Low Calorie Diet on Resting Metabolic Rate and Body Composition. *Int J Obes* 1989;13(Suppl):87.

2. Heshka S, et al. Weight Loss and Change in Resting Metabolic Rate. *Am J Clin Nutr* 1990;52:981.

3. Mole PA, et al. Exercise Reverses Depressed Metabolic Rate Produced by Severe Caloric Restriction. *Med Sci Sports Exerc* 1989;21:29.

4. Finer N, Swan PC, Mitchell FT. Metabolic Rate after Massive Weight Loss in Human Obesity. *Clin Sci* 1986;70:395.

5. Schutz Y, et al. Role of Fat Oxidation in the Long-Term Stabilization of Body Weight in Obese Women. *Am J Clin Nutr* 1992;55:670.

6. Ballor DL, et al. Decrease in Fat Oxidation following a Meal in Weight-Reduced Individuals: A Possible Mechanism for Weight Recidivism. *Metabolism* 1996;45:174.

7. Nicklas BJ, Rogus EM, Goldberg AP. Exercise Blunts Declines in Lipolysis and Fat Oxidation after Dietary-Induced Weight Loss in Obese Older Women. *Am J Physiol* 1997;273:E149.

8. Halaas JL, et al. Weight-Reducing Effects of the Plasma Protein Encoded by the Obese Gene. *Science* 1995;269:543.

9. Pelleymounter MA, et al. Effects of the Obese Gene Product on Body Weight Regulation in Ob/Ob Mice. *Science* 1995;269:540.

10. Niskanen LK, et al. Serum Leptin in Obesity is Related to Gender and Body Fat Topography but does not Predict Successful Weight Loss. *Eur J Endocrinol* 1997;137:61.

11. Rosenbaum M, et al. Effects of Weight Change on Plasma Leptin Concentrations and Energy Expenditure. *J Clin Endocrinol Metab* 1997;82:3647.

12. Rissanen P, et al. Effect of Weight Loss and Regional Fat Distribution on Plasma Leptin Concentration in Obese Women. *Int J Obes Relat Metab Disord* 1999;23:645.

13. Wing RR, et al. Relationship between Weight Loss Maintenance and Changes in Serum Leptin Levels. *Horm Metab Res* 1996;28:698.

14. Torgerson JS, et al. A Low Serum Leptin Level at Baseline and a Large Early Decline in Leptin Predict a Large 1-Year Weight Reduction in Energy-Restricted Obese Humans. *J Clin Endocrinol Metab* 1999;84:4197.

15. Schwartz RS, Brunzell JD. Increase of Adipose Tissue Lipoprotein Lipase Activity with Weight Loss. *J Clin Invest* 1981;67:1425.

16. Kern PA, et al. The Effect of Weight Loss on the Activity and Expression of Adipose Tissue Lipoprotein Lipase in Very Obese Humans. *N Engl J Med* 1990;322:1053.

17. Eckel RH, Yost TJ. Weight Reduction Increases Adipose Tissue Lipoprotein Lipase Responsiveness in Obese Women. *J Clin Invest* 1987;80:992.

18. Chomard P, et al. Serum Concentrations of Total and Free Thyroid Hormones in Moderately Obese Women during a Six-Week Slimming Cure. *Eur J Clin Nutr* 1988;42:285.

19. Robinson HM, Betton H, Jackson AA. Free and Total Triiodothyronine and Thyroxine in Malnourished Jamaican Infants. The Effect of Diet on Plasma Levels of Thyroid Hormones, Insulin and Glucose during Recovery. *Hum Nutr Clin Nutr* 1985;39:245.

20. Visser TJ, et al. Serum Thyroid Hormone Concentrations during Prolonged Reduction of Dietary Intake. *Metabolism* 1978;27:405.

21. Cavallo E, et al. Resting Metabolic Rate, Body Composition and Thyroid Hormones. Short Term Effects of Very Low Calorie Diet. *Horm Metab Res* 1990;22:632.

22. Yang MU, van Itallie TB. Variability in Body Protein Loss during Protracted, Severe Caloric Restriction: Role of Triiodothyronine and other Possible Determinants. *J Clin Nutr* 1984;40:611.

23. Kaptein EM, et al. Relationship between the Changes in Serum Thyroid Hormone Levels and Protein Status during Prolonged Protein Supplemented Caloric Deprivation. *Clin Endocrinol* (Oxf) 1985;22:1.

24. Kiortsis DN, Durack I, Turpin G. Effects of a Low-Calorie Diet on Resting Metabolic Rate and Serum Tri-Iodothyronine Levels in Obese Children. *Eur J Pediatr* 1999;158:446.

25. Henson LC, Heber D. Whole Body Protein Breakdown Rates and Hormonal Adaptation in Fasted Obese Subjects. *J Clin Endocrinol Metab* 1983;57:316.

26. Kmiec Z, et al. Thyroid Hormones Homeostasis in Rats Refed after Short-Term and Prolonged Fasting. *J Endocrinol Invest* 1996;19:304.

27. Penicaud L, Le Magnen J. Recovery of Body Weight Following Starvation or Food Restriction in Rats. *Neurosci Biobehav Rev* 1980;(Suppl)1:47S.

28. Elliot DL, et al. Sustained Depression of the Resting Metabolic Rate after Massive Weight Loss. *Am J Clin Nutr* 1989;49:93.

29. Dengel DR, et al. Effects of Weight Loss by Diet Alone or Combined with Aerobic Exercise on Body Composition in Older Obese Men. *Metabolism* 1994;43:867.

30. Ballor DL, Poehlman ET. Exercise-Training Enhances Fat-Free Mass Preservation during Diet-Induced Weight Loss: A Meta-Analytical Finding. *Int J Obes Relat Metab Disord* 1994;18:35.

31. Garrow JS, Summerbell CD. Meta-Analysis: Effect of Exercise, With or Without Dieting, on the Body Composition of Overweight Subjects. *Eur J Clin Nutr* 1995;49:1.

32. Kraemer WJ, et al. Influence of Exercise Training on Physiological and Performance Changes with Weight Loss in Men. *Med Sci Sports Exerc* 1999;31:1320.

33. Pavlou KN, et al. Effects of Dieting and Exercise on Lean Body Mass, Oxygen Uptake, and Strength. *Med Sci Sports Exerc* 1985;17:466.

34. Gornall J, Villani RG. Short-Term Changes in Body Composition and Metabolism with Severe Dieting and Resistance Exercise. *Int J Sport Nutr* 1996;6:285.

35. Bandini LG, et al. Energy Expenditure during Carbohydrate Overfeeding in Obese and Nonobese Adolescents. *Am J Physiol* 1989;256:E357.

36. Curcio C, et al. Development of Compensatory Thermogenesis in Response to Overfeeding in Hypothyroid Rats. *Endocrinology* 1999;140:3438.

37. Klein S, Goran M. Energy Metabolism in Response to Overfeeding in Young Adult Men. *Metabolism* 1993;42:1201.

38. Yamashita J, Hayashi S. Changes in the Basal Metabolic Rate of a Normal Woman Induced by Short-Term and Long-Term Alterations of Energy Intake. *J Nutr Sci Vitaminol (Tokyo)* 1989;35:371.

39. Welle S, et al. Decreased Free Fraction of Serum Thyroid Hormones during Carbohydrate Overfeeding. *Metabolism* 1984;33:837.

40. Oppert JM, et al. Thyroid Hormones and Thyrotropin Variations during Long Term Overfeeding in Identical Twins. *J Clin Endocrinol Metab* 1994;79:547.

41. Katzeff HL. Increasing Age Impairs the Thyroid Hormone Response to Overfeeding. *Proc Soc Exp Biol Med* 1990;194:198.

42. Garrow JS. Chronic Effects of Over- and Under-Nutrition on Thermogenesis. *Int J Vitam Nutr Res* 1986;56:201.

43. Jequier E. [Thermogenesis Induced by Nutrients in Man: Its Role in Weight Regulation]. *J Physiol (Paris)* 1985;80:129. French.

44. Almeida NG, Levitsky DA, Strupp B. Enhanced Thermogenesis during Recovery from Diet-Induced Weight Gain in the Rat. *Am J Physiol* 1996;271:R1380.

45. Levine JA, Eberhardt NL, Jensen MD. Role of Nonexercise Activity Thermogenesis in Resistance to Fat Gain in Humans. *Science* 1999;283:212.

46. Levine JA, Eberhardt NL, Jensen MD. Leptin Responses to Overfeeding: Relationship with Body Fat and Nonexercise Activity Thermogenesis. *J Clin Endocrinol Metab* 1999;84:2751.

47. Kolaczynski JW, et al. Response of Leptin to Short-Term and Prolonged Overfeeding in Humans. *J Clin Endocrinol Metab* 1996;81:4162.

48. Norgan NG, Durnin JV. The Effect of 6 Weeks of Overfeeding on the Body Weight, Body Composition, and Energy Metabolism of Young Men. *Am J Clin Nutr* 1980;33:978.

49. Bouchard C, et al. The Response to Long-Term Overfeeding in Identical Twins. *N Engl J Med* 1990;322:1477.

50. Levine JA, Eberhardt NL, Jensen M. Role of Nonexercise Activity Thermogenesis in Resistance to Fat Gain in Humans. *Science* 1999;283:212.

51. Webb P, Annis JF. Adaptation to Overeating in Lean and Overweight Men and Women. *Hum Nutr Clin Nutr* 1983;37:117.

52. Tremblay A, et al. Overfeeding and Energy Expenditure in Humans. *Am J Clin Nutr* 1992;56:857.

53. Pasquet P, Apfelbaum M. Recovery of Initial Body Weight and Composition after Long-Term Massive Overfeeding in Men. *Am J Clin Nutr* 1994;60:861.

54. Leibel RL, Rosenbaum M, Hirsch J. Changes in Energy Expenditure Resulting from Altered Body Weight. *N Engl J Med* 1995;332:621.

55. Remington D, Fisher G, Parent E. *How to Lower You Fat Thermostat,* Appendix One: Evidence for a Weight Regulating Mechanism. Utah: Vitality House International 1983.

56. Levine JA, Eberhardt NL, Jensen MD. Role of Nonexercise Activity Thermogenesis in Resistance to Fat Gain in Humans. *Science* 1999;283:212.

57. deCastro J, Paullin S, DeLugas G. Insulin and Glucagon as Determinants of Body Weight Set Point and Microregulation in Rats. *J Comp Physiol Psychol* 1978;92:571.

58. Steffens AB, et al. Neuroendocrine Mechanisms Involved in Regulation of Body Weight, Food Intake and Metabolism. *Neurosci Biobehav Rev* 1990;14:305.

59. Harris RB. Role of Set-Point Theory in Regulation of Body Weight. *FASEB J* 1990;4:3310.

60. Keesey RE. The Body-Weight Set Point. What Can You Tell Your Patients? *Postgrad Med* 1988;83:114.

61. Keesey RE, Hirvonen MD. Body Weight Set-Points: Determination and Adjustment. *J Nutr* 1997;127(Suppl):1875S.

62. Greenwood MR, et al. Adipose Tissue: Cellular Morphology and Development. *Ann Intern Med* 1985;103:996.

63. Pettersson P, et al. Adipocyte Precursor Cells in Obese and Nonobese Humans. *Metabolism* 1985;34:808.

64. Levine JA, et al. Adipocyte Macrophage Colony-Stimulating Factor is a Mediator of Adipose Tissue Growth. *J Clin Invest* 1998;101:1557.

65. Prins JB, O'Rahilly S. Regulation of Adipose Cell Number in Man. *Clin Sci (Colch)* 1997;92:3.

66. Naslund I, Hallgren P, Sjostrom L. Fat Cell Weight and Number before and after Gastric Surgery for Morbid Obesity in Women. *Int J Obes* 1988;12:191.

67. Bjorntorp P, et al. Effect of an Energy-Reduced Dietary Regimen in Relation to Adipose Tissue Cellularity in Obese Women. *Am J Clin Nutr* 1975;28:445.

68. Hager A, et al. Body Fat and Adipose Tissue Cellularity in Infants: A Longitudinal Study. *Metabolism* 1977;26:607.

Natural Hormonal Enhancement

69. McGarry J, Wright PH, Foster DW. Hormonal Control of Ketogenesis. Rapid Activation of Hepatic Ketogenic Capacity in Fed Rats by Anti-Insulin Serum and Glucagon. *J Clin Invest* 1975;55:1202.

70. Alberti KG, et al. Hormonal Regulation of Ketone-Body Metabolism in Man. *Biochem Soc Symp* 1978;:163.

71. Grey NJ, Karl I, Kipnis DM. Physiologic Mechanisms in the Development of Starvation Ketosis in Man. *Diabetes* 1975;24:10.

72. Jones AE, et al. Effect of Fatty Acid Chain Length and Saturation on the Gastrointestinal Handling and Metabolic Disposal of Dietary Fatty Acids in Women. *Br J Nutr* 1999;81:37.

73. Bruce JS, Salter AM. Metabolic Fate of Oleic Acid, Palmitic Acid and Stearic Acid in Cultured Hamster Hepatocytes. *Biochem J* 1996;316:847.

74. Hill JO, et al. Lipid Accumulation and Body Fat Distribution is Influenced by Type of Dietary Fat Fed to Rats. *Int J Obes Relat Metab Disord* 1993;17:223.

75. Okuno M, et al. Perilla Oil Prevents the Excessive Growth of Visceral Adipose Tissue in Rats by Down-Regulating Adipocyte Differentiation. *J Nutr* 1997;127:1752.

76. Bell RR, Spencer MJ, Sherriff JL. Voluntary Exercise and Monounsaturated Canola Oil Reduce Fat Gain in Mice Fed Diets High in Fat. *J Nutr* 1997;127:2006.

77. Jones PJ, Pencharz PB, Clandinin MT. Whole Body Oxidation of Dietary Fatty Acids: Implications for Energy Utilization. *Am J Clin Nutr* 1985;42:769.

78. Baer DJ, et al. Dietary Fiber Decreases the Metabolizable Energy Content and Nutrient Digestibility of Mixed Diets Fed to Humans. *J Nutr* 1997;127:579.

79. Kaneko K, et al. Effect of Fiber on Protein, Fat and Calcium Digestibilities and Fecal Cholesterol Excretion. *J Nutr Sci Vitaminol (Tokyo)* 1986;32:317.

80. Wrick KL, et al. The Influence of Dietary Fiber Source on Human Intestinal Transit and Stool Output. *J Nutr* 1983;113:1464.

81. Stevens J, et al. Comparison of the Effects of Psyllium and Wheat Bran on Gastrointestinal Transit Time and Stool Characteristics. *J Am Diet Assoc* 1988;88:323.

82. Miles CW, Kelsay JL, Wong NP. Effect of Dietary Fiber on the Metabolizable Energy of Human Diets. *J Nutr* 1988;118:1075.

83. Miles CW. The Metabolizable Energy of Diets Differing in Dietary Fat and Fiber Measured in Humans. *J Nutr* 1992;122:306.

84. Gillard ER, et al. Stimulation of Eating by the Second Messenger Camp in the Perifornical and Lateral Hypothalamus. *Am J Physiol* 1997;273:R107.

85. Montgomery RB, Singer G. Functional Relationship of Lateral Hypothalamus and Amygdala in Control of Eating. *Pharmacol Biochem Behav* 1975;3:905.

86. Stanley BG, Chin AS, Leibowitz SF. Feeding and Drinking Elicited by Central Injection of Neuropeptide Y: Evidence for a Hypothalamic Site(s) of Action. *Brain Res Bull* 1985;14:521.

87. Ramirez I, Friedman MI. Dietary Hyperphagia in Rats: Role of Fat, Carbohydrate, and Energy Content. *Physiol Behav* 1990;47:1157.

88. Friedman MI. Insulin-Induced Hyperphagia in Alloxan-Diabetic Rats Fed a High-Fat Diet. *Physiol Behav* 1977;19:597.

89. Blundell JE, et al. Dietary Fat and the Control of Energy Intake: Evaluating the Effects of Fat on Meal Size and Postmeal Satiety. *Am J Clin Nutr* 1993;57(Suppl):772S.

The Hormonal Response to Food

The poorest man would not part with health for money,
but the richest would gladly part with all their money for health.
Charles Caleb Cotton

Execute an effective fat loss plan before excess bodyfat executes you.
Rob Faigin

More people commit suicide with a fork than with a gun.
Unknown

Each time you eat you provoke a storm of hormonal activity, and you prospectively influence the state of your body and mind for the ensuing several hours in four critical respects.

- **Fuel Usage**: Whether you will burn fat or store fat.

- **Mental State**: Whether you will experience an alert, clear-headed state of mind or a sluggish, foggy state of mind - or something in-between. (Mental state is interrelated with *fuel usage* insofar as excessive dependence on sugar for fuel can lead to depressed blood sugar levels which, along with the neurotransmitter disturbances associated with high-carbohydrate meals, can reduce mental productivity and negatively alter mood/outlook.)

- **Energy Level**: Whether you will experience a higher energy level or a lower energy level. (Energy level is interrelated with *fuel usage* insofar as fat yields higher and more stable energy levels than does sugar. Energy level is interrelated with *mental state* insofar as the brain orchestrates all physical activities – hence, a sluggish brain means a sluggish body.)

Prime Your Biochemistry

- **Appetite**: Whether or not you will experience food cravings. (Appetite is interrelated with *fuel usage* insofar as appetite influences what and how much you eat – and therefore what type of fuel your body uses. Appetite therefore indirectly influences *mental state* and *energy levels* since both are influenced by fuel usage.)

For this reason, eating should be viewed. . .

<u>not</u> as an event limited in time to how long it takes to swallow the food comprising a meal, <u>but rather</u> as a means of priming your biochemistry for the ensuing four hours in terms of fat-burning/-storage, mental state, energy levels, and appetite.

Insulin and Glucagon:
Opposing Forces in the Kingdom of Metabolism

Insulin (lipogenic/anabolic) and glucagon (lipolytic/catabolic) are inverse paired hormones, which simply means that when one goes up the other goes down. They are the master controllers of metabolism, and they serve diametrically opposite functions. Before exploring these functions, let's look at the effect of these hormones on fat burning/storage.

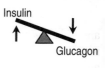

Not only do insulin and glucagon exert a short-term impact on eating behavior and whether you burn fat or store it, [1,2] but also, as you learned in Chapter 9, these hormones can have a long-term impact on your "fat setpoint." The effect of insulin and glucagon on bodyfat is well-illustrated by a study published in the *Journal of Comparative and Physiological Psychology* in 1978.[3] In this appealingly simple study, researchers injected a group of rats with insulin and another group of rats with glucagon. The rats that received insulin injections gained bodyfat; the rats that received glucagon injections lost bodyfat. (Also, the insulin-injected rats ate more, reflecting the hormonal hunger phenomenon described in Chapter 11.)

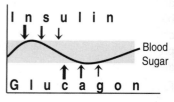

This finding has been corroborated over and over again in humans, in the context of diabetes. It is a well-established clinical observation that the lead-up to adult-onset (Type II) diabetes (characterized by excess insulin produced to compensate for insulin resistance) is highly associated with obesity; whereas the onset of insulin-dependent (Type I) diabetes (in which the pancreas produces insufficient insulin) is marked by uncontrollable drastic weight loss. The fact is that with high insulin levels you can't lose fat, and with insufficient insulin you can't help losing fat (and muscle, too - without anabolic insulin to counterbalance catabolic glucagon, muscle comes off in a hurry). Insulin insufficiency is relevant only as a frame of reference; it does not happen outside the context of diabetes. **Within its normal range of fluctuation, we can manipulate insulin levels to our advantage**.

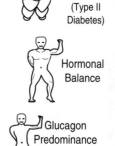

In addition to dictating whether you will burn fat or store it, the insulin/glucagon axis influences other hormones, many of which, too, affect body composition, such as testosterone, growth hormone, cortisol, and IGF-1. Furthermore, in Chapter 8 you learned that the insulin/glucagon axis regulates cholesterol and triglyceride production. Insulin also affects neurotransmitters which, in turn, influence mood, energy levels, and motivation (see Chapter 11).

As you can see, **the insulin/glucagon axis is the pivot-point for body composition, health, energy levels, mental productivity, and emotional well-being**. The NHE Eating Plan focuses on strategically managing insulin/glucagon as a lever for getting your entire hormonal army to work for you in the quest for a fit, healthy body and optimal physical and mental performance.

The Insulin Mechanism: How it Works

Because of the chief importance of insulin, it is crucial to understand what it does and how it works.

Insulin is a hormone produced and secreted into the bloodstream by the pancreas, which is an organ located in the abdominal cavity, behind the stomach. The primary function of insulin is to regulate the level of sugar in the blood. In addition, insulin shuttles amino acids and other nutrients into muscle cells, thereby facilitating protein synthesis and promoting anabolism (see below). Without insulin, consuming carbohydrate would be fatal because blood sugar would rise too high, inducing coma and death. The other side of this coin is that chronically high insulin levels can also lead to death, albeit much more gradually, by promoting heart disease and diabetes (see Chapter 8) and possibly cancer as well.[4,5,6,7,8,9,10,11] In addition to undermining health by directly promoting deadly diseases, excess insulin is a potent fat-building force.

Insulin as Fat-Builder

It is helpful to think of insulin as a storage and locking hormone. In more direct terms, it *makes you fat* (by causing fat storage) and it *keeps you fat* (by barring access to fat stores). Hence, keeping a tight rein on this fat-promoting kingpin is critical to permanent fat loss.

Storage & Locking Hormone

What causes insulin levels to rise relative to glucagon?

    1) carbohydrate consumption

       or

    2) a large quantity of calories consumed at one sitting (protein and/or carbohydrate)

Protein is much less insulinogenic (i.e., insulin-stimulatory) than carbohydrate. Therefore, you have to eat much more protein to get the same insulin response as you would from less carbohydrate (see below). However, a very large meal will (regardless of its composition) stimulate high postprandial (i.e., after a meal) insulin levels. **This is why the "starve and stuff" dietary pattern, all too common among dieters, is hormonally incorrect**. Less frequent, larger meals result in higher insulin levels, more fat storage, and higher cholesterol and triglyceride levels than do more frequent, smaller meals (see Chapter 17).

What happens to the sugar that is removed from the bloodstream by insulin? In sequential order, here's the answer:

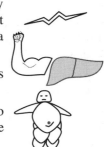

1) Some is utilized by the body - *instead of fat* - for immediate energy needs. Getting rid of excess blood sugar takes precedence, and fat burning is put "on hold," and can remain on hold for hours after a high-carbohydrate meal is consumed.

2) The remainder is converted to glycogen and stored in the muscles and liver for later use.

3) Any remainder, after glycogen synthesis, is converted to triglyceride and transported through the bloodstream to adipose tissue for storage. In other words, TURNED INTO BODYFAT.[12,13,14,15]

NOTE - All carbohydrates are broken down to sugar in the digestive process. Although the human body is efficient at converting sugar into fat, it is not efficient at converting fat into sugar. **Therefore, if you are a sugar-burner, you need a constant supply of incoming sugar which, consequently, keeps you in a sugar-burning mode and hinders fat burning.** When there is an interruption in a sugar-burner's sugar supply (i.e., a skipped meal), the body secretes catabolic hormones to break down glycogen and protein to provide sugar.

Insulin as Muscle-Builder

In addition to being lipogenic, insulin is anabolic. As I mentioned a moment ago, insulin shuttles not only sugar into the muscles, but amino acids and other nutrients too. In this way, insulin enhances muscle growth, recovery, and repair by delivering to the muscles the raw materials needed for protein synthesis. Insulin also benefits muscle by inhibiting protein breakdown.[16,17,18,19,20] Additionally, as discussed in Chapter 11, insulin is necessary for the production of IGF-1, a powerful anabolic hormone-like substance.

Insulin Action
in response to feeding

The Glucagon Mechanism: How it Works

Glucagon, too, is produced and secreted by the pancreas, and it serves the opposite function of insulin. Whereas insulin lowers blood sugar and converts sugar to glycogen, glucagon raises blood sugar by converting glycogen to blood sugar.[21,22,23,24] And whereas insulin promotes fat storage, glucagon promotes fat burning.

Glucagon is, in effect, the "safety valve" for the sugar-burner. When several hours elapse without incoming sugar, liver glycogen is broken down under the direction of glucagon (which activates the glycogen-breakdown enzyme, *phosphorylase*[25,26,27]). The degradation of glycogen yields sugar, which is then released into the bloodstream.[28]

In response to the blood-sugar-raising action of glucagon, insulin is secreted to transport the newly released sugar out of the bloodstream and into the cells of the body. This precipitates a drop in

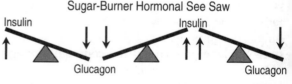

Sugar-Burner Hormonal See Saw

blood sugar, which causes cravings. Consequently, glucagon is secreted to raise blood sugar; consequently insulin is secreted; consequently glucagon is secreted; consequently insulin is secreted, etc.[29,30,31] This hormonal tug-of-war between insulin and glucagon continues indefinitely if you regularly consume carbohydrate-laden meals. Absent incoming carbs, this hormonal see-saw gradually ceases as liver glycogen becomes depleted.* Metabolism switches to fat burning increasingly as liver glycogen dwindles.[32,33,34] Likewise, as reliance on sugar for energy lessens, carbohydrate cravings subside.

---

* Absent incoming food, complete liver glycogen depletion occurs in about 24 hours. The human liver can store approximately 120 grams of glycogen. (Total glycogen storage capacity in adults is 200-500 grams, depending on muscle mass.) Liver glycogen depletion occurs at a rate of about 5 grams per hour. So multiply 5 grams times 24 hours and you get 120, the approximate gram limit of liver glycogen storage. As a practical matter, physical activity influences this rate, with exercise accelerating it considerably.[34a]

The NHE Eating Plan aims to keep liver glycogen low, in order to keep you in a fat-burning state and free from cravings. The Eating Plan accomplishes this in two ways. For one, carbohydrate intake is cycled to prevent liver glycogen accumulation. Second, when carbs are eaten, the emphasis is on starchy carbs rather than sugary carbs. Starchy carbs promote muscle glycogen storage as opposed to liver glycogen storage; the opposite is true for sugary carbs (see Chapter 15).

Glucagon as Fat-Burner

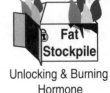

Fat Stockpile

Unlocking & Burning Hormone

Just as insulin is a storage and locking hormone for fat, glucagon is an unlocking and burning hormone. In other words, glucagon mobilizes fat for use as energy.[35,36,37] (However, as noted a moment ago, in order to actualize the fat-burning potential of glucagon, liver glycogen saturation must be avoided.) The NHE Eating Plan, by raising glucagon and lowering insulin, aims to correct the imbalance that causes fat storage and blocks fat burning (and the carbohydrate cycling feature of the Eating Plan precludes liver glycogen saturation). But there is a downside to glucagon, as well.

Glucagon as Muscle-Destroyer

Glucagon Action
in response to fasting

As a fat-burning hormone, glucagon can be a force for good, and it will play an important role in helping you shed bodyfat on the NHE Eating Plan. But just as insulin is a "double-edged sword" so is glucagon, but in reverse. To carry-out its function of raising blood sugar, glucagon in certain instances (i.e., the "sugar-burner-deprived-of-sugar scenario" described in Chapter 11) extracts sugar from muscle as well as from glycogen stores, through a process called gluconeogenesis. Via gluconeogenesis, muscle protein is degraded to provide amino acids for conversion to glucose. This accounts for glucagon's catabolic properties.[38,39,40,41]

The catabolic effects of glucagon are maximized for a sugar-burner and minimized for a fat-burner, because a fat-burner does not need sugar in the same desperate way that a sugar-burner does. The dark side of glucagon is evident in Type I diabetics, who are insulin-deficient due to pancreatic dysfunction. Without insulin to counterbalance glucagon, Type I diabetics suffer precipitous loss of both fat and muscle, until such time as insulin is administered exogenously.[42]

One of the guiding principles of Natural Hormonal Enhancement is that *muscle loss is unacceptable.* Accordingly, the challenge becomes how to get the positive, fat-burning effect of glucagon without the negative, catabolic effect. To understand how to achieve this objective, we must look at what causes glucagon to be secreted. As you may have guessed, the answer is the opposite of what causes insulin to be secreted.

Macronutrient Hormonal Triggers

Whereas carbohydrate is the primary trigger for insulin, protein is the primary trigger for glucagon.[43,44,45] Protein also exerts a weak stimulatory effect on insulin, approximately 30%

Carb triggers insulin
Protein triggers glucagon

of the effect of carbohydrate on insulin.[46,47,48] This explains why if you gorge yourself at one sitting, regardless of whether you ingest carbohydrate, protein, or a combination of both, a strong insulin response will ensue, and you will likely feel sluggish and drowsy as tryptophan rushes into your brain and is converted to serotonin (see Chapter 11). In addition, whereas insulin is triggered by too much food (feasting), glucagon is triggered by too little food (fasting).[49,50,51]

If you are wondering about fat, it does not elicit a response either way when it is consumed alone. When fat is *added* to a

Fat alone triggers neither

protein and/or carbohydrate meal, it either has no effect on insulin response or slightly increases the insulin response (but it does not blunt the insulin response as represented by many authors and commentators*). However, when fat *replaces* an equal caloric quantity of carbohydrate, the insulin response is reduced. For example, if you add butter to a baked potato, you will likely experience an insulin response equal to or slightly greater than if you ate the potato plain. However, if you eat *half a potato with butter*, you will likely experience a significantly lesser insulin response than if you ate *a whole potato plain*. In other words, an isocaloric exchange of carbohydrate for fat yields lower insulin levels.

Immediate Hormonal Response to Macronutrients

	Insulin	Glucagon
Protein**	■	■
Fat	—	—
Carbohydrate	▐	—

---

* Part of the confusion on this subject is a result of a failure to recognize the distinction between adding fat versus substituting fat for carbohydrate. But there is a subtler misapprehension operating, as well. Studies show that adding fat to a meal blunts the postprandial rise in blood sugar. Given that the insulin response generally parallels the rise in blood sugar, it was widely assumed that adding fat to a meal reduces the insulin response to that meal. However, studies show, counter-intuitively, that the insulin response is not attenuated by the addition of fat to a meal [51a,51b,51c] - and in some instances a paradoxical increase in insulin has been observed.[51d,51e] It is not clear why this happens, but it likely relates to *gastric inhibitory polypeptide*, which is secreted in response to fat ingestion and which can augment the insulin response.[51f,51g,51h,51i]

** The insulin response to protein is influenced by three factors. One is the amino acid profile of the protein. For instance, proteins like beef, which contain a high concentration of the amino acid lysine, tend to be more insulinogenic than other protein sources.[51j] The second factor that determines the insulin-raising capacity of a protein source concerns the fat content (see above). The third factor is the extent to which a food has been processed. For instance, ground beef tends to be more insulinogenic than steak, because ground beef does not require as much digestion and thus enters the bloodstream more rapidly.

Chapter 10 - The Hormonal Response to Food

Now that you know what triggers glucagon, we can return to the question of how to offset the catabolic properties of glucagon. The two glucagon triggers can be categorized accordingly:

Active Release: Consuming protein prompts glucagon release.

Passive Release: Not consuming anything for several hours prompts glucagon release to counteract the consequent fall in blood sugar.

The NHE Eating Plan, by prescribing frequent protein feedings, effectuates "active release" and minimizes "passive release." Active release neutralizes the catabolic effect of glucagon by providing amino acids at the same time as glucagon is stimulated so that, with amino acids available in the bloodstream, there is no need to break down muscle tissue to get them. And as a fat-burner, your body will be less dependent on glucose to begin with, which will also minimize the catabolic effect of glucagon.

Avoiding Spillover and the Conveyor belt Problem

Understanding how the insulin mechanism works allows you to avoid two fat-producing pitfalls: "spillover" and the "conveyor belt problem."

Cycle Carbohydrate to Avoid Spillover

On p. 77, we discussed what happens to blood sugar removed from the bloodstream by insulin; and you learned that glycogen stores, in the liver and muscles, are filled before glucose is converted to bodyfat. Hence, there is a direct correlation between glycogen levels and storage of ingested carbohydrate as fat.[52,53,54,55] Therefore, *in order to avoid storing carbohydrate as fat, you must make sure that there is room available in glycogen storage when you consume carbohydrate. Otherwise, any blood sugar that is not immediately used for energy has nowhere else to go but to your hips, butt, midsection, thighs, etc.,- in the form of bodyfat.*

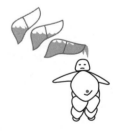

When ingested carbohydrate is channeled to fat stores because glycogen stores have "No Vacancy," I call it "spillover." Frequent high-carbohydrate feedings (exactly what the standard low-fat diet prescribes) promotes fat storage by keeping glycogen depots filled to the brim. The NHE Eating Plan, by contrast, avoids spillover by cycling carbohydrate intake to assure that there is always room available for carbohydrate to be stored as glycogen, rather than as fat.

It is a fundamental fact of human metabolism that the body strives to store that which is in short supply. In Chapter 18, I give several examples of this and discuss the implications of this phenomenon in connection with dietary fat. With carbohydrate, this compensatory mechanism is reflected in the activity of *glycogen synthase*, an enzyme that converts carbohydrate to glycogen and stores it in the liver and muscles. As glycogen stores become depleted, this enzyme becomes more active. And when carbohydrate becomes plentifully available following a period of carbohydrate scarcity, glycogen synthase works "overtime" to store as much carbohydrate as possible as fast as possible.[56,57,58] This translates to an accelerated "loading" of carbohydrate into glycogen depots. For individuals practicing hormonally-intelligent exercise (presumably everyone who reads this book), glycogen loading is of great practical benefit. Other, more general, benefits of glycogen loading are discussed in Chapter 15.

Divide and Conquer to Avoid the Conveyor belt Problem

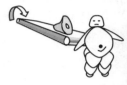

When fat is consumed while your body is in a fat-storage mode (due to a high level of insulin), it is more likely to wind-up as bodyfat.[59,60,61] It is helpful to think of high insulin as turning on a conveyor belt leading to adipose tissue. When the conveyor belt is turned on, everything you put in your mouth has a greater probability of being converted to triglyceride and packed into fat stores. Dietary fat, in particular, has a strong affinity for fat stores when the conveyor belt is on, especially since, as noted above, an upsurge in blood sugar (which turns on the conveyor belt in the first place) causes a temporary suspension of fat burning. The conveyor belt analogy is an image-evocative way of saying: *fat is fattening when you are in a fat-storing state*.

The NHE Eating Plan avoids the conveyor belt problem by keeping dietary fat low when insulin is high (during and after the carb-load), and keeping carbohydrate consumption low at all other times. Thus, the Eating Plan can be viewed as employing a "divide and conquer" strategy that prevents fat and carbohydrate from teaming-up to make you fat.

High Insulin Dropkicks Energy Levels

High insulin can dampen energy levels like a wet rag on a match flame. Because energy is an indispensable ingredient in success - it's the enabling force that bridges the gap between potential and results - all feasible measures should be undertaken to maximize energy levels. Insulin undercuts energy levels in two ways.

Insulin Bars Access to the Supreme Fuel Source

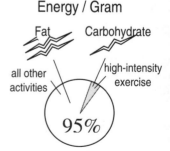

Energy / Gram

Because carbohydrate has been so heavily hyped in recent years as "energy food," people assume that carbohydrate is the best energy source for average daily activities. The fact of the matter is that whereas glycogen is the body's optimal fuel source for high-intensity work like weightlifting, FAT IS THE BODY'S OPTIMAL FUEL SOURCE FOR 95% OF DAILY ACTIVITY. Fat yields 2 1/4 times more energy per gram than carbohydrate, and fat is a much more stable energy source.

Glycogen can be depleted during the course of an athletic event, known as "hitting the wall," whereas the average person weighing 150 pounds has bodyfat containing energy sufficient to enable that person to walk from Ft. Lauderdale, FL to New York City without eating. Furthermore, whereas a sugar-burner's energy level fluctuates and is dependent upon the availability of sugar, a fat-burner has ready access to a steady and practically infinite, superior-quality fuel source.

Elevated insulin makes a person a sugar-burner by directing the body to use glucose for fuel and halting fat burning (see p. 238-239). *Therefore, chronically high insulin forces you to sputter through the day on "low-octane" sugar rather than coasting through the day on premium fuel - fat.*

High Insulin Dulls Mental Acuity

As explained in Chapter 11, high insulin causes tryptophan to flood into the brain inducing a temporary increase in the neurotransmitter serotonin. At moderate levels, serotonin fosters a positive mindset: it enhances feelings of security and well-being, and it helps you concentrate by easing your nerves.

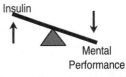

At excessive levels, however, serotonin decreases energy levels and impairs mental performance.

When serotonin is unnaturally elevated relative to other neurotransmitters, it inhibits mental activity by slowing the rate of transmission between the neurons in the brain.[62] As a result, you become drowsy and sluggish[63,64,65] and you experience a mental fuzziness that makes it difficult to concentrate on anything except images of your pillow. Practically everyone has experienced post-meal lethargy (think back to last Thanksgiving). You may have been told that this was because blood had been diverted from your brain to your stomach for digestion - nope; it's serotonin turning-out the lights upstairs. In other words, the drugged, sedated feeling you experience after a large meal is, in fact, of chemical origin and affects brain function in the most basic and profound way - by slowing the rate of neurotransmission (i.e., thought). Cocaine and caffeine, two drugs similar in nature but varying greatly in potency, have the opposite effect - raising levels of serotonin's antagonists, norepinephrine and dopamine.

Your Brain on Carbs

Your Brain on Protein

People who spend their lives on the blood sugar roller coaster spend a minimum of time in neurotransmitter balance. Consequently, they spend a lot of time either struggling to keep their eyes open, or being anxious, irritable, distracted, and craving carbohydrate due to an underlying need to re-boost serotonin levels (see Chapter 11). The intensity of these symptoms varies significantly from person to person depending upon an individual's rate of neurotransmitter synthesis. Nevertheless, **everyone can improve his or her mental state through better diet**.

Because the NHE Eating Plan keeps insulin stable, serotonin can be produced on a regular, steady basis rather than soaring and sagging. This helps eliminate cravings, and results in better neurotransmitter balance - hence, better mood, higher energy levels, and greater mental productivity. As well, the Eating Plan optimizes the body's use of protein (see Chapter 17) thereby providing plentiful raw materials for neurotransmitter synthesis: the amino acid tryptophan for serotonin production, and the amino acids phenylalanine and tyrosine for dopamine and norepinephrine production.

References

1. Galton D. *The Human Adipose Cell*. London: Butterworth and Company 1971, p. 133.

2. Grossman SP. The Role of Glucose, Insulin and Glucagon in the Regulation of Food Intake and Body Weight. *Neurosci Biobehav Rev* 1986;10:295.

3. deCastro J, Paullin S, DeLugas G. Insulin and Glucagon as Determinants of Bodyweight Set Point and Microregulation in Rats. *J Comp Physiol Psychol* 1978;92:571.

4. Brunning PF, et al. Insulin Resistance and Breast Cancer Risk. *Int J Cancer* 1992;52:511.

5. Boutron-Ruault MC, et al. Foods as Risk Factors for Colorectal Cancer: A Case-Control Study in Burgundy (France). *Eur J Cancer Prev* 1999;8:229.

6. Chatenoud L, et al. Refined-Cereal Intake and Risk of Selected Cancers in Italy. *Am J Clin Nutr* 1999;70:1107.

7. Schoen RE, et al. Increased Blood Glucose and Insulin, Body Size, and Incident Colorectal Cancer. *J Natl Cancer Inst* 1999;91:1147.

8. Giovannucci E. Insulin and Colon Cancer. *Cancer Causes Control* 1995;6:164.

9. Hu FB, et al. Prospective Study of Adult Onset Diabetes Mellitus (Type 2) and Risk of Colorectal Cancer in Women. *J Natl Cancer Inst* 1999;91:542.

10. Yamada K, et al. Relation of Serum Total Cholesterol, Serum Triglycerides and Fasting Plasma Glucose to Colorectal Carcinoma in Situ. *Int J Epidemiol* 1998;27:794.

11. Stoll BA. Western Nutrition and the Insulin Resistance Syndrome: A Link to Breast Cancer. *Eur J Clin Nutr* 1999;53:83.

12. Acheson KJ, et al. Glycogen Storage Capacity and De Novo Lipogenesis during Massive Carbohydrate Overfeeding in Man. *Am J Clin Nutr* 1988;48:240.

13. Passmore R, Swindells YE. Observations on the Respiratory Quotients and Weight Gain of Man after Eating Large Quantities of Carbohydrate. *Br J Nutr* 1963;17:331.

14. Acheson KJ, Flatt J-P, Jequier E. Glycogen Synthesis Versus Lipogenesis after a 500 Gram Carbohydrate Meal in Man. *Metabolism* 1982;31:1234.

15. Labayen I, Forga L, Martinez JA. Nutrient Oxidation and Metabolic Rate as Affected by Meals Containing Different Proportions of Carbohydrate and Fat, in Healthy Young Women. *Eur J Nutr* 1999;38:158.

16. Grizard J, et al. Insulin Action on Skeletal Muscle Protein Metabolism during Catabolic States. *Reprod Nutr Dev* 1999;39:61.

17. Gelfand RA, Barrett EJ. Effect of Physiologic Hyperinsulinemia on Skeletal Muscle Protein Synthesis and Breakdown in Man. *J Clin Invest* 1987;80:1.

18. Miers WR, Barrett EJ. The Role of Insulin and other Hormones in the Regulation of Amino Acid and Protein Metabolism in Humans. *J Basic Clin Physiol Pharmacol* 1998;9:235.

19. Fryburg DA, et al. Insulin and Insulin-Like Growth Factor-I Enhance Human Skeletal Muscle Protein Anabolism during Hyperaminoacidemia by Different Mechanisms. *J Clin Invest* 1995;96:1722.

20. Airhart J, et al. Insulin Stimulation of Protein Synthesis in Cultured Skeletal and Cardiac Muscle Cells. *Am J Physiol* 1982;243:C81

21. Wasserman DH, et al. Glucagon is a Primary Controller of Hepatic Glycogenolysis and Gluconeogenesis during Muscular Work. *Am J Physiol* 1989;257:E108.

22. Shiota M, et al. Inability of Hyperglycemia to Counter the Ability of Glucagon to Increase Net Glucose Output and Activate Glycogen Phosphorylase in the Perfused Rat Liver. *Metabolism* 1996;45:481.

23. Dobbins RL, et al. Role of Glucagon in Countering Hypoglycemia Induced by Insulin Infusion in Dogs. *Am J Physiol* 1991;261:E773.

24. Hendrick GK, et al. Importance of Basal Glucagon in Maintaining Hepatic Glucose Production during a Prolonged Fast in Conscious Dogs. *Am J Physiol* 1992;263:E541.

25. Yorek MA, Blair JB, Ray PD. The Influences of Glucagon, Epinephrine and Adrenergic Agents on Glycogen Phosphorylase A and Pyruvate Kinase Activities in Hepatocytes from Juvenile and Adult Rabbits. *Biochim Biophys Acta* 1982;717:143.

26. Brunt ME, McNeill JH. The Effect of Glucagon on Rat Cardiac Cyclic AMP, Phosphorylase A and Force of Contraction. *Arch Int Pharmacodyn Ther* 1978;233:42.

27. Birnbaum MJ, Fain JN. Activation of Protein Kinase and Glycogen Phosphorylase in Isolated Rat Liver Cells by Glucagon and Catecholamines. *J Biol Chem* 1977;252:528.

28. Caprio S, et al. Relationship between Changes in Glucose Production and Gluconeogenesis during Mild Hypoglycemia in Humans. *Metabolism* 1988;37:707.

29. Cryer PE. Glucose Counterregulation: Prevention and Correction of Hypoglycemia in Humans. *Am J Physiol* 1993;264:E149.

30. Cryer PE. Regulation of Glucose Metabolism in Man. *J Intern Med Suppl* 1991;735:31.

31. Genter P, Ipp E. Plasma Glucose Thresholds for Counterregulation after an Oral Glucose Load. *Metabolism* 1994;43:98.

32. Schrauwen P, et al. Fat Balance in Obese Subjects: Role of Glycogen Stores. *Am J Physiol* 1998;274:E1027.

33. Schrauwen P, et al. Role of Glycogen-Lowering Exercise in the Change of Fat Oxidation in Response to a High-Fat Diet. *Am J Physiol* 1997;273:E623.

34. Flatt JP. Glycogen Levels and Obesity. *Int J Obes Relat Metab Disord* 1996;20 (Suppl):S1.

34a. Flatt J-P. Use and Storage of Carbohydrate and Fat. *Am J Clin Nutr* 1995;61:952S

35. Voss KH, Masoro EJ, Anderson W. Modulation of Age-Related Loss of Glucagon-Promoted Lipolysis by Food Restriction. *Mech Ageing Dev* 1982;18:135.

36. Schade DS, Eaton RP. Modulation of Fatty Acid Metabolism by Glucagon in Man. I. Effects in Normal Subjects. *Diabetes* 1975;24:502.

37. Howland RJ, Benning AD. Differential Effects of Noradrenaline and Glucagon on Lipolysis and Fatty-Acid Utilization in Brown Adipose Tissue. *FEBS Lett* 1986;208:128.

38. Maki Y, et al. A Profile of Plasma Branched Chain Amino Acids in a Totally Pancreatectomized Patient: Effects of Glucagon Replacement under a Steady Feeding State. *Horm Metab Res* 1987;19:226.

39. Schworer CM, Mortimore GE. Glucagon-Induced Autophagy and Proteolysis in Rat Liver: Mediation by Selective Deprivation of Intracellular Amino Acids. *Proc Natl Acad Sci U S A* 1979;76:3169.

40. Tessari P, et al. Hyperglucagonemia Stimulates Phenylalanine Oxidation in Humans. *Diabetes* 1996;45:463.

41. Charlton MR, Adey DB, Nair KS. Evidence for a Catabolic Role of Glucagon during an Amino Acid Load. *J Clin Invest* 1996;98:90.

42. Charlton MR, Nair KS. Role of Hyperglucagonemia in Catabolism Associated with Type 1 Diabetes: Effects on Leucine Metabolism and the Resting Metabolic Rate. *Diabetes* 1998;47:1748.

43. Day JL, et al. Factors Governing Insulin and Glucagon Responses during Normal Meals. *Clin Endocrinol (Oxf)* 1978;9:443.

44. Muller WA, et al. The Influence of the Antecedent Diet upon Glucagon and Insulin Secretion. *N Engl J Med* 1971;285:1450.

45. Wolever TM, Bolognesi C. Prediction of Glucose and Insulin Responses of Normal Subjects after Consuming Mixed Meals Varying in Energy, Protein, Fat, Carbohydrate and Glycemic Index. *J Nutr* 1996;126:2807.

46. Krezowski PA, et al. The Effect of Protein Ingestion on the Metabolic Response to Oral Glucose in Normal Individuals. *Am J Clin Nutr* 1986;44:847.

47. Westphal SA, Gannon MC, Nuttall FQ. Metabolic Response to Glucose Ingested with Various Amounts of Protein. *Am J Clin Nutr* 1990;52:267.

48. Capani F, et al. [Insulin Secretion after a Protein and Lipid Meal in Healthy Subjects]. *Boll Soc Ital Biol Sper* 1985;61:351. Italian.

49. Boyle PJ, Shah SD, Cryer PE. Insulin, Glucagon, and Catecholamines in Prevention of Hypoglycemia during Fasting. *Am J Physiol* 1989;256:E651.

50. Boisjoyeux B, et al. Comparison between Starvation and Consumption of a High Protein Diet: Plasma Insulin and Glucagon and Hepatic Activities of Gluconeogenic Enzymes during the First 24 Hours. *Diabete Metab* 1986;12:21.

51. Aguilar-Parada E, Eisentraut AM, Unger RH. Effects of Starvation on Plasma Pancreatic Glucagon in Normal Man. *Diabetes* 1969;18:717.

51a. Collier G, McLean A, O'Dea K. Effect of Co-Ingestion of Fat on the Metabolic Responses to Slowly and Rapidly Absorbed Carbohydrates. *Diabetologia* 1984;26:50.

51b. Ercan N, Gannon MC, Nuttall FQ. Effect of Added Fat on the Plasma Glucose and Insulin Response to Ingested Potato Given in Various Combinations as Two Meals in Normal Individuals. *Diabetes Care* 1994;17:1453.

51c. Collier G, O'Dea K. The Effect of Co-ingestion of Fat on the Glucose, Insulin, and Gastric Inhibitory Polypeptide Responses to Carbohydrate and Protein. *Am J Clin Nutr* 1983;37:941.

51d. Gannon MC, et al. Effect of Added Fat on Plasma Glucose and Insulin Response to Ingested Potato in Individuals with NIDDM. *Diabetes Care* 1993;16:874.

51e. Collier GR, et al. The Acute Effect of Fat on Insulin Secretion. *J Clin Endocrinol Metab* 1988;66:323.

51f. Crockett SE, et al. The Insulinotropic Effect of Endogenous Gastric Inhibitory Polypeptide in Normal Subjects. *J Clin Endocrinol Metab* 1976;42:1098.

51g. Falko JM, et al. Gastric Inhibitory Polypeptide (GIP) Stimulated by Fat Ingestion in Man. *J Clin Endocrinol Metab* 1975;41:260.

51h. Pederson RA, Schubert HE, Brown JC. Gastric Inhibitory Polypeptide. Its Physiologic Release and Insulinotropic Action in the Dog. *Diabetes* 1975;24:1050.

51i. Lardinois CK, Starich GH, Mazzaferri EL. The Postprandial Response of Gastric Inhibitory Polypeptide to Various Dietary Fats in Man. *J Am Coll Nutr* 1988;7:241.

51j. Sener A, et al. Stimulus-Secretion Coupling of Arginine-Induced Insulin Release: Comparison with Lysine-Induced Insulin Secretion. *Endocrinology* 1989;124:2558.

52. Flatt JP. Glycogen Levels and Obesity. *Int J Obes Relat Metab Disord* 1996;20 (Suppl) 2:S1.

53. Flatt JP. The Difference in the Storage Capacities for Carbohydrate and for Fat, and its Implications in the Regulation of Body Weight. *Ann N Y Acad Sci* 1987;499:104.

54. Acheson KJ, et al. Nutritional Influences on Lipogenesis and Thermogenesis after a Carbohydrate Meal. *Am J Physiol* 1984;246:E62.

55. Acheson KJ, et al. Carbohydrate Metabolism and De Novo Lipogenesis in Human Obesity. *Am J Clin Nutr* 1987;45:78.

56. Yan Z, Spencer MK, Katz A. Effect of Low Glycogen on Glycogen Synthase in Human Muscle during and after Exercise. *Acta Physiol Scand* 1992;145:345.

57. Kochan RG, et al. Glycogen Synthase Activation in Human Skeletal Muscle: Effects of Diet and Exercise. *Am J Physiol* 1979;236:E660.

58. Zachwieja JJ, et al. Influence of Muscle Glycogen Depletion on the Rate of Resynthesis. *Med Sci Sports Ex* 1991;23:44.

59. Murphy MC, et al. Postprandial Lipid and Hormone Responses to Meals of Varying Fat Contents: Modulatory Role of Lipoprotein Lipase? *Eur J Clin Nutr* 1995;49:578.

60. Cohen JC, Schall R. Reassessing the Effects of Simple Carbohydrates on the Serum Triglyceride Responses to Fat Meals. *Am J Clin Nutr* 1988;48:1031.

61. Kabir M, et al. A High Glycemic Index Starch Diet Affects Lipid Storage-Related Enzymes in Normal and to a Lesser Extent in Diabetic Rats. *J Nutr* 1998;128:1878.

62. Robertson J. *Peak Performance Living*. San Francisco, CA: Harper Collins 1996.

63. Spring B, et al. Psychobiological Effects of Carbohydrates. *J Clin Psychiatry* 1989;50 (Suppl):27.

64. Lieberman HR, Wurtman JJ, Chew B. Changes in Mood after Carbohydrate Consumption among Obese Individuals. *Am J Clin Nutr* 1986;44:772.

65. Spring B, et al. Effects of Protein and Carbohydrate Meals on Mood and Performance: Interactions with Sex and Age. *J Psychiatr Res* 1983;17:155.

Chapter 11

Dietary Strategies for:
Reshaping Your Body • Combating Aging •
Subduing Cravings • Increasing Energy Levels •
Improving Athletic Performance • Promoting Health

Let thy food be thy medicine.
Hippocrates

Americans have more food to eat than any other people on Earth,
and more diets to keep you from eating it.
Andy Rooney

Reshaping Your Body
and Combating Aging

Maximum Fat Loss Without Sacrificing Lean Body Mass

Most fat loss programs are really weight loss programs, causing indiscriminate loss of body tissue. For example, on a calorie-restrictive diet up to 40% of the weight you lose is muscle (see p. 66). Shedding muscle along with fat is not a good bargain. In fact, it becomes a net loss when, typically, the fat comes back but the muscle does not. This results in a worsening of body composition, by increasing bodyfat percentage. This, in turn, can reduce growth hormone levels because growth hormone release is negatively correlated with "relative adiposity" (a fancy term for bodyfat percentage).[1,2,3]

The association between fatness and growth hormone is very strong. In fact, fatness is a stronger predictor than age of growth hormone status.[4,5,6] The relationship is mutually causative and thus unfavorably reinforcing: reduced growth hormone secretion promotes bodyfat accretion, and bodyfat accretion reduces growth hormone secretion. Abdominal obesity, in particular, is correlated with low growth hormone.[7] Given that abdominal obesity is also correlated with insulin resistance (see p. 101), and given the antagonistic relationship between insulin and growth hormone (discussed later in this chapter), it is probable that insulin resistance underlies the linkage between obesity and reduced growth hormone output.

You may have noticed that neither this book nor any literature about Natural Hormonal Enhancement ever uses the term "weight loss." Weight loss is meaningless: a degenerative disease, a viral infection, or an amputation can each cause plenty of weight loss. But none of these will do anything to improve body composition.

The human body is remarkably efficient at using muscle for energy through a process called *gluconeogenesis,* in which protein from muscle tissue is converted to glucose.[8,9,10] Here's a helpful analogy: when times are bad financially, what is the first thing to go? That which is not necessary and which is the most expensive to maintain. Your body operates on the same basis: when times are tough (i.e., you are on a restrictive diet) your body is quick to ditch muscle tissue.

Beyond minimal levels, muscle is an expensive luxury item. It is expensive in that it requires the most calories to maintain of any kind of tissue. It is a luxury item in that the "extra" muscle necessary to look your best and excel athletically is considered expendable by your body. On your body's list of priorities, survival is number one, and looking good in a swimsuit and performing well at sports and physique competitions are at the bottom of the list.

Your body's readiness to cannibalize muscle tissue in times of stress is graphically illustrated in the case of starvation. If you have ever seen a starving person, you were probably struck by the grotesque deterioration resulting from extreme loss of muscle. THIS IS EXACTLY WHAT YOU ARE DOING TO YOURSELF, TO A LESSER DEGREE, WHEN YOU ENGAGE IN CONVENTIONAL RESTRICTIVE DIETING. Reduced food intake resulting in a calorie and/or protein deficiency stimulates catabolic hormones[11,12] and suppresses anabolic hormones.[13] These hormonal shifts are responsible for the deterioration that attends conventional dieting and other forms of starvation. As you might suspect, in patients with anorexia, catabolic hormone levels are sky-high.[14,15] Because the "muscle axis" (see Chapter 4) of starving people is so drastically out-of-whack, they have a sick, emaciated look - not the lean, sculpted look for which you are aiming.

Using Your Muscles to Turn Back the Hands of Time

Muscle is a powerful ally to both men and women in the fight against fat, the fight against aging, and in the effort to look your best.

- Muscle gives your body form, shape, and contour, which, along with low bodyfat are the characteristics that define a sexy, attractive body.

- Muscle is your hedge against aging. As you get older you tend to lose muscle, thereby becoming a stooped-over, frail, weak person. *People who lose muscle as a result of dieting are, in effect, accelerating a central feature of aging.*

- Muscle is the most metabolically active tissue, so when you lose muscle you reduce your metabolic rate - exactly what you *don't* want if you wish to maintain low bodyfat.

Women and Muscles

It is easy to overlook how precious is muscle. Women, in particular, often fail to appreciate the vital importance muscle plays in having an attractive physique. The fact is that diet-induced muscle loss is a *more* serious problem for women because they have less muscle to begin with, tend to lose it more readily, and are hormonally limited in their ability to build muscle.

Skinny Mini (restrictive dieter)   Sexy Sue (NHE follower)   Beastly Bertha (steroid user)

Most womens' view of muscle is tainted by the unfounded fear of "getting big" or looking unfeminine. Don't worry, as long as you do not take steroids or other anabolic drugs, your female hormonal chemistry will not permit you to look anything like the "female" bodybuilders you may have seen on T.V. or in magazines. To the contrary, a bit of added muscle, when coupled with fat loss, will produce a *smaller* look. The reason for this is that muscle is denser and therefore takes-up less space on your body than does fat. What this means is that shedding bodyfat and building a little bit of muscle (which is all that you, as a female, are capable of building anyway) will make you *leaner, smaller, firmer, healthier,* and *shapelier.* Depending on how much fat you have to begin with, improving your body composition may not be reflected by much of a change in weight due to the fact that muscle weighs more than fat - *but who cares?* As long as you are becoming healthier and feeling and looking better, it should not matter to you what the scale says.

With this in mind, you should begin to deprogram the weight loss mentality that has been relentlessly instilled in you by society, and which guarantees failure. Commit yourself to your new strategy, which is to shed excess bodyfat and to preserve - or even better, to build a bit of muscle - and thereby become leaner, smaller, firmer, healthier, and shapelier.

The Anabolic, "Construction," Effect

Anabolism is a natural process of construction that goes on inside your body. At the cellular level, your body is a work in progress. By means of protein synthesis, the structures of your body are constantly being rebuilt, repaired, and replaced. Anabolic hormones are called upon by the body to carry-out these tasks.

The NHE Eating Plan is anabolic, which means that it optimizes the "big three" anabolic hormones: growth hormone, testosterone, and insulin. This *does not* mean that the Eating Plan will invariably build big muscles. To the contrary, as noted above, women cannot build large muscles without anabolic drugs, regardless of diet or any other natural factor. Similarly, it is unrealistic for men to think that diet alone will build muscle.

Having said that, the anabolic effects of the NHE Eating Plan are significant insofar as they help counteract the muscle loss associated with losing fat and with aging. Furthermore, if you are engaged in a weight-training program, you will find that the Eating Plan complements your efforts to build muscle. In terms of enhancing lean body mass, the Eating Plan is markedly superior to both the high-carbohydrate/low-fat diet and the low-carbohydrate/high-fat diet.

If building muscle mass is your top priority, you should consider the bodybuilders' version NHE Eating Plan, which is designed to maximize anabolic hormonal output (see

Chapter 14). Because of the high calorie consumption that the bodybuilders' version mandates, you will not get the same fat-burning effect that you would from the general NHE Eating Plan. But you will be able to build muscle faster than with any other diet you have ever experienced - and without the accompanying fat gain characteristic of conventional bodybuilding diets.

Anabolic Hormones in Action:
Growth Hormone and Insulin - Adversaries in Partnership

You can think of growth hormone and insulin as partners who do not like each other, and fight a lot, but who need each other to execute their anabolic duties. Whereas growth hormone tells your body to burn fat, insulin tells your body to store fat and directs it to use sugar for energy instead. In this way, insulin directly opposes the lipolytic action of growth hormone;[16,17] and in Chapter 21 we will examine the implications of this for the pre- and post-workout meals. In addition to playing conflicting roles on your "fat axis," these two hormones do not like being in each other's presence. Generally, when growth hormone levels are high, insulin levels are low, and vice versa (see p. 201). One reason why the high-carbohydrate/low-fat diet is hormonally incorrect is because it keeps insulin up, which keeps growth hormone down.

Although these hormones work in opposition to each other on the "fat axis," they work in cooperation on the "muscle axis" by promoting anabolism and by co-regulating production of insulin-like growth factors, also called *somatomedins*, in the liver.[18,19,20] Researchers were tipped-off to the complementary anabolic interaction between growth hormone and insulin in 1951 by an experiment in depancreatized (pancreas removed) cats. Growth hormone had no anabolic effect when the cats were not given insulin.[21] The discovery of growth factors provided the "missing anabolic link" between insulin and growth hormone.

Growth factors are not actually hormones, but rather they are peptides that function like hormones on a more localized level in the body. Science has only recently begun to uncover the critical role played by these substances. The most extensively studied of this family of quasi-hormones is *insulin-like growth factor I* (IGF-1).

IGF-1, the offspring of growth hormone and insulin, is at least as powerful an anabolic agent as either of its parents. The importance of IGF-1 for growth is underscored by a form of growth retardation called Laron dwarfism, a disorder marked by low IGF-I production despite high circulating levels of growth hormone.[22] Recent research suggests that IGF-I, and perhaps other insulin-like growth factors as well, is the "behind-the-scenes-player" responsible for much of the anti-aging benefits for which growth hormone has been accorded credit. Prompted by this hypothesis, researchers have homed-in on growth factors.

The insights acquired by researchers pursuing leads in this area have intensified the excitement surrounding growth factors, and have shed light on their vast potential. Scientists are seeking to ascertain precisely how hormones and growth factors interrelate. At the same time, a race is on among biotech companies to identify, isolate, and use genetic engineering to clone growth factors for use as drugs. Already a growth factor called *erythropoietin*, which stimulates the proliferation of red blood cells, is being used in patients with anemia due to chemotherapy, AZT treatment, or kidney failure. Epidermal growth factor also has been developed and is being used to treat burn victims, with marked success. One individual who is watching the fast-paced developments in this field with keen interest is paralyzed actor Christopher Reeve, who, on the *Today Show* (Aug. 26, 1996), expressed his belief that nerve growth factors will someday enable him to walk again. The current research suggests that Superman's hope is not unrealistic.

While the outer reaches of growth factor potential are yet unmapped, it is clear that IGF-1 is a powerful tool in your body-sculpting/anti-aging arsenal. We also know that without insulin and growth hormone working together to produce IGF-I, neither hormone can accomplish much on the "muscle axis." The close relationship between growth hormone and IGF-I is well established.[23,24] In fact, tests of growth hormone levels actually measure IGF-1 levels, since they are easier to detect and generally reflect growth hormone status.[25] The importance of insulin in the production of IGF-1 is demonstrated by studies of insulin-dependent diabetics, in which injections of growth hormone fail to raise IGF-1 levels when insulin is inadequate.[26] IGF-1 production is also dependent upon adequate dietary protein.[27,28,29]

With the NHE Eating Plan, carbohydrate consumption is restricted to boost baseline growth hormone levels but insulin levels are raised at strategic intervals to allow these two hormones to work together beneficially, while avoiding the fattening properties of insulin. Furthermore, the Eating Plan prescribes ample protein, which is crucial to maintaining optimal IGF-1 levels.

Protecting Protein:
The Anti-Catabolic, Anti-Aging, Effect

Muscle is constantly being built up (anabolism) and broken down (catabolism). Regardless of whether you are a bodybuilder training for maximum muscle mass or a woman trying to get firm and toned (and stay that way even as you get older), it behooves you to curb catabolism. Women, in particular, because they have much less anabolic firepower than men, should be mindful to keep catabolic hormones in check.

As I explained earlier, until recently, scientists viewed the age-related deterioration of the human body as genetically programmed and basically unalterable. We now know that we have much more control over this process than even the most optimistic scientists had previously imagined. Hormones have been found to be the key players in this process, and some scientists go so far as to say that what we call "aging" is nothing more than a symptom of adverse hormonal changes. As the scientific evidence mounts, this theory increasingly gains converts - even within the fusty corridors of conventional medicine.

Specifically, much of the degenerative process we call "aging" is attributable to the increasing predominance of catabolic activity over anabolic activity. The image you have in your mind of an elderly person - frail, weak, stooped-over - is the picture of what happens when catabolic hormones get the upper-hand on anabolic hormones over an extended period of time. *Don't let it happen to you.*

Anabolic   Catabolic
Predominance Predominance

The NHE Eating Plan has a strong anti-catabolic effect, by means of the metabolic shift it causes away from dependence on glucose for fuel and toward fat burning. In effect, fat helps protect muscle tissue. When you are a sugar-burner, your precious muscle tissue is constantly at risk: miss a meal or deplete glycogen stores by exercising, and your body will release the hormone glucagon to break down muscle protein, through a process called gluconeogenesis, in which glucose (sugar) is formed from protein (see p. 88). Doesn't it make much more sense to burn fat than to burn muscle given that 1) fat is ugly whereas muscle is attractive, 2) fat has scant functional value whereas muscle has great functional value, 3) fat is a much better energy source gram for gram, providing 2 1/4 times more energy than protein?

91

Glucagon is not the only hormone that comes into play when blood sugar levels fall. The highly catabolic hormone cortisol is released in response to stress. When a sugar-burner's blood sugar level drops too low (which can happen several times a day) the body perceives this as a traumatic event and releases cortisol from the adrenal cortex.[30,31,32,33,34] As the most catabolic hormone in the body, cortisol is a very efficient muscle-destroyer.[35,36,37,38] In the words of Dr. Michael Colgan, author of *Hormonal Health,* "cortisol will chop-up your muscles faster than a sushi chef."[39] Elevated cortisol levels threaten bone too, with studies showing that higher cortisol levels correspond with a faster rate of bone loss in elderly individuals.[40,41] Moreover, once cortisol is turned loose, not only does it go after muscle and bone but it also promotes insulin resistance[42,43,44,45] and immune suppression.[46,47,48,49]

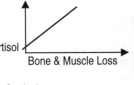

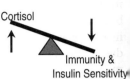

The NHE Eating Plan stabilizes blood sugar, thus averting catabolic blood sugar free-falls. Furthermore, as a fat-burner, with unlimited access to bodyfat stores, a blood sugar drop does not represent the physiologically stressful situation that it does for a sugar-burner. Therefore, cortisol is kept in check and muscle is preserved. For a more in-depth discussion of dietary anti-catabolism, see "The Bodybuilders' NHE Eating Plan" (Chapter 14).

Increasing Energy Levels and Improving Athletic Performance

High Energy Levels while Losing Bodyfat

Conventional dieting is strongly associated with diminished energy levels. With conventional diets, energy levels drop either because of less ingested energy (calorie-restrictive diet), low glycogen and mineral/electrolyte imbalances (low-carbohydrate diet), or blood sugar irregularities and neurotransmitter disturbances (high-carbohydrate/low-fat diet). With the NHE Eating Plan, none of these problems is present. Rather, energy levels increase as you make the metabolic shift to being a fat-burner. If you are an athlete, you will find the Eating Plan to be a blessing, giving you the twin advantages of greater access to fat stores and heightened glycogen use efficiency.

Because carbohydrate has been hyped to death in recent years as "energy food," in an effort to sell you cheap, sugar-loaded drinks and candy bars (marketed as performance supplements or meal replacements), people assume that carbohydrate is the best energy source for average daily activities. In fact, as discussed on p. 82, fat is the body's preferred fuel source for 95% of daily activities. Only during high-intensity activities like weightlifting or sprinting is carbohydrate the optimal fuel source. As a fat-burner, you will be better able to access fat for fuel, which is a much more reliable, stable, and higher-yield energy source.

Paradoxically, cycled carbohydrate intake improves glycogen utilization as compared with consistently high carbohydrate intake. The reason for this is that high carbohydrate intake activates the sugar-burning metabolic pathway and inhibits the fat-burning metabolic pathway (see p. 167, 238-239). Consequently, the body becomes more dependent on sugar for fuel and taps into glycogen stores more heavily for ordinary energy needs as opposed to burning fat. Conversely, a lower intake of carbohydrate coupled with a proportional increase in fat intake promotes glycogen conservation coupled with more liberal use of fat for fuel during both exercise and rest.[50,51,52,53] This *glycogen-sparing effect* means you get more mileage out of less dietary carbohydrate and you burn more fat – this translates to advantages both in terms of exercise performance and body composition. Chapter 18 describes more specifically the role played by dietary fat in effectuating the shift to a fat-burning state, and Chapter 21 discusses the practical implications of fuel utilization patterns for exercise and sport.

The "Metabolic Advantage" in the Gym
- More Fat Loss from Exercise

You may be familiar with the exercise axiom that holds that you must do aerobic exercise for at least twenty minutes before you start burning fat (technically, this is incorrect to begin with because you are always burning *some* fat - the difference is one of percentages, and it can be a very substantial difference). The underlying assumption is that you are in a sugar-burning state when you walk into the gym, and thus you need to exercise for a while as a means of making the transition to a predominately fat-burning state. Given that the NHE Eating Plan is designed to keep you in a predominately fat-burning state around the clock, the standard reasoning does not apply. While aerobic exercise will increase, even more, the amount of fat burned, you will have the "metabolic advantage" from the outset, and thus you will burn more fat during and after each workout.

For Athletes and Bodybuilders: Avoiding the Pitfalls of Cutting Weight, and Making Steady Progress Competition to Competition, Year to Year.

I'm not a doctor, but I'd like to see some research done here. I think, physiologically, when they dry those guys down to the bone, then put the water back in, I think there may be a connection with those problems.
Famed boxing referee, Mills Lane, commenting on the deaths and hospitalizations that have occurred in boxing. *KO Magazine*, Holiday Issue 1997.

You're right Mills, and here's the research you requested . . .

Virtually every sports fan is acquainted with the all-too-common phenomenon of an athlete who has had to cut weight for a competitive event "coming in flat," or wilting prematurely as the competition progresses. Sub-par performances are more the rule than the exception among athletes who resort to drastic measures to make weight. For these athletes, moreover, a decrease in performance is accompanied by an increase in health risks associated with physical competition.

93

Rapid weight loss exacts a considerable toll on the body, especially for the sugar-burner athlete who inevitably suffers catabolic consequences from the crash weight loss process. Furthermore, because of the general ineffectiveness of the high-carb/low-fat diet as a vehicle for fat loss, the athlete who relies on this formula is often forced to resort to extreme calorie restriction *along with* fat restriction. This compromises the athlete's performance by causing muscle loss AND depleting glycogen stores AND creating psychological stress incompatible with optimal pre-contest mental preparation AND reducing the athlete's dietary energy and nutrient intake.

The latter is particularly troubling in view of the fact that vitamin and mineral status is crucial not only to athletic performance, but to health as well. Reduced food intake is a predisposing factor in vitamin deficiency for athletes and non-athletes alike.[54,55] And the reduced nutrient intake that results from reduced food intake is exacerbated in athletes by intense training, which increases nutritional needs. Reflective of these factors and poor nutritional counseling, there are many studies showing vitamin and mineral deficiency in athletes.[56,57,58,59,60,61,62,63,64,65,66] In one study, athletes were found to be deficient in vitamins E, B1, and B6, despite *higher* intake of these vitamins than among control subjects – and even one month of supplementation did not entirely remedy the problem.[67]

Moreover, before a nutrient deficiency deepens to the point of causing overt symptoms, marginal subclinical deficiency can impair athletic performance.[68,69,70,71] The upshot is that athletes who are training hard while on a reduced diet are virtually assured of nutritional deficits unless they undertake vigorous dietary supplementation. Unfortunately, although supplement use is higher among athletes than the general population,[72] most supplementation regimens are unbalanced – favoring the latest overhyped pseudo-nutrient rather than augmenting the full spectrum of nutrients that interact synergistically to enhance health, performance, and physique. Indeed, the "racer's edge" can sometimes be found in pill form when all other training variables are optimized, but not in the worthless pills many athletes are swallowing by the dearly expensive handful.

What is worse, when all else fails, which often happens, the athlete (especially wrestlers, boxers, and bodybuilders) resorts to dehydration to make weight. This eleventh-hour tactic can cause electrolyte imbalance and other problems that undercut performance and endanger health. Whereas an advantage can, in some cases, be gained by hydrating before competition (prehydrating), dehydrating prior to competition places the athlete in a compromised condition at the outset. Once competition begins, depending on exercise intensity and ambient conditions (i.e., temperature, humidity, and wind speed) water loss can range up to 3 liters per hour;[73] and few athletes drink nearly enough water during competition to offset this loss. As the athlete becomes more severely dehydrated, he or she increasingly incurs physiological consequences adverse to performance and perilous to health.

Water lost through sweating derives from all parts of the body, including the blood.[74] Reduced plasma volume increases cardiovascular strain by forcing the heart to work harder.[75,76] This added cardiac burden places the athlete at a decided disadvantage, with studies showing significant decrements in strength and endurance even at modest levels of dehydration.[77,78,79] Furthermore, fluid loss reduces the body's ability to dissipate heat, thus allowing body temperature to rise dangerously.[80,81,82] As thermoregulatory efficiency deteriorates, and core body temperature rises, the risk of heat-related disorders, including life-threatening heat stroke, escalates. Yearly heat-related deaths among high school and college wrestlers and during spring and summer football practice provide tragic testimony of the dangers of exercising in a dehydrated state. Idiot coaches who encourage dehydration tactics or withhold water from players practicing in full pads in summer heat should be shot (or at least fired).

When diuretics (which operate by tampering with the hormones that govern fluid/electrolyte balance) are added to the equation, the risks to performance and health are compounded. Diuretics cause excretion of water and upset electrolyte balance.[83,84,85] Electrolyte imbalance, in turn, can hamper neuromuscular function[86,87,88] and disrupt cardiac rhythm.[89,90,91] It is for these reasons that diuretics are death to performance - and sometimes death to the athlete as well.

Nevertheless, use of diuretics is not uncommon among athletes. Even athletes who are aware of the risks occasionally use them anyway in desperation, reasoning that if they do not make weight they will be disqualified from competing, and the risk of sub-par performance is preferable to the guarantee of no performance. Viewed in light of this dilemma, diuretic use, general dehydration tactics, and restrictive dietary practices can be seen as efforts to compensate for shortcomings in diet and training. By obviating the need for these measures, you can capture an advantage over less-wisely-prepared competitors.

The pre-competition, self-defeating phenomenon is illustrated most strikingly by bodybuilders who "bulk-up" most of the year and then use a low-fat, calorie-restrictive diet, often coupled with a large volume of aerobic exercise, to "cut-up" for a contest. Any bodybuilder who has employed this methodology can testify to the prolonged physical and psychological torture that the cut-up phase entails. What is worse, most, if not all, of the hard-earned muscle gained during the bulk-up phase is lost during the cut-up phase. When all is said and done, the bodybuilder is lucky to have made any net gain for months of effort and self-sacrifice. As you might suspect, diuretic use is particularly common among bodybuilders - and so are post-contest hospitalizations.

The NHE Eating Plan puts a halt to the insanity of having to drop a large amount of weight and/or fat leading up to a competition by allowing you to gain muscle while staying relatively lean, and then reduce bodyfat without losing muscle. In this way, the Eating Plan keeps you "within striking distance" of any contest or competition year-round, making it much easier and less taxing to drop the few extra pounds of fat. This allows you to come into the event on a physical and psychological high, rather than being drained, flat, and weak. It also enables you to make steady progress year to year, and competition to competition, without having to resort to drastic and counterproductive measures to shed bodyfat prior to the contest.

Promoting Health

Avoiding the Health Problems Associated with Conventional Dieting
(While Enjoying the Health Benefits of the NHE Eating Plan)

It seems like each day we hear more about the health problems associated with conventional dieting. Chronically elevated insulin levels, fostered by a diet high in carbohydrate, is a decidedly unhealthy condition and has been implicated in the development and progression of several deadly diseases (see Chapters 8 and 10). Weight cycling (also known as "yo-yo dieting") is suspected of exacerbating metabolic and cardiovascular risk factors for obesity and heart disease.[92,93,94,95] And the safety and net health effects of the unbalanced, extremely low-carbohydrate "ketogenic" diet has long been a subject of intense debate. Where does this leave you? The NHE Eating Plan. . .

- Promotes optimal insulin levels,

- Emphasizes consumption of "good" fat (see Chapter 18),

- Offers a practical, livable plan for a lifetime (thereby protecting you from the psychological and physiological disadvantages of yo-yo dieting),

- Emphasizes consumption of fruits and vegetables within prescribed carbohydrate limits (and fruits and vegetables are strongly associated with reduced risk of cardiovascular disease and cancer),

- Increases potassium intake (vital to growth hormone production*); and decreases intake of unhealthy trans fat by limiting consumption of processed carbohydrate foods, which tend to be virtually devoid of potassium and high in sodium and trans fat,

- Enhances production of "good" hormones like growth hormone, testosterone, IGF-1, and "series 1" eicosanoids; and suppresses "bad" hormones like cortisol and "series 2" eicosanoids.

---

* Medical science has known for quite some time that even modest potassium deficiency can inhibit growth.[95] Recently, though, researchers discovered that this effect is hormonally mediated. Specifically, potassium deficiency has been found to cause growth hormone and IGF-1 suppression.[95b,95c] Although this finding has not received much attention, I believe that it bears profound implications in light of the vast reduction in the mineral content of the food supply caused by food processing and soil degradation.

Of all the alterations that have occurred in the nutritional profile of the human diet since the advent of food processing, the change in the sodium/potassium ratio is among the most dramatic. The diet of Paleolithic man and woman is estimated to have contained 16 times more potassium than sodium[95d] (this makes sense given that unprocessed meat and plant foods contain between 10-20 times as much potassium as sodium). In stark contrast, most refined carbohydrate-/sugar-based foods, the cornerstone of the American diet, contain substantially more sodium than potassium. The radical reversal of the sodium/potassium ratio is likely a significant factor in the differences in the physique and health status of the "ancient warriors" (see Chapter 5) as compared with modern man and woman.

Subduing Cravings
The Psychological Edge

The NHE Eating Plan has a psychological edge over conventional diets, which *put you* psychologically on edge. Conventional diets by their nature are psychologically brutal. What other human endeavor necessitates such a constant application of restraint and willpower in an effort that will almost surely come to failure? Even for those people who are discerning enough to realize the ultimate hopelessness of their struggle, when failure does befall them, it is not any easier to accept. Oftentimes, just the word "diet" is enough to send people running to the refrigerator for a pacifying mouthful of whatever it is they are not supposed to eat.

When you read about "hormonal hunger" (below), you will see that food cravings are a much more subtle and deeply rooted phenomenon than you might imagine. With most diets, cravings are as inevitable as the sunrise, which places the dieter in an impossible situation: either endure the torment and be unhappy, or indulge the craving in which case it's bye-bye diet. No one likes to fail. In fact, psychologists will tell you that along with loss, failure is one of the more difficult events for people to handle. Well, with the NHE Eating Plan you won't experience failure, but you will experience loss - of bodyfat - so prepare yourself.

Later, you will learn the reasons for the mood swings and erratic energy levels associated with hormonally incorrect eating. Conventional diets are hormonally incorrect; so combine mood swings and yo-yo energy levels with the anxiety, stress, and deprivation of dieting and you have the makings of real misery. But this is not the case with the NHE Eating Plan. Unlike restrictive diets, the Eating Plan does not entail monastic austerity, and you are not asked to play the role of a constantly sacrificing martyr.

The NHE Eating Plan is the most flexible dietary plan you have ever encountered. Knowing that no food is absolutely restricted, but must be appropriately cycled into your diet, will have a psychologically soothing effect as you won't feel pressured, tested, or imposed upon. Equally important, the Eating Plan eradicates the physiological/chemical basis of cravings.

Real Hunger vs. Hormonal Hunger:
A Critical Distinction

Our biological drives are several million years older than our intelligence.
Arthur E. Morgan

In trying to adhere to any type of dietary plan, the enemy is hunger/cravings. (It may be helpful to think of "hunger" as a general craving for food, and "craving" as hunger for a particular kind of food.) Giving-in to hunger/cravings does not mean that you are weak; they are immensely powerful biological drives.

97

Willpower has limits, but there are no limits to hunger and cravings. Conventional dieting puts willpower and appetite on a collision course. Unfortunately, this is a case of the irresistible force against the movable object: willpower weakens as the fight wears on, but hunger and cravings become stronger and stronger.

The NHE Eating Plan is an eating-intensive program in which food is utilized to help you burn fat. If eating your way to a lean, fit body strikes you as an oxymoron, it is because, like most people trying to lose fat, you harbor a negative conception of eating. The reasoning underlying the average dieter's mindset goes something like this:

- food contains calories,
- calories make people fat,
- therefore, eating is essentially bad because it is the activity whereby calories enter the body.

This type of thinking is a means to an end: *a dead end.* To change your body, you must first change your mind - about eating. The reality of the matter is this:

- every meal/snack generates a hormonal response,
- some meals/snacks put you in a beneficial, fat-burning state whereas others put you in a detrimental, fat-storing state,
- therefore, eating can be either good or bad depending on the hormonal response it generates.

Once you master the technology of eating for optimal hormonal response, your attitude toward eating will change completely. You will not want to miss a meal, because you will view eating as an opportunity to crank-up fat-burning and muscle-enhancing hormones. Each meal will take you a step forward toward building the body of your dreams.

Because most people trying to lose fat conceive of eating as a necessary evil, they do not eat unless they are hungry. This is a very self-defeating practice. Waiting until you are hungry before eating is like waiting until you are drunk before driving. In the same way that alcohol impairs your judgment at the wheel, hunger and cravings impair your judgment at the dinner table. You cannot make sound eating decisions when you are eating under the influence of hunger or cravings.

Appetite flare-ups stem from either of two sources: "real hunger" or "hormonal hunger."

Real Hunger

Real hunger is the body's response to a food shortage. The human body - a highly evolved, finely tuned, survival machine - is very sensitive to reductions in food supply. When you go several hours during the day without eating, your body (specifically your hypothalamus) responds swiftly and decisively by taking two self-preservation measures, both of which work against your fat loss efforts: 1) it slows your metabolism to conserve energy 2) it puts you in a state of physical discomfort and passionate desire for food called "hunger".

The key to defeating real hunger is simple: don't wait for hunger to strike, strike first by eating before you become hungry. But to eliminate hormonal hunger, you must know *what* to eat. With the NHE Eating Plan, your eating habits will control hunger rather than hunger controlling your eating habits.

Hormonal Hunger

Hormonal hunger results from widely fluctuating insulin levels, and is responsible for the intense hunger pangs and wild, irrational cravings that can overwhelm even the most determined dieter. Insulin naturally ebbs and flows in dynamic tension with glucagon. This dynamic tension is maintained as long as insulin levels remain relatively stable, which was not an issue for most of human existence. However, as explained in Chapter 5, the diet consumed by civilized societies in the modern era is a drastic departure from the diet on which humanity evolved over millions of years.

From the standpoint of evolutionary adaptation, the high-density carbohydrate foods introduced into the human diet by the food processing revolution in the late 19th century are foreign to our metabolism. These foods, especially when consumed in high quantities (as prescribed by the high-carbohydrate diet), induce an aggressive insulin response and a consequent insulin/glucagon imbalance. Furthermore, to the extent that refined carbohydrate displaces protein (recall from Chapter 10 that protein stimulates glucagon release), insulin/glucagon imbalance is exacerbated. Under these dietary conditions, there is no longer dynamic tension between insulin and glucagon, but rather polar dissociation. Instead of yinging and yanging in smooth cooperation these two hormonal regulators begin clinging and clanging – and this turns your hormonal symphony into a cacophony.

When the metabolic control imposed by insulin and glucagon becomes disrupted, blood sugar and the neurotransmitter serotonin go haywire. Unnatural alterations in these two parameters - blood sugar and serotonin - conspire to produce the syndrome I call "hormonal hunger." While carbohydrate craving is the hallmark symptom of hormonal hunger, irregularities in mood, mental outlook, and energy levels, too, are associated with hormonal imbalance; and they can reduce productivity and quality of life.

Hormonal hunger is insidious because, in addition to causing carbohydrate cravings, it, unlike real hunger, has nothing to do with a real need for food. Because of these two factors: 1) overpowering cravings for the kind of food that perpetuates the problem 2) which corrupt hypothalamic food-intake regulation to the extent that you wind-up consuming an excessive amount of 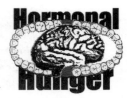 calories; **you must subdue hormonal hunger to have any reasonable hope of succeeding at any fat-loss diet**. Unfortunately, most conventional diets *activate* hormonal hunger. The high-carbohydrate/low-fat diet is a classic example, explaining why for the vast majority of people the low-fat diet is an uphill struggle leading to failure.

Have you ever noticed that sometimes you are hungrier around lunchtime on days when you ate breakfast than on days when you did not? And sometimes you are hungry a few hours after eating, whereas other times you are not hungry even 6 or 7 hours after eating? If you pay attention to these things, you may have wondered why there is not the correlation one would expect between food consumption and appetite. The confounding factor - the joker in the deck, so to speak - is hormonal hunger.

Two 1999 studies, published in the *International Journal of Obesity Related Metabolic Disorders*[96] and *Appetite*[97] illustrate how meal distribution and insulin levels influence food intake. In these studies (the former using obese individuals and the latter using lean individuals as subjects, both yielding virtually identical results), the subjects were fed equivalent caloric-content/macronutrient-composition meals either as one large breakfast or divided into five equal portions served hourly. Result: insulin levels rose higher and fluctuated more widely in response to the single-meal regimen, and the single-meal subjects consumed approximately 25% more food at a subsequent "eat-all-you-want" meal. Meal distribution, through its influence on insulin levels, also affects cholesterol and triglyceride levels, fat burning/storage, and muscle growth/degradation (see Chapter 17).

These two studies are reinforced by another 1999 study, published in *Pediatrics*, demonstrating hormonal hunger. In the *Pediatrics*[98] experiment, using obese teenagers as subjects, the researchers observed an 81% difference in food intake within five hours of a calorie-controlled meal, correlating directly with the magnitude of the insulin response generated by the meal. All three of these studies support the remarkable proposition that lies at the heart of my hormonal hunger theory: **in the short term, appetite is governed chiefly by insulin fluctuations not caloric intake**. (Remember, though, that meal size exerts an influence secondary to meal composition on insulin response - see Chapter 10).

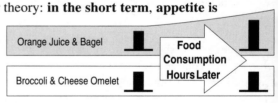

When Blood Sugar Goes South

The problem - hormonal hunger - begins when insulin levels are catapulted skyward by a hormonally incorrect meal. The primary function of insulin is to transport sugar out of the bloodstream and into the cells of the body. A meal high in refined carbohydrate produces a blood sugar spike, which in turn, prompts insulin levels to escalate rapidly.

Like all biological parameters, insulin function spans a continuum of genetic variability.[99] Individuals predisposed to Type II diabetes exhibit a particularly disordered insulin response to a rapid blood sugar elevation. In these individuals, there is some degree of "overreaction" by insulin. Even those individuals who do not have this unlucky genetic draw can develop the condition from years of consuming a diet high in refined carbohydrate.[100,101,102,103,104] This is called insulin resistance, which means the

100

cellular receptors become "less receptive," or desensitized, to insulin and therefore more insulin from the pancreas is required to do the job.[105] As insulin resistance worsens, so does the imbalance between insulin and glucagon. Saturated fat, although largely unproblematic when insulin levels are low (see Chapter 8), aggravates insulin resistance when consumed in the context of a diet high in refined carbohydrate.[106,107,108]

Insulin resistance is strongly correlated with obesity (particularly abdominal obesity),[109,110,111,112,113,114] and cardiovascular disease (see Chapter 8), and is the first step toward adult-onset diabetes.[115,116,117,118,119] Even where insulin resistance is not present, a sharp insulin escalation triggers several unfavorable events. In addition to encouraging fat storage, an insulin surge forces blood sugar down too low, while locking you into a sugar-burning state.

When blood sugar plummets, the body is faced with the "sugar-burner-deprived-of-sugar" predicament that I described on p. 78. In this scenario, the blood sugar derived from the last meal has been chased from the bloodstream by the stiff dose of insulin that came rushing forth from the pancreas in response to a high-carbohydrate meal or an overly large mixed meal. Insulin, however, has a longer "half-life" than blood sugar, which means it lingers in your bloodstream for a longer period of time - and herein lies the problem.

In addition to being lipogenic, insulin exerts an anti-lipolytic effect (see "The Pre-Workout Meal," in Chapter 21), which means it blocks fat burning and directs the body to use sugar for energy instead. So insulin remains in circulation after its purpose, to lower blood sugar, has been accomplished; and all this time insulin limits access to fat stores. The other fuel source, glucose, is not readily available either, because insulin escorted it out of the bloodstream. At this point, the sugar-burner is likely to experience unpleasant symptoms including any or a combination of the following: anxiety, bad mood, light-headedness, poor concentration, cognitive impairment, or "tense tiredness." Starving for sugar, the brain sends a resounding message to the body: EAT - *hormonal hunger has struck.*[120,121,123,124,125,126,127,128]

Hormonal hunger manifests itself as a craving for cookies, cake, candy, french fries, or any other high-sugar/high-starch food (note that these foods can also be very high in fat). What is more, under the influence of these intense cravings you are likely to overeat carbohydrates, causing insulin to soar and restarting the whole vicious cycle. In this way, and helped along by the infinite assortment of refined-carbohydrate-laden foods that have become a part of American culture, many people go through their entire life yanked from pillar to post by hormonal hunger and the cravings it produces. *They may never realize that what they perceive to be hunger is really a symptom of hormonal imbalance, and has nothing to do with a real need for calories or nutrients.*
Hence, when a sugar-burner-deprived-of-sugar reaches for a carbohydrate snack it has as much to do with hunger as an alcoholic reaching for a bottle of liquor has to do with thirst.

Serotonin Confusion: That Which Goes Up Must Come Down

There is another dimension to hormonal hunger. This one relates to the effect of insulin on the neurotransmitter serotonin. A rise in insulin prompts a temporary increase in the rate at which serotonin is synthesized in the brain. Among the several noteworthy effects of serotonin is its effect on appetite: it promotes a feeling of satiety.[129,130]

Insulin increases serotonin levels by increasing the amount of the amino acid tryptophan, a precursor to serotonin, that enters the brain.[131,132] The inescapable conclusion would appear to be that eating foods like chicken, rich in tryptophan, would increase tryptophan levels in your brain. But that elusive thing called truth has an annoying habit of escaping from the inescapable. The fact is that a protein-rich meal limits tryptophan passage into the brain.[133,134]

The reason for this paradox stems from the fact that tryptophan competes with five other amino acids for attachment to a single species of carrier molecule responsible for facilitating passage across the blood-brain barrier.[135,136] Furthermore, the five other "large neutral" amino acids (tyrosine, phenylalanine, leucine, isoleucine, and valine) are more plentiful in most protein foods. A protein-rich meal, therefore, reduces the ratio of tryptophan to the competing amino acids in the bloodstream.

A carbohydrate-rich meal has the opposite effect, causing a relative elevation in serum tryptophan and, consequently, raising brain serotonin levels. One reason for this is that after a carbohydrate meal there are fewer competing amino acids in the bloodstream than after a protein meal. Additionally, insulin shuttles amino acids into the cells of the body. Tryptophan, though, because it circulates bound to the plasma protein *albumin,* is resistant to the effect of insulin.[137,138] Thus, when insulin is secreted in response to a carbohydrate-rich meal, the freely circulating large neutral aminos get pulled into the cells, but tryptophan remains in the bloodstream. With competition eliminated, tryptophan wins by default and is able to cross the blood-brain barrier in high concentration.

The fact that insulin increases serotonin and serotonin decreases appetite seems to point to the conclusion that you should raise insulin levels. In fact, there are several popular diet books that recommend consuming a high-carbohydrate diet based on this reasoning. Unfortunately, once again, as is the case with the calorie restriction theory, the fat makes you fat theory, and so many other fat loss ideas, this one looks good on paper but does not work in practice. The problem here is something you learned prior to your first birthday: that which goes up, must come down.

You can raise baseline serotonin levels through sound nutrition, exposure to sunlight, and hormonally-intelligent exercise, but if you send serotonin soaring by creating a hormonal imbalance - look out below. Like blood sugar, serotonin rises sharply in response to a carbohydrate-rich meal and then falls. The research in this area is ongoing, but it appears that the relative drop in serotonin provokes carbohydrate cravings[139,140,141,142] and mood irregularities.[143,144,145,146] Thus, if you frequently launch serotonin with high-

102

carbohydrate meals, serotonin will frequently be on a decline and your brain will activate carbohydrate cravings in order to re-boost serotonin to unnaturally high levels. You can see that this has the features of an addiction, and I think "addiction" is an apt description for this phenomenon.

Can a High-Carbohydrate Diet Lead to Serotonin Depletion?

Whereas a protein meal supplies the raw materials to make neurotransmitters, a carbohydrate meal does not. Rather, a high-carbohydrate meal artificially boosts serotonin by means of inducing a temporary hormonal imbalance that forces a disproportionate amount of tryptophan into the brain. This raises the question whether chronic high-carbohydrate, low-protein eating can, over time, reduce serotonin levels. It is indisputable that a diet high in refined carbohydrates is unnatural from an evolutionary perspective (see Chapter 5), and that a meal rich in refined carbohydrates profoundly impacts upon brain chemistry. I suspect that chronic high-refined-carbohydrate eating does, indeed, have a long-term adverse effect on brain function by means of impairing serotonin synthesis.

Investigation of my hypothesis is warranted in light of its explosive implications. For one, *might the prevailing high-carbohydrate/low-fat/low-protein dietary prescription, by causing serotonin depletion, be partly responsible for the exceedingly high incidence of depression and other psychological and emotional disorders in the United States?* We know that serotonin plays a role in many types of depression[147,148,149] as well as other emotional disorders;[150] and we know that tryptophan deficiency can cause depression.[151,152,153] Secondly, *might diet-induced serotonin depletion be instrumental in the high incidence of obesity in the United States?* We know that obese individuals exhibit a markedly lower rate of serotonin synthesis;[154,155] and we know that low serotonin can cause carbohydrate cravings (see above), which, in turn, promotes obesity. We also know that both lean and obese carbohydrate cravers (who presumably consume more carbohydrate than non-cravers) have lower baseline levels of serotonin.[156] The circumstantial evidence is strong and the logic compelling. I hope to see some studies directed at my hypothesis - and soon.

When serotonin is moderately high and in balance with other neurotransmitters, you feel relaxed, composed, and clear-headed. But when serotonin is sky-high and your neurotransmitter balance is upset, which is the typical neurochemical aftermath of a carbohydrate-rich meal, you tend to feel drowsy, lethargic, and mentally fuzzy (see Chapter 10) - not a mindset associated with success or productivity. The ensuing drop in serotonin hours after a carbohydrate-rich meal coupled with a hypoglycemic-induced surge in norepinephrine[157,158,159,160] causes a neurotransmitter imbalance of the opposite nature, with norepinephrine too high relative to serotonin. This can produce anxiety, irritability, and depression.

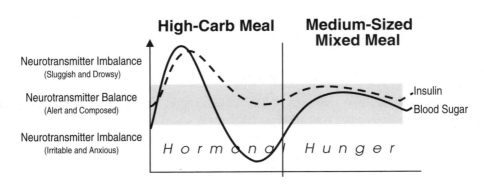

Natural Hormonal Enhancement

It has long been observed that people tend to reach for sweets when they are upset or anxious. We now understand from studies of P.M.S.[161,162] and seasonal affective disorder[163,164] that the craving is not so much for the sweet food itself, but rather for the tranquilizing serotonin-boost elicited by eating the food. (Although many people do not have conscious knowledge of the carbohydrate/serotonin connection, subconsciously they know from a lifetime of conditioned response that a sweet snack will make them feel better.) But it is often low serotonin that makes them upset or anxious to begin with; and, as explained above, carbohydrate-induced serotonin peaks can lead to a temporary, and possibly chronic, reduction in serotonin levels. Therefore, the school of thought that recommends medicating food cravings, or depression, by eating carbohydrate-laden foods is merely perpetuating a vicious cycle that makes both conditions worse.

As you can see, hormonal hunger is a condition with chemical, psychological, and physiological roots. Specifically, hormonal hunger results from neurotransmitter disturbances and exaggerated blood sugar fluctuations. Both of these problems are of hormonal origin, caused by excessive insulin, which in turn is a direct result of what and how much you eat.

References

1. Weltman A, et al. Relationship between Age, Percentage Body Fat, Fitness, and 24-Hour Growth Hormone Release in Healthy Young Adults: Effects of Gender. *J Clin Endocrinol Metab* 1994;78:543.

2. Iranmanesh A, Lizarralde G, Veldhuis JD. Age and Relative Adiposity are Specific Negative Determinants of the Frequency and Amplitude of Growth Hormone (GH) Secretory Bursts and the Half-Life of Endogenous GH in Healthy Men. *J Clin Endocrinol Metab* 1991;73:1081

3. Veldhuis JD, et al. Dual Defects in Pulsatile Growth Hormone Secretion and Clearance Subserve the Hyposomatotropism of Obesity in Man. *J Clin Endocrinol Metab* 1991;72:51.

4. Vahl N, et al. Abdominal Adiposity and Physical Fitness are Major Determinants of the Age Associated Decline in Stimulated GH Secretion in Healthy Adults. *J Clin Endocrinol Metab* 1996;81:2209.

5. Vahl N, et al. Abdominal Adiposity Rather than Age and Sex Predicts Mass and Regularity of GH Secretion in Healthy Adults. *Am J Physiol* 1997;272:E1108.

6. Veldhuis JD, Iranmanesh A. Physiological Regulation of the Human Growth Hormone (GH)-Insulin-Like Growth Factor Type I (IGF-I) Axis: Predominant Impact of Age, Obesity, Gonadal Function, and Sleep. *Sleep* 1996;19(Suppl):S221.

7. See, supra, notes 4 and 5.

8. Tsalikian E, et al. Increased Leucine Flux in Short-Term Fasted Human Subjects: Evidence for Increased Proteolysis. *Am J Physiol* 1984;247:E323.

9. Frizzell RT, et al. Role of Gluconeogenesis in Sustaining Glucose Production during Hypoglycemia Caused by Continuous Insulin Infusion in Conscious Dogs. *Diabetes* 1988;37:749.

10. Jungas RL, Halperin ML, Brosnan JT. Quantitative Analysis of Amino Acid Oxidation and Related Gluconeogenesis in Humans. *Physiol Rev* 1992;72:419.

11. Smith SR, Bledsoe T, Chetri MK. Cortisol Metabolism and the Pituitary-Adrenal Axis in Adults with Protein-Calorie Malnutrition. *J Clin Endocrinol Metab* 1975;40:43.

12. Bergendahl M, et al. Fasting as a Metabolic Stress Paradigm Selectively Amplifies Cortisol Secretory Burst Mass and Delays the Time of Maximal Nyctohemeral Cortisol Concentrations in Healthy Men. *J Clin Endocrinol Metab* 1996;81:692.

13. Griffin JE, Ojeda SR, eds. *Textbook of Endocrine Physiology*. NY: Oxford University Press 1988, p. 214.

14. Gold PW, et al. Abnormal Hypothalmic-Pituitary-Adrenal Function in Anorexia Nervosa. Pathophysiologic Mechanisms in Underweight and Weight-Corrected Patients. *N Engl J Med* 1986;314:1335.

15. Casper RC, Chatterton RT Jr, Davis JM. Alterations in Serum Cortisol and its Binding Characteristics in Anorexia Nervosa. *J Clin Endocrinol Metab* 1979;49:406.

16. Campbell RM, Scanes CG. Inhibition of Growth Hormone-Stimulated Lipolysis by Somatostatin, Insulin, and Insulin-Like Growth Factors (Somatomedins) In Vitro. *Proc Soc Exp Biol Med* 1988;189:362.

17. Gerich JE, et al. Effects of Physiologic Levels of Glucagon and Growth Hormone on Human Carbohydrate and Lipid Metabolism. Studies Involving Administration of Exogenous Hormone during Suppression of Endogenous Hormone Secretion with Somatostatin. *J Clin Invest* 1976;57:875.

18. Houston B, O'Neill IE. Insulin and Growth Hormone Act Synergistically to Stimulate Insulin-Like Growth Factor-I Production by Cultured Chicken Hepatocytes. *J Endocrinol* 1991;128:389.

19. Johnson TR, et al. Expression of Insulin-Like Growth Factor I in Cultured Rat Hepatocytes: Effects of Insulin and Growth Hormone. *Mol Endocrinol* 1989;3:580.

20. Boni-Schnetzler M, et al. Insulin Regulates Insulin-Like Growth Factor I mRNA in Rat Hepatocytes. *Am J Physiol* 1991;260:E846.

21. Milman AE, DeMoor P, Lukens FDW. Relation of Purified Pituitary Growth Hormone and Insulin in Regulation of Nitrogen Balance. *Am J Physiol* 1951;166:354.

22. Griffin JE, Ojeda SR, eds. *Textbook of Endocrine Physiology.* NY: Oxford University Press 1988, p. 214.

23. Mathews LS, Norstedt G, Palmiter RD. Regulation of Insulin-Like Growth Factor I Gene Expression by Growth Hormone. *Proc Natl Acad Sci U S A* 1986;83:9343.

24. Bichell DP, Kikuchi K, Rotwein P. Growth Hormone Rapidly Activates Insulin-Like Growth Factor I Gene Transcription In Vivo. *Mol Endocrinol* 1992;6:1899.

25. Furlanetto RW. Insulin-Like Growth Factor Measurements in the Evaluation of Growth Hormone Secretion. *Horm Res* 1990;33 (Suppl):25S.

26. Scheiwiller E, et al. Growth Restoration of Insulin-Deficient Diabetic Rats by Recombinant Human Insulin-Like Growth Factor I. *Nature* 1986;323:169.

27. Wheelhouse NM, et al. Growth Hormone and Amino Acid Supply Interact Synergistically to Control Insulin-Like Growth Factor-I Production and Gene Expression in Cultured Ovine Hepatocytes. *J Endocrinol* 1999;163:353.

28. Thissen JP, et al. Evidence that Pretranslational and Translational Defects Decrease Serum Insulin-Like Growth Factor-I Concentrations during Dietary Protein Restriction. *Endocrinology* 1991;129:429.

29. Maiter D, et al. Dietary Protein Restriction Decreases Insulin-Like Growth Factor I Independent of Insulin and Liver Growth Hormone Binding. *Endocrinology* 1989;124:2604.

30. Davis SN, et al. Role of Cortisol in the Pathogenesis of Deficient Counterregulation after Antecedent Hypoglycemia in Normal Humans. *J Clin Invest* 1996;98:680.

31. Carnes M, et al. Pulsatile ACTH and Cortisol in Goats: Effects of Insulin-Induced Hypoglycemia and Dexamethasone. *Neuroendocrinology* 1992;55:97.

32. Lins PE, et al. The Role of Glucagon, Catecholamines and Cortisol in Counterregulation of Insulin-Induced Hypoglycemia in Normal Man. *Acta Med Scand* 1986;220:39.

33. Lecavalier L, Bolli G, Gerich J. Glucagon-Cortisol Interactions on Glucose Turnover and Lactate Gluconeogenesis in Normal Humans. *Am J Physiol* 1990;258:E569.

34. De Feo P, et al. Contribution of Cortisol to Glucose Counterregulation in Humans. *Am J Physiol* 1989;257:E35.

35. Hasselgren PO. Glucocorticoids and Muscle Catabolism. *Curr Opin Clin Nutr Metab Care* 1999;2:201.

36. Ferrando AA, et al. Inactivity Amplifies the Catabolic Response of Skeletal Muscle to Cortisol. *J Clin Endocrinol Metab* 1999;84:3515.

37. Darmaun D, Matthews DE, Bier DM. Physiological Hypercortisolemia Increases Proteolysis, Glutamine, and Alanine Production. *Am J Physiol* 1988;255:E366.

38. Simmons PS, et al. Increased Proteolysis. An Effect of Increases in Plasma Cortisol within the Physiologic Range. *J Clin Invest* 1984;73:412.

39. Colgan M. "Cortisol: Grinch of Muscle," *Muscular Development Fitness and Health*, June 1995.

40. Dennison E, et al. Profiles of Endogenous Circulating Cortisol and Bone Mineral Density in Healthy Elderly Men. *J Clin Endocrinol Metab* 1999;84:3058.

41. Raff H, et al. Elevated Salivary Cortisol in the Evening in Healthy Elderly Men and Women: Correlation with Bone Mineral Density. *J Gerontol A Biol Sci Med Sci* 1999;54:M479.

42. Rizza RA, Mandarino LJ, Gerich JE. Cortisol-Induced Insulin Resistance in Man: Impaired Suppression of Glucose Production and Stimulation of Glucose Utilization Due to a Post-Receptor Defect of Insulin Action. *J Clin Endocrinol Metab* 1982;54:131.

43. Rooney DP, et al. The Effect of Cortisol on Glucose/Glucose-6-Phosphate Cycle Activity and Insulin Action. *J Clin Endocrinol Metab* 1993;77:1180.

44. Holmang A, Bjorntorp P. The Effects of Cortisol on Insulin Sensitivity in Muscle. *Acta Physiol Scand* 1992;144:425.

45. Andrews RC, Walker BR. Glucocorticoids and Insulin Resistance: Old Hormones, New Targets. *Clin Sci (Colch)* 1999;96:513.

46. Norbiato G, et al. Glucocorticoids and the Immune Function in the Human Immunodeficiency Virus Infection: A Study in Hypercortisolemic and Cortisol-Resistant Patients. *J Clin Endocrinol Metab* 1997;82:3260.

47. May M, et al. Protection from Glucocorticoid Induced Thymic Involution by Dehydroepiandrosterone. *Life Sci* 1990;46:1627.

48. Nakamura M, Brown J, Miller WC. Glycogen Depletion Patterns in Trained Rats Adapted to a High-Fat or High-Carbohydrate Diet. *Int J Sports Med* 1998;19:419.

49. Saitoh S, et al. Effects of Short-Term Dietary Change from High Fat to High Carbohydrate Diets on the Storage and Utilization of Glycogen and Triacylglycerol in Untrained Rats. *Eur J Appl Physiol* 1996;74:13.

50. Simi B, et al. Additive Effects of Training and High-Fat Diet on Energy Metabolism during Exercise. *J Appl Physiol* 1991;71:197.

51. Rennie MJ, et al. A Sparing Effect of Increased Plasma Fatty Acids on Muscle and Liver Glycogen Content in the Exercising Rat. *Biochem J* 1976;156:647.

52. Schmidt M, et al. Glucocorticoids Induce Apoptosis in Human Monocytes: Potential Role of IL-1 Beta. *J Immunol* 1999;163:3484.

53. Oehling AG, et al. Suppression of the Immune System by Oral Glucocorticoid Therapy in Bronchial Asthma. *Allergy* 1997;52:144.

54. Carbajal A, Nunez C, Moreiras. Energy Intake as a Determinant Factor of Vitamin Status in Healthy Young Women. *Nutr Res* 1996;66:227.

55. van Erp-Baart AM, Saris WM, Binkhorst RA, Vos JA, Elvers JW. Nationwide Survey on Nutritional Habits in Elite Athletes. Part II. Mineral and Vitamin Intake. *Int J Sports Med* 1989;10 (Suppl):S11.

56. Podorozhnyi PG, Kononenko AI. [Vitamin B1, PP and C Allowances of Weight Lifters and their Requirements during Training and Competition Periods]. *Vopr Pitan* 1979;4:27. Russian.

57. Keith RE, et al. Dietary Status of Trained Female Cyclists. *J Am Diet Assoc* 1989;89:1620.

58. Dam BV. Vitamins and Sport. *Br J Sports Med* 1978;12:74.

59. Berning JR, The Nutritional Habits of Young Adolescent Swimmers. *Int J Sport Nutr* 1991;1:240.

60. Faber M, Benade AJ. Mineral and Vitamin Intake in Field Athletes (Discus-, Hammer-, Javelin-Throwers and Shotputters). *Int J Sports Med* 1991;12:324.

61. Moffatt RJ. Dietary Status of Elite Female High School Gymnasts: Inadequacy of Vitamin and Mineral Intake. *J Am Diet Assoc* 1984;84:1361.

62. Bauer S, Jakob E, Berg A, Keul J. [Energy and Nutritional Intake in Young Weight Lifters Before and after Nutritional Counseling]. *Schweiz Z Med Traumatol* 1994;3:35. German.

63. Steen SN, et al. Dietary Intake of Female Collegiate Heavyweight Rowers. *Int J Sport Nutr* 1995;5:225.

64. Sugiura K, Suzuki I, Kobayashi K. Nutritional Intake of Elite Japanese Track-and-Field Athletes. *Int J Sport Nutr* 1999;9:202.

65. Frentsos JA, Baer JT. Increased Energy and Nutrient Intake during Training and Competition Improves Elite Triathletes' Endurance Performance. *Int J Sport Nutr* 1997;7:61.

66. Jonnalagadda SS, Bernadot D, Nelson M. Energy and Nutrient Intakes of the United States National Women's Artistic Gymnastics Team. *Int J Sport Nutr* 1998;8:331.

67. Guilland JC, et al. Vitamin Status of Young Athletes Including the Effects of Supplementation. *Med Sci Sports Exerc* 1989;21:441.

68. van der Beek EJ, et al. Thiamin, Riboflavin and Vitamin B6: Impact of Restricted Intake on Physical Performance in Man. *J Am Coll Nutr* 1994;13:629.

69. Colgan M. *Optimum Sports Nutrition.* NY: Advanced Research Press 1993.

70. van der Beek EJ, et al. Thiamin, Riboflavin, and Vitamins B-6 and C: Impact of Combined Restricted Intake on Functional Performance in Man. *Am J Clin Nutr* 1988;48:1451.

71. Williams MH. Vitamin Supplementation and Athletic Performance. *Int J Vitam Nutr Res Suppl* 1989;30:163.

72. Sobal J, Marquart LF. Vitamin/Mineral Supplement Use among Athletes: A Review of the Literature. *Int J Sport Nutr* 1994;4:320.

73. McArdle WD, Katch FI, Katch VL. *Exercise Physiology.* Baltimore, MD: Williams and Wilkins 1996, p. 508.

74. Nose H, et al. Shift in Body Fluid Compartments after Dehydration in Humans. *J Appl Physiol* 1988;65:318.

75. Coyle EF. Cardiovascular Drift during Prolonged Exercise and the Effects of Dehydration. *Int J Sports Med* 1998;19 (Suppl):S121.

76. Gonzalez-Alonso J, et al. Dehydration Markedly Impairs Cardiovascular Function in Hyperthermic Endurance Athletes during Exercise. *J Appl Physiol* 1997;82:1229.

77. Burge CM, Carey MF, Payne WR. Rowing Performance, Fluid Balance, and Metabolic Function following Dehydration and Rehydration. *Med Sci Sports Exerc* 1993;25:1358.

78. Sawka MN. Physiological Consequences of Hypohydration: Exercise Performance and Thermoregulation. *Med Sci Sports Exerc* 1992;24:657.

79. Sawka MN, et al. Influence of Hydration Level and Body Fluids on Exercise Performance in the Heat. *JAMA* 1984;252:1165.

80. Sawka MN, et al. Hydration Effects on Temperature Regulation. *Int J Sports Med* 1998;19 (Suppl):S108.

81. Sawka MN, et al. Thermoregulatory and Blood Responses during Exercise at Graded Hypohydration Levels. *J Appl Physiol* 1985;59:1394.

82. Candas V, et al. Thermal and Circulatory Responses during Prolonged Exercise at Different Levels of Hydration. *J Physiol (Paris)* 1988;83:11.

83. Armstrong LE, Costill DL, Fink WJ. Influence of Diuretic-Induced Dehydration on Competitive Running Experience. *Med Sci Sports Exerc* 1985;17:456.

84. Mendyka BE. Fluid and Electrolyte Disorders Caused by Diuretic Therapy. *AACN Clin Issues Crit Care Nurs* 1992;3:672.

85. Melby JC. Selected Mechanisms of Diuretic-Induced Electrolyte Changes. *Am J Cardiol* 1986;58:1A.

86. Chhabra A, et al. Neuromuscular Manifestations of Diarrhea Related Hypokalemia. *Indian Pediatr* 1995;32:409.

87. Haralambie G, Senser L, Sierra-Chavez R. Physiological and Metabolic Effects of a 25 Km Race in Female Athletes. *Eur J Appl Physiol* 1981;47:123.

88. Stewart GW. Serum Potassium, Hydrogen Ion and Magnesium: Neuromuscular Regulation by Variation of Cation Concentration in the Extracellular Fluid? *Magnes Res* 1994;7:117.

89. Olsson SB. Nature of Cardiac Arrhythmias and Electrolyte Disturbances. Role of Potassium in Atrial Fibrillation. *Acta Med Scand Suppl* 1981;647:33.

90. Siegel D, et al. Diuretics, Serum and Intracellular Electrolyte Levels, and Ventricular Arrhythmias in Hypertensive Men. *JAMA* 1992;267:1083.

91. Hollifield JW. Potassium and Magnesium Abnormalities: Diuretics and Arrhythmias in Hypertension. *Am J Med* 1984;77:28.

92. Stein LJ. Repeated Weight Fluctuation Increases Plasma Insulin in the Obese Wistar Fatty Diabetic Rat. *Physiol Behav* 1992;52:345.

93. Rodin J, et al. Weight Cycling and Fat Distribution. *Int J Obes* 1990;14:303.

94. Archambault CM, et al. Effects of Weight Cycling in Female Rats. *Physiol Behav* 1989;46:417.

95. Guagnano MT, et al. Weight Fluctuations Could Increase Blood Pressure in Android Obese Women. *Clin Sci (Colch)* 1999;96:677.

95a. Dorup I, Clausen T. Effects of Potassium Deficiency on Growth and Protein Synthesis in Skeletal Muscle and the Heart. *Brit J Nutr* 1970;24:205.

95b. Flyvbjerg A, et al. Evidence that Potassium Deficiency Induces Growth Retardation through Reduced Circulating Levels of Growth Hormone and Insulin-Like Growth Factor I. *Metabolism* 1991;40:769.

95c. Hochberg Z, et al. Growth Hormone (GH) Receptor and GH-Binding Protein Deficiency in the Growth Failure of Potassium-Depleted Rats. *J Endocrinol* 1995;147:253.

95d. Eaton S, Konner M. Paleolithic Nutrition. *N Engl J Med* 1985;312:283.

96. Speechly DP, Rogers GG, Buffenstein R. Acute Appetite Reduction Associated with an Increased Frequency of Eating in Obese Males. *Int J Obes Relat Metab Disord* 1999;23:1151.

97. Speechly DP, Buffenstein R. Greater Appetite Control Associated with an Increased Frequency of Eating in Lean Males. *Appetite* 1999;33:285.

98. Ludwig DS, et al. High Glycemic Index Foods, Overeating, and Obesity. *Pediatrics* 1999;103:E26.

99. Hollenbeck C, Reaven GM. Variations in Insulin-Stimulated Glucose Uptake in Healthy Individuals with Normal Glucose Tolerance. *J Clin Endocrinol Metab* 1987;64:1169.

100. Barnard RJ, et al. Diet-Induced Insulin Resistance Precedes other Aspects of the Metabolic Syndrome. *J Appl Physiol* 1998;84:1311.

101. Barnard RJ, Youngren JF, Martin DA. Diet, Not Aging, Causes Skeletal Muscle Insulin Resistance. *Gerontology* 1995;41:205.

102. Grimditch GK, et al. Peripheral Insulin Sensitivity as Modified by Diet and Exercise Training. *Am J Clin Nutr* 1988;48:38.

103. Kim JY, et al. Insulin Resistance of Muscle Glucose Transport in Male and Female Rats Fed a High-Sucrose Diet. *Am J Physiol* 1999;276:R665.

104. Marangou AG, et al. Metabolic Consequences of Prolonged Hyperinsulinemia in Humans. Evidence for Induction of Insulin Insensitivity. *Diabetes* 1986;35:1383.

105. Olefsky JM, Kolterman OG. Mechanisms of Insulin Resistance in Obesity and Noninsulin-Dependent (Type II) Diabetes. *Am J Med* 1981;70:151.

106. Maron DJ, Fair JM, Haskell WL. Saturated Fat Intake and Insulin Resistance in Men with Coronary Artery Disease. The Stanford Coronary Risk Intervention Project Investigators and Staff. *Circulation* 1991;84:2020.

107. Parker DR, et al. Relationship of Dietary Saturated Fatty Acids and Body Habitus to Serum Insulin Concentrations: The Normative Aging Study. *Am J Clin Nutr* 1993;58:129.

108. Folsom AR, et al. Relation between Plasma Phospholipid Saturated Fatty Acids and Hyperinsulinemia. *Metabolism* 1996;45:223.

109. Lockwood DH. Insulin Resistance in Obesity. *Hosp Pract* 1976;11:79.

110. Kelley DE, et al. Skeletal Muscle Fatty Acid Metabolism in Association with Insulin Resistance, Obesity, and Weight Loss. *Am J Physiol* 1999;277:E1130.

111. Karter AJ, et al. Insulin Sensitivity and Abdominal Obesity in African-American, Hispanic, and Non-Hispanic White Men and Women. The Insulin Resistance and Atherosclerosis Study. *Diabetes* 1996;45:1547.

112. Despres JP. Abdominal Obesity as Important Component of Insulin-Resistance Syndrome. *Nutrition* 1993;9:452.

113. Pedersen SB, et al. Abdominal Obesity is Associated with Insulin Resistance and Reduced Glycogen Synthetase Activity in Skeletal Muscle. *Metabolism* 1993;42:998.

114. Lemieux S, et al. Seven-Year Changes in Body Fat and Visceral Adipose Tissue in Women. Association with Indexes of Plasma Glucose-Insulin Homeostasis. *Diabetes Care* 1996;19:983.

115. Haffner SM, Miettinen H. Insulin Resistance Implications for Type II Diabetes Mellitus and Coronary Heart Disease. *Am J Med* 1997;103:152.

116. Zavaroni I, et al. Hyperinsulinemia in a Normal Population as a Predictor of Non-Insulin-Dependent Diabetes Mellitus, Hypertension, and Coronary Heart Disease: The Barilla Factory Revisited. *Metabolism* 1999;48:989.

117. Kekalainen P, et al. Hyperinsulinemia Cluster Predicts the Development of Type 2 Diabetes Independently of Family History of Diabetes. *Diabetes Care* 1999;22:86.

118. Weyer C, et al. The Natural History of Insulin Secretory Dysfunction and Insulin Resistance in the Pathogenesis of Type 2 Diabetes Mellitus. *J Clin Invest* 1999;104:787.

119. Nijpels G. Determinants for the Progression from Impaired Glucose Tolerance to Non-Insulin-Dependent Diabetes Mellitus. *Eur J Clin Invest* 1998;28 (Suppl):8S.

120. Hvidberg A, et al. Impact of Recent Antecedent Hypoglycemia on Hypoglycemic Cognitive Dysfunction in Nondiabetic Humans. *Diabetes* 1996;45:1030.

121. Gold AE, et al. Changes in Mood during Acute Hypoglycemia in Healthy Participants. *J Pers Soc Psychol* 1995;68:498.

122. Blackman JD, et al. Hypoglycemic Thresholds for Cognitive Dysfunction in Humans. *Diabetes* 1990;39:828.

123. Cox DJ, et al. Disruptive Effects of Acute Hypoglycemia on Speed of Cognitive and Motor Performance. *Diabetes Care* 1993;16:1391.

124. McCrimmon RJ, et al. Appraisal of Mood and Personality during Hypoglycaemia in Human Subjects. *Physiol Behav* 1999;67:27.

125. Merbis MA, et al. Hypoglycaemia Induces Emotional Disruption. *Patient Educ Couns* 1996;29:117.

126. Cryer PE. Symptoms of Hypoglycemia, Thresholds for their Occurrence, and Hypoglycemia Unawareness. *Endocrinol Metab Clin North Am* 1999;28:495.

127. Johnson WG, et al. Repeated Binge/Purge Cycles in Bulimia Nervosa: Role of Glucose and Insulin. *Int J Eat Disord* 1994;15:331.

128. Larue-Achagiotis C, Le Magnen J. Feeding Rate and Responses to Food Deprivation as a Function of Fasting-Induced Hypoglycemia. *Behav Neurosci* 1985;99:1176.

129. Edwards S, Stevens R. Peripherally Administered 5-Hydroxytryptamine Elicits the Full Behavioural Sequence of Satiety. *Physiol Behav* 1991;50:1075.

130. Simansky KJ. Serotonergic Control of the Organization of Feeding and Satiety. *Behav Brain Res* 1996;73:37.

131. Lyons PM, Truswell AS. Serotonin Precursor Influenced by Type of Carbohydrate Meal in Healthy Adults. *Am J Clin Nutr* 1988;47:433.

132. Blum I, et al. The Influence of Meal Composition on Plasma Serotonin and Norepinephrine Concentrations. *Metabolism* 1992;41:137.

133. Yokogoshi H, Wurtman RJ. Meal Composition and Plasma Amino Acid Ratios: Effect of Various Proteins or Carbohydrates, and of Various Protein Concentrations. *Metabolism* 1986;35:837.

134. Moller SE. Effect of Various Oral Protein Doses on Plasma Neutral Amino Acid Levels. *J Neural Transm* 1985;61:183.

135. Pratt OE. Kinetics of Tryptophan Transport across the Blood-Brain Barrier. *J Neural Transm Suppl* 1979;15:29.

136. Fernstrom JD. Diet-Induced Changes in Plasma Amino Acid Pattern: Effects on the Brain Uptake of Large Neutral Amino Acids, and on Brain Serotonin Synthesis. *J Neural Transm Suppl* 1979;15:55.

137. Wurtman RJ. Nutrients that Modify Brain Function. In: Wurtman JJ. *The Carbohydrate Craver's Diet.* Boston, MA: Houghton Mifflin Company 1983, p. 233.

138. Pardridge WM. The Role of Blood-Brain Barrier Transport of Tryptophan and other Neutral Amino Acids in the Regulation of Substrate-Limited Pathways of Brain Amino Acid Metabolism. *J Neural Transm Suppl* 1979;15:43.

139. Wurtman JJ. The Involvement of Brain Serotonin in Excessive Carbohydrate Snacking by Obese Carbohydrate Cravers. *J Am Diet Assoc* 1984;84:1004.

140. Wurtman RJ, Wurtman JJ. Carbohydrate Craving, Obesity and Brain Serotonin. *Appetite* 1986;7(Suppl):99.

141. Wurtman RJ, Wurtman JJ. Brain Serotonin, Carbohydrate-Craving, Obesity and Depression. *Obes Res* 1995;3(Suppl):477S.

142. Stallone D, Nicolaidis S. Increased Food Intake and Carbohydrate Preference in the Rat Following Treatment with the Serotonin Antagonist Metergoline. *Neurosci Lett* 1989;102:319.

143. Christensen L. The Effect of Carbohydrates on Affect. *Nutrition* 1997;13:503.

144. Wurtman JJ. Depression and Weight Gain: the Serotonin Connection. *J Affect Disord* 1993;29:183.

145. Wurtman JJ. Carbohydrate Craving. Relationship between Carbohydrate Intake and Disorders of Mood. *Drugs* 1990;39 (Suppl):S49.

146. Wurtman JJ. Carbohydrate Cravings: A Disorder of Food Intake and Mood. *Clin Neuropharmacol* 1988;11(Suppl):S139.

147. Roy A. Suicidal Behavior in Depression: Relationship to Platelet Serotonin Transporter. *Neuropsychobiology* 1999;39:71.

148. Malison RT, et al. Reduced Brain Serotonin Transporter Availability in Major Depression as Measured by [123I]-2 Beta-Carbomethoxy-3 Beta-(4-Iodophenyl)Tropane and Single Photon Emission Computed Tomography. *Biol Psychiatry* 1998;44:1090.

149. Alvarez JC, et al. Decreased Platelet Serotonin Transporter Sites and Increased Platelet Inositol Triphosphate Levels in Patients with Unipolar Depression: Effects of Clomipramine and Fluoxetine. *Clin Pharmacol Ther* 1999;66:617.

150. Moller SE. Serotonin, Carbohydrates, and Atypical Depression. *Pharmacol Toxicol* 1992;71(Suppl):61S.

151. Smith KA, Fairburn CG, Cowen PJ. Relapse of Depression after Rapid Depletion of Tryptophan. *Lancet* 1997;349:915.

152. Delgado PL, et al. Serotonin Function and the Mechanism of Antidepressant Action. Reversal of Antidepressant-Induced Remission by Rapid Depletion of Plasma Tryptophan. *Arch Gen Psychiatry* 1990;47:411.

153. Neumeister A, et al. Effects of Tryptophan Depletion on Drug-Free Patients with Seasonal Affective Disorder During a Stable Response to Bright Light Therapy. *Arch Gen Psychiatry* 1997;54:133.

154. Ashley DV, et al. Evidence for Diminished Brain 5-Hydroxytryptamine Biosynthesis in Obese Diabetic and Non-Diabetic Humans. *Am J Clin Nutr* 1985;42:1240 .

155. Caballero B, Finer N, Wurtman RJ. Plasma Amino Acids and Insulin Levels in Obesity: Response to Carbohydrate Intake and Tryptophan Supplements. *Metabolism* 1988;37:672.

156. Blum H, et al. Food Preferences, Body Weight, and Platelet-Poor Plasma Serotonin and Catecholamines. *Am J Clin Nutr* 1993;57:486.

157. Boyle PJ, Shah SD, Cryer PE. Insulin, Glucagon, and Catecholamines in Prevention of Hypoglycemia during Fasting. *Am J Physiol* 1989;256:E651.

158. Yamaguchi N, Briand R, Brassard M. Direct Evidence that an Increase in Aortic Norepinephrine Level in Response to Insulin-Induced Hypoglycemia is Due to Increased Adrenal Norepinephrine Output. *Can J Physiol Pharmacol* 1989;67:499.

159. Hilsted J, Christensen NJ, Larsen S. Norepinephrine Kinetics during Insulin-Induced Hypoglycemia. *Metabolism* 1985;34:300.

160. Voorhess ML, MacGillivray MH. Low Plasma Norepinephrine Responses to Acute Hypoglycemia in Children with Isolated Growth Hormone Deficiency. *J Clin Endocrinol Metab* 1984;59:790.

161. Wurtman JJ, et al. Effect of Nutrient Intake on Premenstrual Depression. *Am J Obstet Gynecol* 1989;161:1228.

162. Sayegh R, et al. The Effect of a Carbohydrate-Rich Beverage on Mood, Appetite, and Cognitive Function in Women with Premenstrual Syndrome. *Obstet Gynecol* 1995;86:520.

163. Arbisi PA, et al. Seasonal Alteration in Taste Detection and Recognition Threshold in Seasonal Affective Disorder: The Proximate Source of Carbohydrate Craving. *Psychiatry Res* 1996;59:171.

164. Rosenthal NE, et al. Psychobiological Effects of Carbohydrate- and Protein-Rich Meals in Patients with Seasonal Affective Disorder and Normal Controls. *Biol Psychiatry*. 1989;25:1029.

Chapter 12

Monitoring Your Progress

It is not so much where we are, but in what direction we are moving, that matters.
Unknown

Just as all movement is not forward, all change is not improvement.
Unknown

I recommend that you carefully keep track of your results so that the progress you make does not go unappreciated by you. It is important to keep enthusiasm high so you will persevere and remain committed to the NHE Eating Plan. No matter how effective a dietary program is, if you don't stick to it, it can't work. With this in mind, here are a few suggestions.

First, it is difficult to perceive changes in your own body because you see yourself constantly. From one day to the next the results are not visibly noticeable, and over a longer period it is easy to lose sight of exactly how you looked in the beginning. This is why you must be more scientific in monitoring your progress than regularly looking in the mirror. (But the mirror is a more accurate gauge of progress than the scale, which can be downright misleading. When evaluating yourself naked in the mirror, keep a running inventory of what flexes and what jiggles.) In addition to the mirror, the following are important barometers of progress: how your clothes fit, how you feel, comparison of "before" pictures, and bodyfat testing.

Bodyfat Testing

Bodyfat testing addresses the all-important issue of body composition, and it can be a useful gauge of progress. However, there is wide variation in the reliability of different methods of testing.

Hydrostatic Weighing

The most accurate method of bodyfat testing is hydrostatic weighing, which involves submergence in a tank filled with water. Fat is more buoyant than muscle, and the buoyancy differential is the principle governing this method of testing. After the dunking procedure is concluded, the tester uses a mathematical formula to arrive at a calculation of the ratio of lean tissue to bodyfat. While underwater weighing is the "gold standard" of bodyfat testing, it is generally performed at human performance labs, not at gyms and health clubs.

Caliper Testing

A more accessible method of bodyfat testing involves the use of calipers to measure subcutaneous fat at selected sites on the body. This method, although more convenient and less expensive than hydrostatic weighing, bears the problems of human error and variability. Using calipers to measure fatfolds requires skill and knowledge. Specifically, the tester must place the calipers in precisely the correct areas, and must apply the right amount of force when pinching with the calipers. Where the tester uses the calipers too aggressively, too much tissue will be picked-up and this will lead to an exaggerated bodyfat measurement. The opposite problem arises where the calipers are used too reservedly.

Even where fatfold measurements are accurately obtained, the data must be properly processed through a mathematical formula to arrive at bodyfat percentage. There are several different such equations, some more accurately predictive of bodyfat percentage than others. To minimize these variables, use the same proficient tester each time to administer the test and rely on the "sum of the fatfolds" to reflect changes in bodyfat over time. Although the sum of the fatfolds will not tell you your bodyfat percentage, it will eliminate the need for the mathematical formula and, assuming an adept tester, it will disclose changes in fatness. Also, have the test done in the morning, before eating or drinking, to minimize fluctuation in water retention from one testing occasion to another.

Bioelectric Impedance

This method of testing is based on the differing electrical conductivity of fat versus lean tissue. Noninvasive, easy, and safe, bioelectric impedance is an effective means of roughly estimating body composition. It has proven useful in clinical settings, but it is of minimal utility for individuals seeking to monitor subtle changes in body composition resulting from a fat-reduction/bodybuilding program.

The accuracy of bioelectric impedance is overrated. In actuality, the margin of error with this method is considerable.[1,2,3,4,5] For instance, in one study bioelectric impedance predicted bodyfat in only 72% of subjects within 4% of values obtained by hydrostatic weighing.[6] Even within this group, the values generated lacked the pinpoint accuracy that people assume they are getting when they solicit body composition feedback from a technologically impressive device like this one.

The confounding variables with this method include hydration level (water retention)[7,8] and skin temperature.[9] Both of these factors can alter the impedance of the electric current used in the test, and thereby skew the results. Although the accuracy of bioelectric impedance currently leaves much to be desired, the technological concept is a good one and newer applications, such as segmental and multifrequency analyzers, promise to expand the utility of this electrical technique.

112

Near-Infrared Interactance

Another high-tech method, near-infrared interactance, which uses principles of light absorption and reflection to assess body composition, is used by the USDA to measure the fat content of beef. The commercial version used with humans, Futrex-5000, has become popular in health clubs, hospitals, and weight loss centers because it is safe, portable, and requires minimal training to use.

In terms of accuracy and reliability, near-infrared interactance runs a distant last, teetering precariously on the verge of being a complete farce. The best thing that can be said about this method of bodyfat testing is that it is consistently inconsistent. One of the problems is its tendency to overestimate bodyfat in lean individuals and to underestimate bodyfat in fatter subjects.[10,11] The questionable capability of this technology to yield accurate measurements across a broad range of bodyfat levels renders it of limited value. Moreover, even when used on individuals at the middle of the bodyfat continuum, it is not unusual for repeated tests with this method to produce varying results, and for the results to diverge substantially from results obtained by hydrostatic weighing and caliper testing.[12,13,14,15]

The Clothes Knows

How your clothes fit can be a good barometer of progress, because it gives you an idea of size changes of particular bodyparts and overall body shape changes. For instance, if you are employing the NHE Eating Plan in conjunction with hormonally-intelligent exercise (which you should be), you may find that although your body weight is dropping only modestly, or not at all, your clothes are fitting better and you feel good about your appearance in clothes that previously made you feel self-conscious. This signifies that fat is coming off while you are firming up and maybe putting on some muscle.

One drawback to this unscientific method of assessing body shape changes is that it will indicate that you have become fatter every time you wear an article of clothing that just came out of the dryer. Be sure to factor this into your analysis. Better yet, set aside a pair of jeans and a shirt that are dispensable to your wardrobe, and use them exclusively for testing purposes. As with weighing and self-evaluation in the mirror, don't drive yourself crazy searching for day-to-day changes.

The Way to Weigh

Monitor your weight if you must, but don't be an obsessive scale-watcher. The aim of the NHE Eating Plan is to reduce bodyfat percentage, and I have yet to encounter a weight scale that measures this. If weight is your preoccupation, you have the wrong mindset at the outset. Remember, the Eating Plan is concerned with fat loss, not weight loss. There are many crash diets that produce much greater weight loss than the Eating Plan. Muscle weighs substantially more than fat; therefore, *the higher the ratio of muscle loss to fat loss, the faster you lose weight.*

113

Accordingly, the most effective way to lose a lot of weight is to drop muscle along with fat (exactly the result produced by most diets) - you'll be lighter, but also weaker and mushier, and you will have lost some of the contour and shapeliness that defines a great-looking body. You will also burn fewer calories at rest, and you will have given the aging process a boost (see "Using Your Muscles to Turn Back the Hands of Time," in Chapter 11). The NHE Eating Plan, by contrast, minimizes muscle loss and does not cause much water loss, either. Thus, the weight you lose will be practically all pure, unadulterated blubber. Keep this in mind when you weigh yourself.

I know from years of experience as a fitness trainer that no matter how vehemently I denounce the scale as a device for measuring your success at losing fat and improving your body, my advice to disregard the scale will fall on deaf ears in most cases. I sympathize with your desire to obtain definitive, quantitative feedback on the success of your efforts. But if you allow yourself to be seduced by the numeric allure of the bathroom scale, you are likely to be led astray.

For years, you have been exposed to fad diets that cause substantial water and muscle loss. The purveyors of these diets, sometimes ignorant themselves but often exploiting the public's misunderstanding of the difference between weight loss and fat loss, have created an intense emphasis on losing weight which, I believe, represents one of the greatest obstacles to teaching people how to improve their bodies. *Until we root-out the term "weight loss" from the vocabulary of health and fitness, widespread misunderstanding of the true path to physical improvement will reign, and the American public will continue to be easy pickings for the fad diet scamsters.*

In my experience as a fitness trainer, I have witnessed many instances of women who, utilizing hormonally correct diet and exercise, have gone down several dress sizes, and have transformed themselves from being "overweight" and out-of-shape to being a spectacularly attractive physical specimen, *while losing only six or seven pounds.* Similarly, I have known of women who have lost forty pounds crash dieting only to become a smaller, flabbier version of their heavier selves. Moreover, the crash-dieter-woman almost always puts the fat back on in relatively short order, while the woman who improves her body composition and her hormonal and metabolic status can stay in great shape for years even while consuming more calories than her crash-dieter counterpart.

This reasoning applies even more emphatically to men, who can gain and lose many more pounds of muscle than can women. Many of our great male athletes are overweight according to life insurance height/weight tables. Barry Sanders, arguably the best running back in NFL history, is very overweight by height/weight standards. But Sanders also has a great-looking body capable of performing amazing athletic feats. Evander Holyfield is another "overweight" guy with a fantastic physique who has done pretty well for himself in the athletic arena.

Although I wish you would ignore the scale altogether, I know you probably won't. So here are two suggestions to mitigate its misleading potential. First, be sure to use the same scale each time you weigh yourself. Based on my observations, it seems that a large percentage of scales are off by a few pounds. An erroneous swing in the wrong direction from one slightly-off scale to another can cause you unwarranted frustration. Be alert to the ever-present threat of mechanical error when weighing yourself.

Secondly, don't weigh yourself more than once every two weeks. Few people understand that body water content normally fluctuates within a range of a few percentage points. Given that the human body is approximately 60% water, a few percentage points translates to a few pounds. For example, a person weighing 150 pounds would lose or gain about 3 pounds as a result of a 3% fluctuation in water retention.

Because transient increases and decreases in weight are normal from day to day, the only meaningful weight assessment is one that looks at a trend over a period of time. The difference in your weight from May 15 to June 15 is worth noting, but the difference from Monday to Thursday is statistically insignificant because neither fat loss nor muscle gain has had a chance to surpass the "margin of error" (i.e., the average 3-pound water weight fluctuation). Also, to minimize the water retention variable, always weigh yourself at the same time of the day: after waking in the morning, before eating or drinking.

How You Feel

Time and again, people on the Natural Hormonal Enhancement program report feeling better than ever. This "great" feeling is a result of living in harmony with the natural eating drives of the body, better nutrient intake and absorption, stable blood sugar and neurotransmitter levels, and the far-reaching hormonal, enzymatic, and metabolic changes that occur with this program.

In addition to physiological improvements, people on the NHE program report less guilt and more self-esteem. The psychological uplift created by Natural Hormonal Enhancement is not difficult to explain: people who feel in control of their life and feel that they are making steady progress toward worthy goals tend to have higher self-esteem, while people who feel that they are not in control of their life and are not making progress tend to have lower self-esteem. With Natural Hormonal Enhancement, you have a comprehensive system that empowers you to gain control of your health and fitness. You will know exactly what to do in all areas - diet, exercise, and lifestyle - to achieve the results you want. And you will make steady progress toward your goals.

References

1. Schroeder D, Christie PM, Hill GL. Bioelectrical Impedance Analysis for Body Composition: Clinical Evaluation in General Surgical Patients. *JPEN J Parenter Enteral Nutr* 1990;14:129.

2. Kaminsky LA, Whaley MH. Differences in Estimates of Percent Body Fat Using Bioelectrical Impedance. *J Sports Med Phys Fitness* 1993;33:172.

3. Kremer MM, et al. Validity of Bioelectrical Impedance Analysis to Measure Body Fat in Air Force Members. *Mil Med* 1998;163:781.

4. Paijmans IJ, Wilmore KM, Wilmore JH. Use of Skinfolds and Bioelectrical Impedance for Body Composition Assessment after Weight Reduction. *J Am Coll Nutr* 1992;11:145.

5. Tagliabue A, How Reliable is Bio-Electrical Impedance Analysis for Individual Patients? *Int J Obes Relat Metab Disord* 1992;16:649.

6. Wilmore KM, McBride PJ, Wilmore JH. Comparison of Bioelectric Impedance and Near-Infrared Interactance for Body Composition Assessment in a Population of Self-Perceived Overweight Adults. *Int J Obes Relat Metab Disord* 1994;18:375.

7. Thompson DL, et al. Effects of Hydration and Dehydration on Body Composition Analysis: a Comparative Study of Bioelectric Impedance Analysis and Hydrodensitometry. *J Sports Med Phys Fitness* 1991;31:565.

8. Brodie DA, et al. Effect of Changes of Water and Electrolytes on the Validity of Conventional Methods of Measuring Fat-Free Mass. *Ann Nutr Metab* 1991;35:89.

9. Caton JR, et al. Body Composition by Bioelectrical Impedence: Effect of Skin Temperature. *Med Sci Sports Exerc* 1988;20:489.

10. McLean KP, Skinner JS. Validity of Futrex-5000 for Body Composition Determination. *Med Sci Sports Exerc* 1992;24:253.

11. Thomas DW, et al. The Performance of an Infra-Red Interactance Instrument for Assessing Total Body Fat. *Physiol Meas* 1997;18:305.

12. See, supra, notes 6 and 10.

13. Israel RG, et al. Validity of a Near-Infrared Spectrophotometry Device for Estimating Human Body Composition. *Res Q Exerc Sport* 1989;60:379.

14. Cassady SL, et al. Validity of Near Infrared Body Composition Analysis in Children and Adolescents. *Med Sci Sports Exerc* 1993;25:1185.

15. Smith DB, et al. Validity of Near-Infrared Interactance for Estimating Relative Body Fat in Female High School Gymnasts. *Int J Sports Med* 1997;18:531.

The Metabolic U-Turn

Energy levels will increase after the first four days and cravings will disappear, as you make the metabolic shift. However, during the first 4 days you will likely experience some version of the "sugar-burner-deprived-of-sugar" syndrome that I described in Chapter 11. Energy levels may sag, and you will probably experience some degree of carbohydrate craving, possibly intense. And then, you will make the metabolic shift and these symptoms will disappear.

Think of the 7-day metabolic shift period as making a sudden U-turn in your car at a high rate of speed. All of a sudden you slam on the breaks and cut the wheel sharply. There is a lot of screeching and friction. Then, before you know it, you have regained control and you are cruising in the opposite direction. In effect, your metabolism is going to make a similar U-turn. The screeching and friction may or may not be as bad as I have portrayed it. In either case, you'll overcome it - *I know you will.*

Sugar- Fat-
Burner Burner

How Much Carbohydrate?

During the 7-day metabolic shift period, you should aim for *fewer than* 20 grams of active carbohydrate each day. (For a definition of "active carbohydrate" see p. 124.) In addition to initial cravings, this period will be difficult from a practical standpoint because

	during shift	cycling begins	
active carb	< 20	30-60	carb-load
day	1-7	8 & 9	10

carbohydrates are ubiquitous in our sweet-tooth society. *Be sure to read:* "Don't Get Nickeled and Dimed to Death by Hidden Carbs," in Chapter 19, before embarking on the metabolic shift. Also in Chapter 19, the discussion of "eating to prevent hunger rather than eating in response to hunger" will be particularly helpful. By consuming smaller meals more frequently, rather than larger meals less frequently, you will go a long way toward defeating the cravings that will likely arise during the first few days of the metabolic shift period (but smaller meals consumed *less frequently* can aggravate cravings, so make sure to eat enough food).

What to Eat during the First Seven Days

Basically, you should focus on meat during this period: steak, fish, shrimp, ribs (without barbecue sauce), lobster, chicken, etc. As well, cheese, eggs, and cottage/ricotta cheese are good choices during the first 7 days. Don't worry about fat consumption during this period - eat as much fat as you want. In fact, fat will facilitate the metabolic shift to fat burning and it will help quell cravings (see Chapter 18). The key factor here is the carbs. If you stay under 20 grams, you will make the metabolic shift; if you don't, you won't.

118

In order to stay under the 20-gram carbohydrate limit, I recommend that you limit yourself to the following vegetables, eaten in moderation: cabbage, celery, broccoli, lettuce, carrots, spinach, onions, garlic, asparagus, radicchio, mushrooms, cucumbers, cauliflower, peppers, avocado, and radishes. Although it is not necessary to eat vegetables in order to make the metabolic shift, I recommend that you eat at least one serving per day of fresh vegetables during the metabolic shift period. Otherwise, you may find yourself constipated from the switch to a protein- and fat-based diet.

If none of the vegetables listed above appeals to you, try melting some butter or cheese on them. It's amazing what melted butter or melted cheese can do to spruce-up the taste of an otherwise unappealing food. You may wish to snack on pieces of fresh broccoli, celery, or cauliflower dipped in high-fat, *low-carb* dressing. French dressing is out of the question, while most blue cheese dressings are fine. Check the label and be wary of "hidden carbs."

What Not to Eat

Essentially, everything except those foods mentioned in this chapter are to be avoided during the metabolic shift period. Starchy or sugary foods, obviously, should be forsaken. Less obviously, fruits, while not nearly as high in carbohydrate as starches and dessert foods, are off-limits during this period. Remember, we are trying to *totally reverse your metabolism* in 7 days, and this requires eliminating incoming carbohydrate and depleting internal sugar stores (i.e., glycogen). To achieve this feat, you must be strict and vigilant about what you eat.

I cannot emphasize strongly enough how important these first 7 days are to your success on the NHE Eating Plan. It will reset your metabolism, give you fat-burning momentum, and subdue your appetite making it easier to get into the groove of macronutrient cycling which begins on the 8th day.

Changing Your Body Requires Changing Your Mind

In addition to the metabolic benefits, there is a psychological advantage to the first 7 days. After this 7-day "boot camp," the moderate carbohydrate restriction of the NHE Eating Plan will be a breeze. On the other hand, after a period of eating whatever you want (which is the mode that most Americans are in when they are not dieting) *any* structured dietary program, *no matter how flexible,* would seem like an imposition by comparison. In addition to changing your metabolism, I want to change *your perspective* about what, in terms of diet, constitutes "difficult." As you can see, you are about to embark on a dietary program that attacks bodyfat from every conceivable angle.

I will now go one step further in transforming your perspective on eating. Before I do, let me assure you, you will *never* have to eat any food that you dislike on the NHE Eating Plan. Having said that, the prevailing outlook on eating in the U.S. and other Western nations is a strange anomaly, caused in large part by the billions of dollars spent by the food industry to promote their products. Somewhere along the way, people have acquired the notion that *every meal* has to be a source of great pleasure.

I do not dispute that everything one eats should be palatable, but a source of great pleasure? *Every meal?* Do you derive great pleasure from every minute you spend at your job? Hopefully, you find your job "palatable" and at least sometimes pleasurable, but few people hold the view that every minute of work, including Monday mornings, should be a source of great pleasure.

Outside of Western culture - in rural India, China, and Africa, for instance - eating is viewed primarily as a source of nourishment, not pleasure. Sure eating is one of the pleasures of life, but that's not the *purpose* of eating. Few people realize how completely they have been brainwashed by powerful market forces in society; but the fact is that many Americans subconsciously hold every meal to the standards of an orgy. Long-term success requires that you replace this self-defeating mindset with a self-empowering one. Toward this end, you may find the following affirmations helpful for programming your mind for dietary success.

Eating Affirmations

♦   Eating happens to be one of the pleasures of life, but attainment of pleasure is not the primary reason why I eat.

♦   Food is a tremendously powerful vehicle for improving my body, my health, and my energy levels. I will use food to my advantage.

♦   I will never, ever, eat any food that I dislike.

♦   I will readily eat foods that I neither like nor dislike if it will help me to achieve my goals.

♦   The concept that pleasure is the central purpose of eating is a propaganda tactic used by a multi-billion dollar industry that cares nothing about my health and well-being, and simply wants to extract money from me.

♦   The pleasure I will derive from optimal health and well being will be infinitely greater than the pleasure that can possibly be derived from eating the most delicious foods every day of my life.

Chapter 14

The Natural Hormonal Enhancement Eating Plan: A Lifetime Dietary Strategy

No crash diet or fad diet can solve the obesity problem, because these diets are so disagreeable and such a continuing nuisance that the obese person soon gives up. A successful treatment is one that will be adhered to year after year.
Dr. Linus Pauling, *How to Live Longer and Feel Better*

Make everything simple as possible - but not simpler.
Albert Einstein

There are two versions of the NHE Eating Plan: 1) general 2) bodybuilders'. The basic principles of Natural Hormonal Enhancement apply to both versions. In order to decide which version is best for you, you must evaluate your health and physique objectives.

The general Eating Plan is an optimal health, fat-reducing dietary program and has much wider appeal than the bodybuilders' Eating Plan. The general Eating Plan is recommended for fat individuals, health/anti-aging enthusiasts, and athletes for whom minimizing bodyfat is a higher priority than maximizing muscle mass. In terms of its physique objectives, the general Eating Plan aims to maximize fat loss while preserving or enhancing muscle mass. This is in contrast to conventional reducing diets, which adversely alter hormone levels (by increasing the catabolic/anabolic ratio), cause muscle loss, and reduce metabolic rate.

The bodybuilders' Eating Plan is recommended for healthy athletes/bodybuilders who are primarily concerned with building as much muscle as possible. The bodybuilders' Eating Plan aims to maximize muscle growth while maintaining or reducing fat mass. This is in contrast to conventional mass-building diets, which adversely alter hormone levels (by increasing the lipogenic/lipolytic ratio), cause fat gain, and diminish health status.

Introduction to Macronutrient Cycling

After you have made the metabolic shift discussed in Chapter 13, you will begin a dietary program based on a technology called **macronutrient cycling**. Macronutrients are fat, protein, and carbohydrate. Fat stays more or less constant while protein and carbohydrate are inversely cycled such that protein intake is high (as a percentage of total caloric intake) when carbohydrate intake is low, and vice versa. The period of carbohydrate

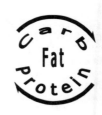

restriction is called the "downcycle." The meals/snacks that comprise the downcycle are called **standard fat-burning** meals. The carbohydrate "upcycle" consists of the **carb-load** meals.

In effect, with the NHE Eating Plan you will be following a diet with a split personality. You will be consuming a carbohydrate-restricted diet punctuated by periodic high-carbohydrate/low-protein meals. Because of the hormonal and metabolic effects of protein (discussed in Chapter 17), it will be the central element of most of your meals.

The cyclical nature of the NHE Eating Plan affords variety and allows you to eat your favorite "pleasure food," provided you eat it at the right time in your cycle. There are many other features of the Eating Plan, which will be introduced in the following chapters. They include: maximizing the thermogenic effect of food, protein optimization, meal frequency, and using dietary fat to burn bodyfat.

Enter the Third Dimension

As you can see, the NHE Eating Plan is a departure from conventional diets, most of which are based on a two-dimensional sort of reasoning: they condemn and restrict one category of food across the board, while extolling another category of food. For instance, the low-fat diet restricts your consumption of fat for as long as you are on the diet (thereby assuring that you won't be on the diet for very long) and exalts carbohydrate as the great ally to humankind in its fight against fat. The low-carbohydrate diet does the opposite, portraying carbohydrate as a source of evil to be eradicated from your diet with the fervor of an exorcism while elevating meat and other protein foods to idol-like status.

There is a natural tendency to try to distill problems down to a good vs. bad dichotomy, and when it comes to food, what is today's dietary darling is tomorrow's dietary devil. It's not that the media and the "experts" are *trying* to confuse you, it's that until recently even the most knowledgeable experts did not understand the crucial role played by hormones in body composition. Many still don't.

The whole metabolic picture cannot be accurately reduced to a two-dimensional dietary formula. Nevertheless, most diets employ such simplistic reductivism, directing us to shun one category of food as if it were dietary kryptonite. Fruit, meat, pasta, eggs, and bread have each been on either side of the condemnation/commendation ledger at different times during the last decade. Which is in the doghouse these days? It depends on which authority you listen to.

The general calorie-restrictive diet is a notable exception to the good food/bad food approach. It, in effect, declares war on *all food* by way of indicting calories, an evil thing which, if it were not for that nemesis called food, would never be able to insinuate its way into our bodies. But as you learned in Chapter 9, excessive caloric intake is symptomatic of a larger problem; specifically, a hormonal state that generates cravings and directs the body to store fat. With the NHE Eating Plan, there is no need to count calories and there are no categorically good or bad foods.

Standard Fat-Burning Meals (Downcycle)

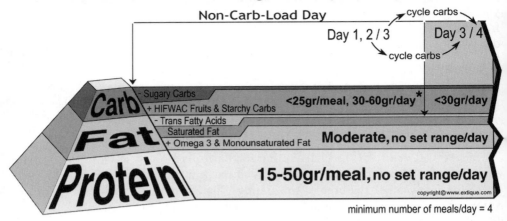

minimum number of meals/day = 4

Functions of Standard Fat-Burning Meals

- stimulate fat-burning enzymes [see Chapter 18]

- stimulate lipolytic hormones (growth hormone and glucagon) [see Chapters 10, 17]

- stimulate anabolic hormones (growth hormone, IGF-1, testosterone) [see Chapters 11, 17, 22]

- confer a thermogenic effect [see Chapter 16]

- keep amino acid pool "topped-off," which affords maximum availability of raw materials for 1) protein synthesis (for muscle growth/enhancement) and 2) neurotransmitter synthesis (for mental productivity) [see Chapter 17]

---

* Carbohydrate values above refer to quantity of *active* carbohydrate. The active carbohydrate content of a food can be determined by subtracting dietary fiber from total carbohydrate, or, for unlabeled foods consult the Extique Pocket Active Carb Counter.

Active Carbohydrate = Total Carbohydrate - Dietary Fiber

Fiber does not act like a carbohydrate in your body - in fact, it has the opposite effect. Active carbohydrates (sugars and starches) contain 4 calories per gram and stimulate insulin release. Fiber, by contrast, is non-caloric since it is not digested. Moreover, whereas active carbohydrates stimulate insulin, fiber blunts the insulin response to a meal by slowing the release of digested food into the bloodstream (see p. 28). Because the carbohydrate values above refer to active carbohydrate, they appear slightly more restrictive than if total carbohydrate were used (which is what you are accustomed to seeing).

For some foods, like white bread and frozen yogurt, which contain virtually zero fiber, the active carbohydrate distinction makes no difference because all of the carbohydrate is active. The total carb/active carb distinction becomes significant with foods like fruits, oatmeal, and nuts. I believe that active carbohydrate is a more helpful and meaningful measure because, when dealing with a carbohydrate limit, it, in effect, rewards you for eating fiber by allowing you to eat more food. By contrast, employing an undifferentiated definition of carbohydrate in effect penalizes you for eating fiber. Given that fiber is healthy and facilitates bodyfat reduction (both by increasing thermogenesis [see Chapter 16] and by reducing insulin levels), it makes no sense to give people an incentive to avoid it.

Although carbohydrate intake is tightly regulated during the downcycle to keep insulin/glucagon primed for fat burning, you will have more leeway in regard to fat than you would on a low-fat diet. So the only thing you are giving up is being able to frequently eat carbohydrate-dominated meals; and once your carbohydrate cravings disappear, you won't have any urge to do so anyway. Nonetheless, a high-carbohydrate "pig-out" meal is always right around the corner! (The actual timing of the carb-load meal is discussed in the next chapter.)

Carb-Load Meals (Upcycle)

During a carb-load meal there is no prescribed carbohydrate limit;* however, there is a limit for protein and fat (fewer than 20 grams each) at these meals.

NOTE - On carb-load days, prior to carb-loading, keep active carbs under 30 grams.

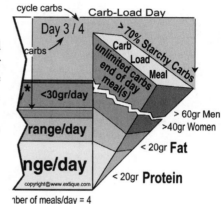

Functions of Carb-Load Meals

- Refuels glycogen stores, and glycogen is crucial to performance of hormonally-intelligent exercise

- Prevents decline in thyroid activity, thereby preventing decline in metabolic rate

- Provides variety and pleasure

- Facilitates anabolism (muscular enhancement) by inducing uptake of amino acids by muscles and driving IGF-1 production

- Causes a transient increase in bioavailable testosterone in men

For a more in-depth discussion of the functions and benefits of the carb-load meal, see Chapter 15.

* While there is no limit, there is a minimum for this meal. Women should aim for *at least* 40 grams and men *at least* 60 grams of active carbohydrate - so get ready to do some serious carbohydrate eating! You should not feel restrained at this meal regarding how much carbohydrate to eat. Should you wish to eat 200 grams of carbs, go right ahead. While there are no quantitative carbohydrate restraints applicable to this meal, starchy carbs - like potatoes, rice, and pasta - are favored over sugary carbs for reasons discussed in the next chapter.

NHE Eating Plan (general)

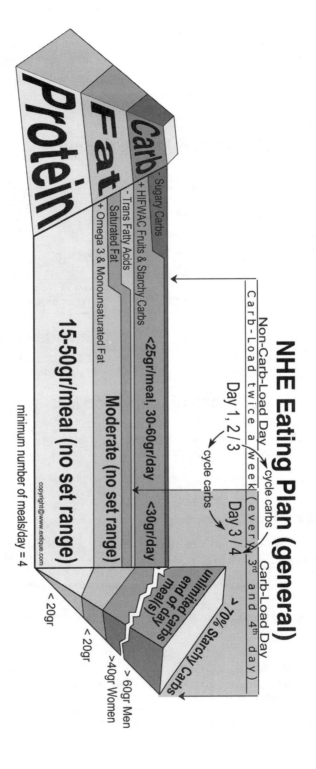

Carb		Fat		Protein
- Sugary Carbs	+ HIFWAC Fruits & Starchy Carbs	- Trans Fatty Acids	+ Omega 3 & Monounsaturated Fat	
		Saturated Fat		

Non-Carb-Load Day

Carb-Load twice a week (every 3rd and 4th day)

Day 1, 2 / 3 — cycle carbs

Day 3 / 4 — cycle carbs

Carb-Load Day

<25gr/meal, 30-60gr/day

<30gr/day

> 70% Starchy Carbs

unlimited carbs end of day meal(s)

> 60gr Men
>40gr Women

< 20gr

< 20gr

15-50gr/meal (no set range)

Moderate (no set range)

minimum number of meals/day = 4

copyright@www.exlique.com

* See footnote p. 124

What to Eat and When to Eat

As you can see, the basic framework of the NHE Eating Plan is simple. But there is much more to the Eating Plan than what you have read so far. The following chapters will give you specific guidance concerning what to eat and when to eat. Your food selections will be governed by several dietary technologies that are designed to work in synergy with each other and within the basic macronutrient cycling framework outlined above, to maximize fat burning, energy levels, mental productivity, muscular enhancement, and health. *The following five chapters are critical.* Study them carefully, and follow them diligently.

In the next chapter, we will discuss the carb-load meals (Chapter 15). We will then shift our focus to the standard fat-burning meals, which will comprise the majority of your eating (Chapters 16, 17, 18). Chapter 19 discusses snacking, and it provides important tips to ensure that you achieve your fat loss goals. Keep in mind that, throughout this book, the term "meal" is used loosely to refer to anytime you eat, i.e., actual meals eaten while sitting at a table with a napkin on your lap, as well as "snacking," "noshing," "grabbing a bite," etc.

The Standard Fat-Burning Meals

There are five dietary strategies that will guide your eating during the downcycle. They are:

- *Daily and Per-Meal Carbohydrate Gram Limits* (see above)

- *Thermogenesis* (Chapter 16)

- *Protein Optimization/Meal Frequency* (Chapter 17)

- *Using Dietary Fat to Burn Bodyfat* (Chapter 18)

- *Favoring Starchy Carbs over Sugary Carbs* (Chapter 15)
  Note - This strategy applies mainly to the carb-load meals, which is why it is discussed in the carb-load chapter. It is a consideration during the downcycle; but it is of limited importance then, due to the low overall amount of carbohydrate consumed.

These five strategies work together within the context of macronutrient cycling. As you learn about these strategies, you may perceive some conflict between them - I want to clear up this matter at the outset. Where such a conflict appears (as it will, for instance, between thermogenesis and using dietary fat to burn bodyfat), the dilemma can be resolved by consulting the Hierarchy of Eating Priorities, below. Your goal is to apply all five of these technologies every day.

127

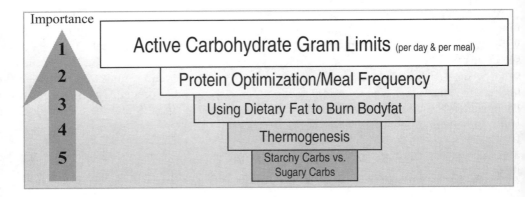

Importance

1 — **Active Carbohydrate Gram Limits** (per day & per meal)

2 — Protein Optimization/Meal Frequency

3 — Using Dietary Fat to Burn Bodyfat

4 — Thermogenesis

5 — Starchy Carbs vs. Sugary Carbs

Drink a Lot of Water

I know you've heard this before, and it is one of the few bits of conventional wisdom on fat loss that is actually correct. You lose about two liters of water per day through the skin, urine, feces, and breath. This loss of water is offset by water contained in ingested food and liquids. In addition, water and carbon dioxide are formed when food molecules are broken down for energy.

As explained in Chapter 11, depending on exercise intensity and ambient conditions, water loss during exercise can exceed two liters *per hour*. Also in Chapter 11, I explained how dehydration impairs athletic performance. Not only does sub-optimal hydration result in sub-optimal performance, it also results in sub-optimal fat loss, sub-optimal muscular development, and sub-optimal health.

Warriors Don't Drink Soda Pop

For the overwhelming majority of our existence, thirsty humans drank water. After reading Chapter 5, you know that this is only one of many points of divergence between the dietary practices of the "ancient warriors" and those of modern man and woman. Water was the uncontested beverage of choice up until the food processing/soda pop revolution in the late 1800's unseated water from its position of supremacy and relegated it to disfavored status.

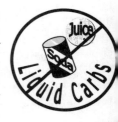

Although water appears to be making a comeback these days, it now competes against liquids of every hue and flavor. In fact, however, water has no competition.

Most beverage ingredients do not add to, but rather detract from, the quality of the drink. Simply put, **calorie-containing fluids have no place in the diet of someone striving for optimal fitness and health** (except for low/moderate red wine consumption as discussed in Chapter 20 and protein shakes as discussed in Chapter 21). This rule applies not only to soda, but to fruit juice as well.

A few years ago "juicing" became a national sensation, and even today juicing devices are strong sellers. For many natural food enthusiasts, juicing has quasi-spiritual overtones. I find it curious that people so opposed to buying processed foods are so fond of processing food themselves. I don't deny that fruit juice is nutritious, and if it were the only available source of vitamins, minerals, and antioxidants, I would heartily endorse its consumption; but this is not the case. The NHE Eating Plan advocates consumption of fruits and vegetables in their natural form, not in their degraded form. The concept of fruit juice as unnatural runs counter to its reputation. But as is the case with soda, juice is a very recent addition to the human diet. The "ancient warriors" drank juice as often as they drank soda - never.

"Unnaturalness," in and of itself, does not render a food unworthy. Vitamin supplements are "unnatural" in a sense, but they can also be very beneficial. Poisonous mushrooms, on the other hand, are "natural" but will kill you instantly. The problem with juice is that it has been unnaturally altered in such a way as to make it hormonally disadvantageous. Specifically, it has been stripped of most of its fiber content. Because the removal of fiber greatly increases both the caloric density of a food and the rate at which sugar from that food enters the bloodstream, fruit juice provokes a much sharper insulin response than does whole fruit. Furthermore, "juicing" a fruit or vegetable vastly diminishes its thermogenic, or metabolism-raising, value. In effect, drinking juice is like intravenously administering sugar into your body (not a helpful practice for someone striving to be a fat-burner rather than a sugar-burner).

Water for Fat Loss and Health

Water serves many beneficial purposes. For one, water promotes a physical feeling of fullness, which helps reduce appetite (see p. 151). Secondly, *ketones,* a natural byproduct of fat burning, are excreted via urine (see p. 68). Water flushes-out ketones, thereby facilitating the fat-burning process. From a broader perspective, water transports nutrients and plays an instrumental role in all biochemical processes that occur within the body, including fat burning. Studies confirm that liberal ingestion of water can enhance fat burning,[1,2] and this enhanced utilization of fat for energy is associated with a reduction in utilization of glycogen.[3,4] Recall from Chapter 11 that glycogen conservation is a key concept of the NHE Eating Plan. (To review, we compensate for a reduced carbohydrate intake by increasing carbohydrate use efficiency.)

Water is particularly important for individuals on a protein-rich diet because elimination of *urea*, the chief metabolic byproduct of protein metabolism, requires water.[5,6] The more protein you consume, the more urea you produce; and the more urea you produce, the more water leaves your body as urine. The dehydrating effect of protein is one reason why I advise athletes to reduce protein intake in favor of lipids 24 hours before competing in the heat.

Is Water Anabolic?

With all the expensive, high-tech-sounding bodybuilding supplements on the market, who would ever think of *water* as an anabolic agent? The fact of the matter is that water possesses some very interesting muscle-enhancing properties. In recent years, scientists have learned that changes in cell volume regulate cell function. In fact, the emerging view is that hormones and nutrients exert their controlling influence on cellular activities by altering cell volume.[7,8,9] Cell volume is a function of the hydration state of the cell – and that brings us to water.

Protein synthesis and protein degradation are affected in opposite directions by cell swelling and shrinking. An increase in cellular hydration (swelling) acts as an anabolic stimulus, whereas a decrease in cellular hydration (shrinkage) acts as a catabolic stimulus.[10,11,12,13,14] Consistent with that, dehydration has been shown to increase cortisol levels.[15,16]

Cellular hydration, however, is more complex than simply guzzling water. Fluid is constantly moving in and out of the cell across an electrical gradient bisected by the cell membrane. The key to obtaining the anabolic benefits of "cell volumization" is to maximize intracellular fluid. Drinking water will improve your overall hydration status, but it will not significantly alter the ratio of intracellular to extracellular fluid. Rather, fluid exchange is transacted by electrically charged particles called ions.

Electrolytes are ions. The mineral sodium is the chief extracellular electrolyte, whereas the mineral potassium is the chief intracellular electrolyte. (Remember on p. 96 I stressed the importance of the sodium/potassium ratio in connection with growth hormone? – well, important concepts just don't go away.) By increasing your potassium intake and reducing your sodium intake, you can shift water from the extracellular compartments of your body into the cells.[17,18] Because potassium levels decline with age and track the age-related decline in growth hormone[19,20] and because cellular dehydration/shrinkage has been strongly linked to several disease states and to cell death,[21,22,23,24,25] I predict that sodium/potassium will become a focal point of nutritional anti-aging research in coming years.

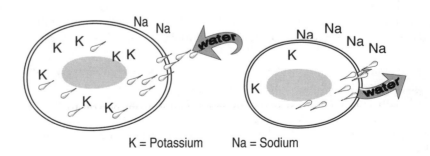

K = Potassium   Na = Sodium

What is the best way to improve your sodium/potassium ratio? Answer: follow the NHE Eating Plan. By limiting consumption of processed carbohydrate foods (most of which contain barely a trace of potassium and a truckload of sodium) and encouraging consumption of unprocessed plant and animal foods (which are high in potassium and low in sodium), the Eating Plan goes a long way toward improving your mineral-electrolyte status. A high water intake coupled with a diet high in potassium-rich foods is a sound strategy for hydrating the trillions of cells that comprise your body.

Water consumption is especially important during exercise. Dehydration hampers performance (see Chapter 11), and accentuates the cortisol response to exercise.[26] Even if you are not sweating much due to a cool environment, a higher respiration rate during exercise causes more water to exit your body via breath. So don't forget the water bottle next time you go to the gym.

There are two practical points to bear in mind concerning hydration:

1) **Hydration is a continuum**. There is no exact point at which you go from being well-hydrated to being "dehydrated." In fact, technically, dehydration is not a state at all. Rather, dehydration and rehydration are relative terms referring to becoming less or more hydrated, respectively. Most people don't drink enough water, and thus they are perpetually in a state of sub-optimal hydration - called hypohydration. Hypohydration can raise cortisol levels.[27,28] Accordingly, to achieve the objective of minimizing cortisol levels, you should avoid hypohydration – and that means drinking a lot of water.

2) **Thirst is not an accurate indicator of hydration**. You can be hypohydrated without being the least bit thirsty. Conversely, if you wait until you are thirsty before drinking water, you will always be hypohydrated.

In summary, there is no substitute for water. Without it, life is not possible. Without enough of it, optimal health is not possible.

The Bodybuilders' NHE Eating Plan:
A Dietary Strategy for MAXIMUM Muscle Growth

IMPORTANT: THE BODYBUILDERS' NHE EATING PLAN IS DESIGNED FOR <u>HEALTHY ATHLETES</u>. A COMPLETE PHYSICAL PRIOR TO BEGINNING THE DIET, AND REGULAR BLOODWORK THEREAFTER, IS REQUIRED. Although there is 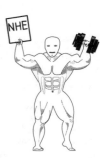 evidence that this version of the NHE Eating Plan, too, can favorably affect serum cholesterol and triglyceride levels, due to a reduction in insulin levels, lipid metabolism varies to some degree from person to person. Therefore, it is important to be vigilant with respect to your blood lipid profile when experimenting with a different diet. And the bodybuilders' NHE Eating Plan is *definitely* different.

The bodybuilders' NHE Eating Plan is designed to maximize muscle growth while minimizing the fat gain that typically accompanies building muscle. Unlike the general Eating Plan, the bodybuilders' Eating Plan is not designed to be a fat-reducing diet. But depending on your current diet, you may nevertheless lose fat as a result of the bodybuilders' Eating Plan. It is also stricter and more demanding than the general Eating Plan. Presumably, athletes have higher fitness objectives, and they are willing to exert commensurately greater effort and undergo greater sacrifice, to achieve their objectives.

From a practical standpoint, the difference between the general Eating Plan and the bodybuilders' Eating Plan boils down to this: more calories overall, more fat in the downcycle, fewer carbs in the downcycle, and more carbs in the upcycle. All other NHE principles, including the frequency and timing of the carb-load meals, are the same except as noted below. Certain topics, like protein optimization/meal frequency (Chapter 17) and starchy carbs vs. sugary carbs (Chapter 15), apply with added force to bodybuilders. In effect, the bodybuilders' Eating Plan is an exaggerated version of macronutrient cycling as compared with the general Eating Plan - the lows are lower and the highs are higher. During the downcycle, the bodybuilders' Eating Plan is a high-fat diet. To explain fully the reasoning and evidence supporting the cyclical high-fat diet would entail repeating large portions of this book.

In reading *Natural Hormonal Enhancement*, you will learn how high-fat/low-carb eating punctuated by high-carb/low-fat "loading" enhances anabolism by maximizing production of GH, IGF-1, and testosterone, and optimizing insulin. You will also learn how high-fat/low-carb eating promotes fat burning, and why fat burning is anti-catabolic as compared with sugar burning. And you will come to appreciate that anti-catabolism is critical to achieving maximum muscle mass.

Although I am deferring to the foregoing and following chapters to provide the theoretical and scientific foundation for the bodybuilders' Eating Plan, I will share with you a few studies that support this dietary approach (you'll find hundreds more supporting studies sprinkled throughout the book). First, as a threshold matter, it is important to understand that a low-fat diet is catabolic as compared with a higher-fat diet. Millions of earnest and committed bodybuilders, obediently following the bodybuilding establishment's instructions, are practicing a dietary regimen that tears down muscle. To illustrate, controlled (equal calories, equal protein) studies comparing intravenous feeding of high-carbohydrate/low-fat versus lower-carbohydrate/higher-fat mixtures find that muscle loss is greater on the low-fat feeding regimen.[29,30]

You may be skeptical because you know people who have built an impressively muscular physique on a low-fat diet. I submit to you that any muscle gains made while on a high-carb/low-fat diet are achieved in spite of, not because of, diet. And those individuals who have succeeded in overcoming dietary errors by virtue of

132

some combination of smart training, sound nutritional supplementation, exceptional genetics, and/or anabolic steroid use, would have an even better physique had they been eating a proper diet. And let's not lose sight of the fact that for every bodybuilder who succeeds on a low-fat diet, there are hundreds who identify themselves as "hardgainers" and complain that they can't make significant gains no matter how hard they try.

Animal studies comparing a high-fat diet to a high-carbohydrate diet show that a high-fat diet increases nitrogen retention (an indicator of anabolism) AND increases fat burning.[31,32] The positive connection between fat burning and protein sparing is a central premise of the NHE Eating Plan and is expounded in Chapter 11, p. 91, "Protecting Protein: The Anti-Catabolic, Anti-Aging, Effect." This principle is illustrated by human studies involving the anti-lipolytic drug acipimox. This drug, by suppressing lipolysis, forces the body to use glucose for fuel. Stated differently, it makes the person taking it a sugar-burner rather than a fat-burner, thus mimicking the effect of a high-carb/low-fat diet. In acipimox-treated subjects, cortisol levels rise and significant protein breakdown occurs.[33,34]

UPCYCLE (Carb-Load Meals)

Split the carb-load into two meals (second-to-last and last of the day) separated by 2-4 hours. Aim for at least 100 grams of active carbohydrate at each meal. Some bodybuilders will consume 200 carbs or more at each carb-load meal; that's fine if you can handle it. Within reason, the more carbs the better. With this in mind, keep protein, fat, and liquids low at these meals in order to max-out the carbs. Fluid intake should also be minimized immediately before and immediately after carb-loading. (Why after? Because starchy carbs absorb water and expand in your stomach – if you carb-load then drink a lot of water while the carbs are still in your stomach, you will find yourself in a state of bloated discomfort.) However, I do recommend sipping water during and after carb-loading because adequate hydration is necessary for optimal glycogen storage. After you have digested the carb-load, resume liberal ingestion of water, as indicated above. See Chapter 15 for further instructions on the carb-load, and pay particular attention to the distinction between sugary carbs and starchy carbs.

DOWNCYCLE (Standard Fat-Burning Meals)

Carbohydrate

During the downcycle, carbohydrate is restricted to a considerably greater extent than with the general NHE Eating Plan. Active carbohydrate intake should be kept under 30 grams on non-carb-load days and on the carb-load day prior to carb-loading.

Protein

You should consume an ample amount of protein during the downcycle. But as explained in Chapter 17, while protein is crucial for bodybuilders, more is not necessarily better. Additionally, by making you into a fat-burner, the bodybuilders' Eating Plan exerts a protein-sparing effect, which means you get more use out of less protein (see above). Keep portion sizes moderate and aim to maximize meal frequency. If you are not feeding at least five times per day, it is unlikely that you are consuming enough calories to support muscle growth. Consuming fat with every meal is a good way to bolster caloric intake. Eating for mass is like training: you must be disciplined and sometimes you've got to do it even when you don't feel like it. Protein shakes can be helpful in attaining your five-meal-a-day minimum requirement, and they are especially valuable when you lack desire to eat.

Fat

During the downcycle, the bodybuilders' NHE Eating Plan is a high-fat diet. To preclude ambiguity, let me clarify: during the downcycle, you should make a special effort to eat a lot of fat. With carbohydrate restricted, fat will be your chief source of calories, and without sufficient calories you can't build muscle – so don't hold back. However, while quantity of fat intake is unlimited, there are qualitative considerations that must be taken into account. Specifically, read and follow Chapter 18's and Chapter 22's instructions concerning what kind of fat to eat - this is a very important aspect of this diet.

Consuming enough fat to fill the caloric void left by carbohydrate is not easy. Some individuals following the bodybuilders' Eating Plan have resorted to an occasional swig of olive oil, and there's nothing wrong with doing this - except for the possibility that you will vomit. For bodybuilders, puking is bad because it represents a moving of valuable calories in the wrong direction. A more palatable way to get lipids into your system is through protein shakes, see p. 243, and by liberally adding butter or olive oil to vegetables and adding mayonnaise to chicken, turkey, or tuna.

134

NHE Eating Plan (bodybuilders')

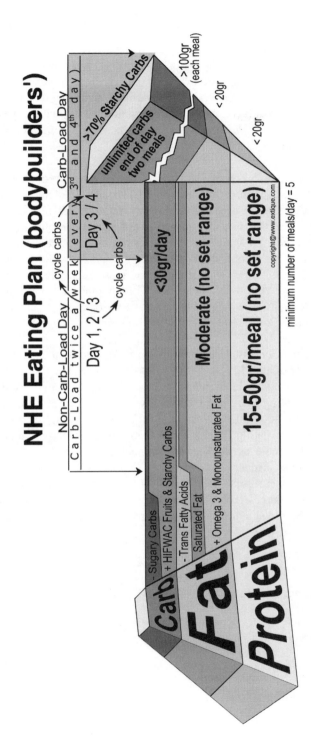

Non-Carb-Load Day — cycle carbs

Carb-Load twice a week (every 3rd and 4th day)

Carb-Load Day

Day 1, 2 / 3 — cycle carbs

Day 3 / 4 — cycle carbs

>70% Starchy Carbs

unlimited carbs
end of day
two meals

>100gr (each meal)

<20gr

<20gr

Carb
- Sugary Carbs
+ HiFWAC Fruits & Starchy Carbs

<30gr/day

Fat
- Trans Fatty Acids
- Saturated Fat
+ Omega 3 & Monounsaturated Fat

Moderate (no set range)

Protein
15-50gr/meal (no set range)

minimum number of meals/day = 5

copyright@www.extique.com

* See footnote p.124

** Whereas the 50 gram per-meal protein limit is mandatory on the general NHE Eating Plan
it is highly recommended on the bodybuilders' NHE Eating Plan. For an explanation of this
distinction and the relationship between per-meal and per-day protein intake, go to extique.com
and click on 'Ask Rob'.

The Cyclical High-Fat Diet in Historical Context

The bodybuilders' NHE Eating Plan is a radical departure from the dietary strategy followed by most bodybuilders and athletes. I believe that after reading this entire book, you will find the reasoning and scientific evidence underlying the cyclical high-fat diet to be compelling. And you will find the results you achieve with this diet to be even more compelling. Not only can you build mass while remaining lean with the bodybuilders' Eating Plan, but the improvement in energy levels on this diet as compared with the high-carb/low-fat diet is dramatic.

As revolutionary as the bodybuilders' Eating Plan may seem, its roots have been around for a long time. However, because of the prevailing bias against dietary fat coupled with commercial considerations (there is no money to be made selling fat which has a short shelf-life and is relatively expensive, as opposed to processed carbohydrate which is dirt cheap and has a virtually eternal shelf-life), the cyclical high-fat diet is not currently, and likely never will be, in favor among the bodybuilding magazine editors and supplement manufactures that control the flow of information on these issues (see "You Can't Trust What You Read in the Bodybuilding Magazines," in Chapter 21). Nonetheless, the late Vince Gironda, Arnold Schwarzenneger's trainer, was a passionate advocate, from the 1960's to the 1990's, of a high-fat, reduced-carbohydrate diet.

If Gironda's endorsement of a high-fat diet does not assuage your misgivings, consider the fact that Mauro Di Pasquale M.D., arguably the world's foremost sports nutritionist and himself a former powerlifting world champion, advocates a cyclical high-fat diet similar to the bodybuilders' NHE Eating Plan.[35] There are, however, significant differences between the bodybuilders' Eating Plan and Dr. Di Pasquale's "Anabolic Diet." And while I believe that the bodybuilders' NHE Eating Plan is considerably more effective than the Anabolic Diet, I credit Dr. Di Pasquale as the leading pioneer of the cyclical high-fat diet for bodybuilding and sports performance. In closing, I can't promise results because metabolic individuality can render general principles inapplicable to a particular person. Having said that, I recommend to individuals embarking on the bodybuilders' Eating Plan that if you don't have much money, start saving-up now because you may soon be forced to buy a new wardrobe of clothes several sizes bigger.

References

1. Berneis K, et al. Effects of Hyper- and Hypoosmolality on Whole Body Protein and Glucose Kinetics in Humans. *Am J Physiol* 1999;276:E188.

2. Bilz S, Ninnis R, Keller U. Effects of Hypoosmolality on Whole-Body Lipolysis in Man. *Metabolism* 1999;48:472.

3. Fallowfield JL, et al. Effect of Water Ingestion on Endurance Capacity during Prolonged Running. *J Sports Sci* 1996;14:497.

4. Hargreaves M, et al. Effect of Fluid Ingestion on Muscle Metabolism during Prolonged Exercise. *J Appl Physiol* 1996;80:363.

5. Bankir L, et al. Direct and Indirect Cost of Urea Excretion. *Kidney Int* 1996;49:1598.

6. Neuhaus OW, Orten JM. *Human Biochemistry*, tenth edition. St. Louis, MO: Mosby Company 1982, p. 567.

7. Lang F, et al. Functional Significance of Cell Volume Regulatory Mechanisms. *Physiol Rev* 1998;78:247.

8. Graf J, Haussinger D. Ion Transport in Hepatocytes: Mechanisms and Correlations to Cell Volume, Hormone Actions and Metabolism. *J Hepatol* 1996;24 (Suppl):53S.

9. vom Dahl S, et al. Regulation of Cell Volume in the Perfused Rat Liver by Hormones. *Biochem J* 1991;280:105.

10. Waldegger S, et al. Effect of Cellular Hydration on Protein Metabolism. *Miner Electrolyte Metab* 1997;23:201.

11. Haussinger D, et al. Cellular Hydration State: An Important Determinant of Protein Catabolism in Health and Disease. *Lancet* 1993;341:1330.

12. Millar ID, et al. Mammary Protein Synthesis is Acutely Regulated by the Cellular Hydration State. *Biochem Biophys Res Commun* 1997;230:351.

13. Haussinger D, et al. Cell Volume is a Major Determinant of Proteolysis Control in Liver. *FEBS Lett* 1991;283:70.

14. Haussinger D. Control of Protein Turnover by the Cellular Hydratation State. *Ital J Gastroenterol* 1993;25:42.

15. Castellani JW, et al. Endocrine Responses during Exercise-Heat Stress: Effects of Prior Isotonic and Hypotonic Intravenous Rehydration. *Eur J Appl Physiol* 1998;77:242.

16. See, infra, notes 26-28.

17. Carlmark B, et al. Intracellular Potassium in Man. A Comparison of In Vivo and In Vitro Measurement Techniques. *Scand J Clin Lab Invest* 1982;42:245.

18. Yawata T. Effect of Potassium Solution on Rehydration in Rats: Comparison with Sodium Solution and Water. *Jpn J Physiol* 1990;40:369.

19. Kehayias JJ, et al. Total Body Potassium and Body Fat: Relevance to Aging. *Am J Clin Nutr* 1997;66:904.

20. Flynn MA, et al. Total Body Potassium in Aging Humans: A Longitudinal Study. *Am J Clin Nutr* 1989;50:713.

21. Waldegger S, et al. Mechanisms and Clinical Significance of Cell Volume Regulation. *Nephrol Dial Transplant* 1998;13:867.

22. Bortner CD, Cidlowski JA. A Necessary Role for Cell Shrinkage in Apoptosis. *Biochem Pharmacol* 1998;56:1549.

23. Bortner CD, Hughes FM Jr, Cidlowski JA. A Primary Role for K+ and Na+ Efflux in the Activation of Apoptosis. *J Biol Chem* 1997;272:32436.

24. Montague JW, et al. A Necessary Role for Reduced Intracellular Potassium during the DNA Degradation Phase of Apoptosis. *Steroids* 1999;64:563.

25. Hughes FM Jr, Cidlowski JA. Potassium is a Critical Regulator of Apoptotic Enzymes In Vitro and In Vivo. *Adv Enzyme Regul* 1999;39:157.

26. Francis KT. Effect of Water and Electrolyte Replacement during Exercise in the Heat on Biochemical Indices of Stress and Performance. *Aviat Space Environ Med* 1979;50:115.

27. Francesconi RP, Sawka MN, Pandolf KB. Hypohydration and Acclimation: Effects on Hormone Responses to Exercise/Heat Stress. *Aviat Space Environ Med* 1984;55:365.

28. Francesconi RP, et al. Plasma Hormonal Responses at Graded Hypohydration Levels during Exercise-Heat Stress. *J Appl Physiol* 1985;59:1855.

29. Martins FM, et al. Total Parenteral Nutrition with Different Ratios of Fat/Carbohydrate at Two Energy Levels: An Animal Study. *JPEN J Parenter Enteral Nutr* 1985;9:47.

30. Bresson JL, et al. Protein-Metabolism Kinetics and Energy-Substrate Utilization in Infants Fed Parenteral Solutions with Different Glucose-Fat Ratios. *Am J Clin Nutr* 1991;54:370.

31. McCargar LJ, et al. Dietary Carbohydrate-to-Fat Ratio: Influence on Whole-Body Nitrogen Retention, Substrate Utilization, and Hormone Response in Healthy Male Subjects. *Am J Clin Nutr* 1989;49:1169.

32. McCargar LJ, Baracos VE, Clandinin MT. Influence of Dietary Carbohydrate-to-Fat Ratio on Whole Body Nitrogen Retention and Body Composition in Adult Rats. *J Nutr* 1989;119:1240.

33. Fery F, et al. Role of Fat-Derived Substrates in the Regulation of Gluconeogenesis during Fasting. *Am J Physiol* 1996;270:E822.

34. Fery F, et al. Inhibition of Lipolysis Stimulates Whole Body Glucose Production and Disposal in Normal Postabsorptive Subjects. *J Clin Endocrinol Metab* 1997;82:825.

35. Di Pasquale M. *The Anabolic Diet*. Optimum Training Systems 1995.

Natural Hormonal Enhancement

Chapter 15

The Carb-Load

There are more old drunkards than old doctors.
Benjamin Franklin

He who has health has hope, and he who has hope has everything.
Arabian proverb

I know a man who gave up smoking, drinking, sex, and rich food.
He was healthy right up to the time he killed himself.
Johnny Carson

The only difference between poison and drugs is the intent of the person administering them.
Unknown

Although the carb-load meals comprise a small percentage of your eating on the NHE Eating Plan, they are essential to your success. Because much of this book seems to have an anti-carbohydrate tone, it is easy to acquire an unduly negative disposition toward carbohydrate. If you allow such a mindset to inhibit you from executing the carb-load, you will not achieve the lasting success that you are looking for from the Eating Plan.

Carbohydrate is problematic only when it is consumed in large quantities, frequently. This is exactly the role that carbohydrate plays in the average American diet, with a preponderance coming in the form of refined carbohydrates – such as sucrose, white flour, and corn syrup - the worst kinds. As demonstrated in Chapter 8, it is this carbohydrate-dominated diet that is largely responsible for the frightful levels of obesity and degenerative disease in the United States. Chronic high-carbohydrate consumption becomes addicting (see Chapter 11); unbalances insulin/glucagon in the short term (see Chapter 10); and in some cases in the long term by promoting insulin resistance (see Chapter 11); [which, besides being a remarkably unhealthy condition (see Chapter 8), can negatively shift your "fat setpoint" (see Chapter 9)]; and locks you into a sugar-burning, muscle-burning, fat-storing, low-energy, state. It's like metabolic prison; and although there is a ready escape, the catch is - you have to eat your way out! The NHE Eating Plan shows you how.

You will have the best of all worlds in terms of eating variety. Between the standard fat-burning meals and the carb-load meals, every food on earth is permissible. Because the NHE Eating Plan allows you to eat all foods (albeit at the right times) with no obligation to restrict overall calories, it is the most flexible and livable dietary plan ever. And rather than being a slave to carbohydrate and having your food desires dictated by hormonal hunger, you will be strategically scheduling carbohydrate feedings to refuel glycogen stores, add variety and pleasure to your diet, and generate advantageous insulin bursts. Then, before carbs have a chance to cause bodyfat storage and drag you back into a sugar-burning state, you cut them off and revert to the standard fat-burning meals. It's very simple - but it's also very effective.

Benefits of the Carb-Load

I. Metabolic Benefits

You learned in Chapter 9 that a thyroid hormone called *triiodothyronine* (T3) is a key regulator of metabolic rate, and that calorie restriction causes a decline in T3. Studies also show that diets that continuously restrict carbohydrate (like the Atkins diet, for instance) cause a reduction in T3, and that administering carbohydrate can restore T3 levels after they have declined.[1,2,3,4,5,6,7,8,9,10] This is one of the reasons why progress screeches to a halt after a few weeks on a low-carbohydrate diet; it also explains why the fat comes piling back on once you quit such a diet. Simply put, any dietary program that causes a reduction in T3 levels is not a viable means of achieving lasting fat loss. Periodic carb-loading prevents a fall in T3 production on the NHE Eating Plan, thereby enabling continued fat loss.

II. Exercise Performance

The carb-load replenishes muscle glycogen stores. Glycogen is crucial to generating intensity when working-out. And as discussed in Chapter 21, intensity is a vital element of hormonally intelligent exercise. Therefore, any dietary program (like the Atkins diet, for instance) that results in continuously low glycogen levels will impair performance of hormonally intelligent exercise. And any dietary program that impairs performance of hormonally intelligent exercise is an enemy of anyone seeking true and lasting physique improvement (as distinguished from temporary weight loss). Moreover, there is specific evidence suggesting that carbohydrate cycling, as prescribed by the NHE Eating Plan, is the most effective dietary strategy for maximizing athletic performance (see p. 241-242).

III. Anabolic Benefits

A. The insulin surge generated by the carb-load speeds amino acids and other nutrients into the muscles, thereby promoting protein synthesis and inhibiting catabolism.[11,12] Periodic carb-loading allows you to capitalize on the acute anabolic effect of insulin while avoiding the lipogenic (fat-producing) effect of chronically elevated insulin. This strategy of maximizing the good while minimizing the bad is called *optimization*. And because insulin is a "double-edged-sword" hormone, our goal is to optimize rather than enhance or suppress it (see "Natural Hormonal Enhancement Strategy in a Nutshell," p. 20).

B. Recall from Chapter 11 that insulin is necessary for production of IGF-1, a powerful anabolic/anti-aging hormone-like substance. The insulin surge generated by the carb-load drives production of IGF-1.

C. Whereas chronic high-carbohydrate intake can lower testosterone levels (by promoting insulin resistance and causing cortisol escalations), periodic high-carbohydrate feedings can boost testosterone by reducing sex-hormone-binding globulin (SHBG).[13,14,15,16] This has the effect of increasing "free" or bioavailable testosterone (see Chapter 22). Periodic high-carbohydrate feedings may also enhance testosterone production at the testicular level.[17]

When to Carb-Load

The formula for when to carb-load is 3 / 4, meaning you carb-load every third day, then every fourth day, then every third day, then every fourth day, etc. For reference, the 3-day cycle is the "short cycle" and the 4-day cycle is the "long cycle." Thus, you are not only cycling your macronutrient intake, but you are also cycling your cycles to prevent your body from fully adapting. In addition, the carb-load should always be the *last meal of the day*. (Note - although the carb-load is the last meal of the day, be sure to observe the guidelines in Chapter 20 pertaining to how much time to allow between consuming carbohydrate and sleeping for purposes of growth hormone release.)

The carb-load should be the last meal of the day for two reasons. For one, to allow a "buffer period" of several hours, without food, for insulin levels to stabilize. Remember, all food is fattening when insulin levels are high. Secondly, recall from our discussion of hormonal hunger in Chapter 11 that an insulin surge tends to evoke cravings a few hours later. Executing the carb-load as the last meal of the day, before going to sleep, counters the threat of hormonal hunger by arranging for you not to be awake to act on any cravings that may arise. (As a corollary to the "tree falls in the forest and no one is there to hear it" question, if a food craving strikes but you are not conscious of it because you are sleeping, is it actually a craving?)

All philosophizing aside, when you wake-up the next morning the carb-load will be a distant memory, and the intervening hours between your carb-load dinner on day 1 and your standard fat-burning breakfast on day 2 will have nullified the carb-load-induced insulin surge. You will be ready to jump back into the standard fat-burning game plan, and to initiate a new cycle of fat loss. Even if cake, cookies, or pizza was part of your carb-load, you will not experience the guilt you ordinarily would from eating these foods while on a fat-loss program, nor will you pay the price you ordinarily would in terms of fat storage.

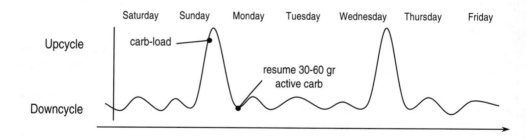

Splitting the Carb-Load

You may wish to split the carb-load into two separate meals. The only difference here relates to the timing and distribution of the ingested carbs. (The two carb-loads should be eaten successively as the second-to-last and last meals of the day; there is no limit on how many carbs you are permitted to eat at either meal; and the carb minimum applies to both meals combined not each meal individually.) The decision whether to split the carb-load is yours to make.

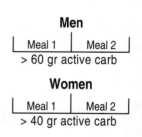

If, when the time comes to carb-load, you have a desire to feast, then you will not want to split. If, on the other hand, your appetite is more modest, then you may wish to split.

Some people will find that they have a low tolerance for a large carbohydrate meal after a few days of carbohydrate restriction. You may find that you get light-headed or nauseous if you consume a lot of carbs at one sitting for your carb-load meal. If so, then you should split the carb-load; and doing so will eliminate the problem. Especially when you are carb-loading on the fourth day (the "long-cycle"), splitting is a good idea because your carbohydrate and particularly your sugar tolerance, will be lower than on the third day. Others will delight in the change of pace of devouring 100 grams of carbohydrate or more at the carb-load meal and, even on the fourth day, will suffer no ill effects from doing so. Personal preference and metabolic individuality dictate whether to split the carb-load.

The Maintenance Plan

Once you have lost as much fat as you wish to lose, you can shift into a maintenance mode. If you wish to indulge more frequently, first try all 3-day cycles instead of the 3 / 4 format. If that does not cause a problem, you can try a 2 / 3 formula, combining 2- and 3-day cycles in the same way described for the 3 / 4 formula. A 2-day cycle (carb-loading every other day) is the furthest you should go. Carb-loading more often than that does not allow for sufficient glycogen depletion between carb-loads to maintain the predominance of the fat-burning metabolic pathway.

The key is to test your way down. Metabolic individuality determines how much indulging you can get away with before you start regaining fat. Whatever your "indulgence threshold" is, you can get away with more if you cycle your indulgences than if you don't. However, be aware that *the more frequently you carb-load, the further you regress into a sugar-burning mode.* Remember, fat burning vs. sugar burning is not a black-and-white issue. Rather, it is a matter of degree. If you are merely trying to keep bodyfat off, it is not necessary to burn as much fat as when you are trying to reduce bodyfat. Accordingly, you can indulge more frequently when you are merely "protecting your losses" as opposed to pursuing fat loss. But during the period in which your objective is to burn as much fat as possible (while preserving muscle mass, of course), the 3 / 4 format is where you should be.

What to Eat When You Carb-Load

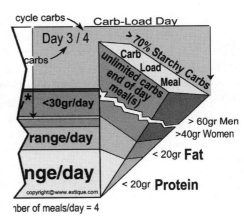

Having addressed *when* to carb-load, the next question is *what* to eat for your carb-load meal(s).

What about Fat?

You should restrict fat at carb-load meals; however, you need not eliminate it entirely. A modest amount of fat will add

141

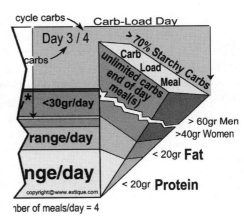inside image: cycle carbs — Carb-Load Day — Day 3 / 4 — carbs — <30gr/day — range/day — nge/day — copyright©www.extique.com — Carb Load — 70% Starchy Carbs — unlimited carbs end of day meal(s) — Carb Load Meal — > 60gr Men — >40gr Women — < 20gr Fat — < 20gr Protein — nber of meals/day = 4

taste, slow the release of sugar into the bloodstream, and help offset the post-meal unpleasantness that sometimes ensues upon a sudden, large influx of carbohydrate. High fat, though, while permissible occasionally during the downcycle, is not appropriate for carb-load meals - at least not in the beginning.

Once you have shifted into a fat-burning mode and have lost a significant amount of bodyfat, you can experiment with a high-fat/high-carb, carb-load. This will open the door to a legion of high-pleasure foods like pizza, ice cream, cake, cookies, and many other such foods from which the conventional dieter would recoil in stark horror. A majority of people will not suffer adverse effects, in terms of fat storage, from a high-fat carb-load once a fat-burning state has been established.[18]

This is an exception to the "conveyor belt" rule discussed in Chapter 10, which states that fat is fattening when eaten in the presence of high insulin levels. While this is the general rule, one high-carb meal is not enough to cause a reversion to a sugar-burning/fat-storing state once a fat-burning state has been established. Therefore, most people can get away with an occasional high-carb/high-fat meal, provided such a meal is properly cycled (i.e., follows and precedes a period of carbohydrate restriction). But you cannot get away with committing this dietary transgression for long. Your reprieve is rescinded if you continue consuming meals high in carbohydrate; the "conveyor belt" is turned back on, and you revert to being a sugar-burner/fat-storer - so be careful.

You are probably wondering how many high-carbohydrate meals can be eaten in succession before your metabolism reverts to sugar-burning/fat-storing. There are too many variables in this equation to give an exact answer. For instance, it depends on the type of carbohydrate eaten (sugary carbs being worse than starchy carbs); how solidly in the fat-burning state you were before going on the carb kick; and individual metabolic factors. The NHE Eating Plan is calculated to avert reversion to a sugar-burning state. Carbohydrate is promptly cut-off after the carb-load meal(s), before your metabolism reverts to sugar burning.

Be prudent when adding fat to carb-load meals. During the first few weeks, at least, keep fat moderate/low at the carb-load. After that, you can experiment with a higher-fat carb-load if you wish. But watch for adverse effects, like a slowing of fat loss or an unfavorable change in blood lipid levels (HDL/LDL cholesterol and triglyceride). While it is generally a good idea to get regular bloodwork done because blood lipid profile is a telling indicator of coronary risk, it is particularly important to keep a watchful eye on blood lipids when you are tinkering with your diet.

Remember, as discussed in Chapters 8 and 10, high insulin coupled with high dietary fat is never a good combination. Having said that, a few unhealthy meals per month may not be so terrible. The NHE Eating Plan is not about turning people into

142

ascetics - it's about losing fat, and keeping it off, while indulging intelligently. This formula allows for lifetime adherence rather than a quick fix that doesn't fix anything, which describes conventional dieting.

During the course of a lifetime on the NHE Eating Plan, all NHE followers will stumble occasionally – including myself. To think otherwise is to be unrealistic (which books are that propose 40:30:30 at every meal, or severe fat or calorie restriction, or perpetual abstention from carbohydrate foods that have become a part of American culture). So rather than intensely striving for perfection in the short-term and then becoming disheartened and quitting when you err, commit yourself to a steady and consistent application of effort in the service of your long-term health and physique objectives. Resolve not to eat an entire cheesecake or drink a twelve-pack of beer. But if it happens, it's not the end of the world. Healthy eating is a lifetime endeavor, one which will likely influence both the length and quality of your life. And like life itself, we will falter occasionally in our efforts to eat right. But if we get back up each time, renew our commitment, and keep moving forward - we cannot fail.

Decisions regarding health, like most decisions, involve a balancing of countervailing considerations. And you must make these decisions - like whether to occasionally depart from a dietary plan - for yourself. With these thoughts in mind, I make the following recommendation: for optimal health, steer clear of high-fat, high-carb meals whenever possible. But if you do combine high fat with high carb, do it in a calculated fashion as outlined above in order to avoid, or at least minimize, the negative effects. In addition, use a technique called *carbohydrate partitioning* to indulge strategically.

Carbohydrate Partitioning

Keeping fat low/moderate at carb-load meals does not necessarily entail avoiding high-fat, high-carb foods like ice cream, cake, and pizza. The key to enjoying these foods as part of the carb-load is just that - make it *part* of the carb-load. I call this technique carbohydrate partitioning. The way it works is that you include a low-fat carbohydrate food and *accompany it with* or *follow it by* (the latter phrase referring to meal-two of a split carb-load, or dessert following a single-meal carb-load) a high-fat, carbohydrate food like cake, pizza, or ice

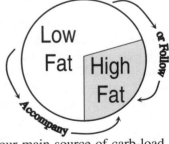

Total Meal is Low-Moderate Fat

cream. For example, you eat pasta with tomato sauce as your main source of carb-load calories and accompany it with buttered garlic bread or follow it by a couple scoops of ice cream. By making a low-fat food the bulk of your carb-load, you limit fat consumption. The key point is that however you distribute the carbohydrate, within one meal or spread-out over two, be sure that *overall* carb-load fat content is low/moderate. As you will see below, carbohydrate partitioning also can be employed in relation to sugar.

143

What about Protein?

Like fat, protein should be restricted at carb-load meals. Protein serves no useful purpose at the carb-load and can cause problems. Specifically, there are two difficulties associated with a substantial amount of protein in the carb-load. For one, the more non-carbohydrate bulk you eat at the carb-load, the less space you will have available in your stomach for carbohydrate. Of course, there are many people who will have no trouble meeting or exceeding the carb-load minimum. But even if protein is not literally getting in the way, it can cause a problem of a different nature at the carb-load; and the problem relates to food combining.

Food combining is a controversial topic. At one extreme, there are several diet books that advocate a complex and highly restrictive set of food combining rules that reads like the bylaws of a multinational corporation. After reading one such book, and wading through and hashing out all the food combining rules it contained, I arrived at the dumbfounding conclusion that we are not supposed to eat anything with anything! In my opinion, this school of thought is, for the most part, silly.

However, existing research and practical experience, including unpleasant recollections of the aftermath of Thanksgiving dinner, indicate that protein and carbohydrate don't mix well. In small to moderate quantities, a mixed protein/carb meal does not present a problem for most people. In large quantities, though, carbohydrate plus protein can impede digestion and elimination, and cause gastrointestinal distress. This is not a problem on the NHE Eating Plan, because during the downcycle carbohydrate is kept low and during the upcycle protein is kept low. In this way, the Eating Plan promotes optimal digestion.

Starchy Carbs vs. Sugary Carbs

The final issue pertaining to the carb-load is what kind of carbohydrate to eat. Aim for at least 70 percent of your carb-load carbohydrate to be of a starchy variety, as opposed to sugary. Should you find that your sweet-tooth has disappeared, which may happen after a few weeks on the NHE Eating Plan, do not feel obligated to eat sugary foods at all. But if you desire a "dessert food," feel free to indulge, using the technique of

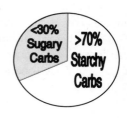

carbohydrate partitioning described above, to ensure that most of your carb-load consists of starchy carbs. Ideal carb-load carbohydrate foods, high in starch and low in sugar, include sweet potatoes, white potatoes, pasta, rice, beans, and oatmeal.

The reason for the distinction between starchy carbs and sugary carbs has nothing to do with insulin response or the glycemic index. Rather, it concerns the relative distribution of glycogen storage from each type of carbohydrate. As you know by now, all carbohydrate is broken down to sugar during digestion. More specifically, starches

144

are broken down to glucose whereas sucrose (the sugar contained in cake, cookies, and ice cream) is a disaccharide consisting of part glucose and part fructose. *Fructose is preferentially used to refill liver glycogen stores, whereas glucose is preferentially used to refill muscle glycogen stores.*[19,20,21]

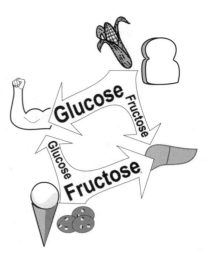

This distinction, and its implications for fat burning and craving control, has been overlooked by just about everyone. Instead, books and magazines have popularized the flawed, misleading, and marginally meaningful glycemic index (see p. 239). Whereas muscle glycogen is a more efficient fuel source for high-intensity muscular activity, liver glycogen is more efficient at raising blood sugar levels under the influence of the hormone glucagon when carbohydrate intake is restricted (which, of course, it will be during the ensuing downcycle). In effect, this means that even after you have resumed carbohydrate restriction after carb-loading, blood sugar, and therefore insulin, will continue to rise and fall for hours as stored sugar is released from the liver into the bloodstream (see p. 78). Fluctuating blood sugar and insulin levels hamper fat burning, decrease energy levels and mental productivity, and give rise to "hormonal hunger" (see Chapters 10, 11).

In addition, sugar, and particularly fructose, when consumed in the large quantities typical of the American diet, stimulate lipogenic enzymes,[22,23,24,25,26] raise serum triglyceride levels and promote insulin resistance,[27,28,29,30,31,32,33,34,35,36,37] and raise LDL cholesterol.[38,39,40] Sadly, diabetics are often advised to consume fructose because of its extremely low glycemic index. This demonstrates the flawed nature of the glycemic index. And, along with the evidence in Chapter 8 concerning the diabetes-worsening effect of the commonly prescribed high-carbohydrate/low-fat diet, it explains why so many Type II diabetics are dying painfully rather than improving their highly treatable condition. Bottom line: **emphasize starchy carbs over sugary carbs when you carb-load**.

Having said all that, don't be deterred from eating fruit because it contains fructose. Although fruit contains a *high percentage* of fructose, the *total amount* is relatively low because the total amount of carbohydrate is relatively low (at least for the HIFWAC fruits listed in Chapter 16). This is in contrast to cake or cookies, which contain a tremendous amount of sucrose (remember, sucrose is a disaccharide made up of half glucose and half fructose). Therefore, although dessert foods may contain a lower percentage of fructose than does fruit, they yield a greater total amount of fructose per ounce.

Misapprehension of this percentage sugar vs. total sugar distinction has prompted some diet "experts" to point an accusatory finger at fruit and to urge avoidance of "fruit

145

Natural Hormonal Enhancement

sugar." When you consider that fruit is a rich source of vitamins, fiber, and disease-combating antioxidants, you realize that, like so many other erroneous instructions that we hear amid the cacophony of health and fitness misinformation, this advice is a disservice. In short, a certain amount of fructose is an unavoidable element of a healthy diet. If you adhere to the carb-limits of the NHE Eating Plan, you will be immunized from the unhealthy effects of high fructose intake – so don't worry about fruit.

Another reason why we limit sugary foods at the carb-load is because sugar will make you sicker quicker if you consume large doses of it after a period of carbohydrate restriction. Individuals involved in activities entailing high-intensity muscular output, like athletes and bodybuilders, should be particularly concerned with maximizing muscle glycogen.

Review: What to Eat When You Carb-Load

♦ During the first few weeks, at least, keep the fat content of the carb-load in the low/moderate range. After a fat-burning state is established, and you have lost a significant amount of bodyfat, you can experiment with adding more fat to the carb-load.

♦ For optimal health, avoid meals containing a high quantity of both fat and carbohydrate.

♦ Protein content of the carb-load should be kept low.

♦ Aim for at least 70% starchy carbs. The higher the ratio of starchy carbs to sugary carbs, the better for fat loss and craving control.

♦ Athletes and bodybuilders should aim for an even higher starchy-carb/sugary-carb ratio to maximize muscle glycogen levels.

♦ Employ carbohydrate partitioning to indulge intelligently. This technique can be used in relation to both sugar and fat.

References

1. Otten MH. The Role of Dietary Fat in Peripheral Thyroid Hormone Metabolism. *Metabolism* 1980;29:930.

2. Madsen M, et al. Effects of Portal Glucose Infusion on Thyroid Hormone Concentrations in Serum after High Energy Trauma in Pigs. *Acta Chir Scand* 1986;152:487.

3. Glade MJ, Luba NK. Serum Triiodothyronine and Thyroxine Concentrations in Weanling Horses Fed Carbohydrate by Direct Gastric Infusion. *Am J Vet Res* 1987;48:578.

4. Spaulding SW, et al. Effect of Caloric Restriction and Dietary Composition of Serum T3 and Reverse T3 in Man. *J Clin Endocrinol Metab* 1976;42:197.

5. Mathieson RA, et al. The Effect of Varying Carbohydrate Content of a Very-Low-Caloric Diet on Resting Metabolic Rate and Thyroid Hormones. *Metabolism* 1986;35:394.

6. Serog P, et al. Effects of Slimming and Composition of Diets on VO2 and Thyroid Hormones in Healthy Subjects. *Am J Clin Nutr* 1982;35:24.

7. Danforth E Jr, Burger AG, Wimpfheimer C. Nutritionally-Induced Alterations in Thyroid Hormone Metabolism and Thermogenesis. *Experientia Suppl* 1978;32:213.

8. Johannessen A, Hagen C, Galbo H. Prolactin, Growth Hormone, Thyrotropin, 3,5,3'-Triiodothyronine, and Thyroxine Responses to Exercise after Fat- and Carbohydrate-Enriched Diet. *J Clin Endocrinol Metab* 1981;52:56.

9. Glass AR, et al. Serum Triiodothyronine in Undernourished Rats: Dependence on Dietary Composition Rather than Total Calorie or Protein Intake. *Endocrinology* 1978;102:1925.

10. Pasquali R, et al. Effect of Dietary Carbohydrates during Hypocaloric Treatment of Obesity on Peripheral Thyroid Hormone Metabolism. *J Endocrinol Invest* 1982;5:47.

11. Biolo G, et al. Physiologic Hyperinsulinemia Stimulates Protein Synthesis and Enhances Transport of Selected Amino Acids in Human Skeletal Muscle. *J Clin Invest* 1995;95:811.

12. See Chapter 10, notes 16-20.

13. Pasquali R, et al. Insulin Regulates Testosterone and Sex Hormone-Binding Globulin Concentrations in Adult Normal Weight and Obese Men. *J Clin Endocrinol Metab* 1995;80:654.

14. Pasquali R, et al. Effects of Acute Hyperinsulinemia on Testosterone Serum Concentrations in Adult Obese and Normal-Weight Men. *Metabolism* 1997;46:526.

15. Peiris AN, et al. The Relationship of Insulin to Sex Hormone-Binding Globulin: Role of Adiposity. *Fertil Steril* 1989;52:69.

16. Strain G, et al. The Relationship between Serum Levels of Insulin and Sex Hormone-Binding Globulin in Men: The Effect of Weight Loss. *J Clin Endocrinol Metab* 1994;79:1173.

17. Adashi EY, et al. Insulin Augmentation of Testosterone Production in a Primary Culture of Rat Testicular Cells. *Biol Reprod* 1982;26:270.

18. Saitoh S, et al. Effects of Short-Term Dietary Change from High Fat to High Carbohydrate Diets on the Storage and Utilization of Glycogen and Triacylglycerol in Untrained Rats. *Eur J Appl Physiol* 1996;74:13.

19. Van Den Bergh AJ, et al. Muscle Glycogen Recovery after Exercise during Glucose and Fructose Intake Monitored by 13C-NMR. *J Appl Physiol* 1996;81:1495.

20. Morikofer-Zwez S, et al. Refeeding of Rats Fasted 36 Hours with Five Different Carbohydrates and with Malt Extract: Differential Effects on Glycogen Deposition in Liver and Muscle, on Plasma Insulin and on Plasma Triglyceride Levels. *J Nutr* 1991;121:302.

21. Ivy JL. Glycogen Resynthesis after Exercise: Effect of Carbohydrate Intake. *Int J Sports Med* 1998;19(Suppl):S142.

22. Fiebig R, et al. Exercise Training Down-Regulates Hepatic Lipogenic Enzymes in Meal-Fed Rats: Fructose versus Complex-Carbohydrate Diets. *J Nutr* 1998;128:810.

23. Katsurada A, et al. Induction of Rat Liver Malic Enzyme Messenger RNA Activity by Insulin and by Fructose. *Biochem Biophys Res Commun* 1983;112:176.

24. Sugawa-Katayama Y, Morita N. Effect of a High Fructose Diet on Lipogenic Enzyme Activities of Meal-Fed Rats. *J Nutr* 1977;107:534.

25. Kazumi T, et al. Effects of Dietary Fructose or Glucose on Triglyceride Production and Lipogenic Enzyme Activities in the Liver of Wistar Fatty Rats, an Animal Model of NIDDM. *Endocr J* 1997;44:239.

26. Carmona A, Freedland RA. Comparison among the Lipogenic Potential of Various Substrates in Rat Hepatocytes: The Differential Effects of Fructose-Containing Diets on Hepatic Lipogenesis. *J Nutr* 1989;119:1304.

27. Zavaroni I, et al. Effect of Fructose Feeding on Insulin Secretion and Insulin Action in the Rat. *Metabolism* 1980;29:970.

28. Thorburn AW, et al. Fructose-Induced In Vivo Insulin Resistance and Elevated Plasma Triglyceride Levels in Rats. *Am J Clin Nutr* 1989;49:1155.

29. Zavaroni I, Chen YD, Reaven GM. Studies of the Mechanism of Fructose-Induced Hypertriglyceridemia in the Rat. *Metabolism* 1982;31:1077.

30. Sleder J, et al. Hyperinsulinemia in Fructose-Induced Hypertriglyceridemia in the Rat. *Metabolism* 1980;29:303.

31. Tuovinen CG, Bender AE. Effect on Dietary Sucrose and Fructose on the Metabolism and Lipid Fractions in Liver in the Rat. *Nutr Metab* 1975;19:1.

32. Tobey TA, et al. Mechanism of Insulin Resistance in Fructose-Fed Rats. *Metabolism* 1982;31:608.

33. Kazumi T, Vranic M, Steiner G. Triglyceride Kinetics: Effects of Dietary Glucose, Sucrose, or Fructose Alone or with Hyperinsulinemia. *Am J Physiol* 1986;250:E325.

34. Hallfrisch J, et al. Effects of Dietary Fructose on Plasma Glucose and Hormone Responses in Normal and Hyperinsulinemic Men. *J Nutr* 1983;113:1819.

35. Reaven GM, Ho H, Hoffman BB. Effects of a Fructose-Enriched Diet on Plasma Insulin and Triglyceride Concentration in SHR and WKY Rats. *Horm Metab Res* 1990;22:363.

36. Coulston AM, et al. Metabolic Effects of Added Dietary Sucrose in Individuals with Noninsulin-Dependent Diabetes Mellitus (NIDDM). *Metabolism* 1985;34:962.

37. Pamies-Andreu E, et al. High-fructose Feeding Elicits Insulin Resistance without Hypertension In Normal Mongrel Dogs. *Am J Hypertens* 1995;8:732.

38. Swanson JE, et al. Metabolic Effects of Dietary Fructose in Healthy Subjects. *Am J Clin Nutr* 1992;55:851.

39. Bantle JP, et al. Metabolic Effects of Dietary Fructose in Diabetic Subjects. *Diabetes Care* 1992;15:1468.

40. Hallfrisch J, Reiser S, Prather ES. Blood Lipid Distribution of Hyperinsulinemic Men Consuming Three Levels of Fructose. *Am J Clin Nutr* 1983;37:740.

Chapter 16

Thermogenesis:
The Science of Using Food to Increase Metabolism

My doctor saved my life. I called him over to my house, and he never showed up.
Unknown

*What society needs is practitioners with more practice in prevention,
not a medical practice with more practitioners.*
Rob Faigin

Conventional thinking conceives of eating in fattening terms, focusing disproportionately on the potential of food to be converted into bodyfat. Just as a knife can injure or help mend injury, and a gun can destroy or defend from destruction, food can make you fat or make you lose fat. Thermogenesis is a central feature of the intrinsic fat-burning potential of food. Specifically, the "thermogenic" or "thermic" effect refers to the calorie-burn associated with digestion and assimilation of food.[1,2,3] In other words, every food contains energy but also *requires an expenditure of energy* when eaten and digested.

Have you ever found yourself sweating after a big meal? This is dietary-induced thermogenesis in action. In effect, you are exercising - not by moving your limbs, but by the activity that is going on inside your body to break down and process the food you ate.

The thermogenic effect of food peaks within one hour after a meal is consumed, and can be quite substantial in terms of the amount of energy dissipated. The magnitude of the thermogenic effect of food ranges 10%-35% of ingested calories, and varies depending on the type of food eaten and individual metabolic differences. Of the three macronutrients, protein outdistances both fat and carbohydrate as a thermogenic stimulant due to the caloric cost incurred in processing amino acids.[4] This is one reason why protein is the centerpiece of the NHE Eating Plan. A meal of pure protein elicits a thermogenic effect amounting to approximately 30% of the meal's total calories, about twice as much as carbohydrate, and more than three times as much as fat.[5,6,7,8,9] In other words, next time you look at the label on a package of lean meat, you can automatically subtract 30% of the calories.

Reducing "Actual" Calories

The *actual* caloric content of a food can be determined by subtracting the caloric "cost" of a food from the total amount of calories that it "pays" into your system. The concept here is a simple one: any calories that get burned-up as a result of eating no longer exist, and thus cannot be turned into bodyfat. These "disappearing calories" must be accounted for - and should be maximized.

Actual Calories = Total Calories* - Caloric "Cost" of Digestion/Assimilation**

* The amount shown on the package label
** Thermogenic effect

Just as accepting a lot of large money payments will fatten your wallet, accepting a lot of large calorie "payments" can fatten your body. Recall from Chapter 9 that deliberate calorie restriction is prohibited on the NHE Eating Plan (although it often happens as a natural result of eliminating hormonal hunger). Therefore, you will not be intentionally altering the "total calories" part of the equation. Rather, the Eating Plan targets the "cost" part of the equation, by increasing it. Returning to the money analogy, if you increase your costs (expenses) while keeping your income constant, your "actual money" decreases in the same way that "actual calories" decreases on the Eating Plan.

One obvious way to increase caloric "costs" is to exercise, but let's defer that topic until Chapter 21 and confine our focus to eating for now. With the NHE Eating Plan, thermogenesis complements lipolytic hormonal enhancement to maximize fat burning. The complementary relationship between thermogenesis and hormonal enhancement works in the following way: as your lipolytic hormones are telling your body to burn fat for fuel instead of sugar, thermogenesis is increasing the overall amount of fuel (calories) burned. It's a very effective one-two punch.

Thus, instead of reducing the total amount of calories consumed like conventional diets, the NHE Eating Plan reduces "actual calories" by increasing thermogenesis. This is a much sounder approach because, whereas reducing total calories slows your metabolism (see Chapter 9), reducing actual calories by means of increasing thermogenesis speeds-up your metabolism. In effect, this approach allows you to avoid the deprivation and metabolic disadvantages of calorie restriction while reducing the amount of food energy available to be converted to bodyfat.

So which foods are highly thermogenic? This question brings us back to "You Can Learn a Lot from an Ancient Warrior" (Chapter 5). All of the "ancient warrior foods" were highly thermogenic. By contrast, processed high-density carbohydrate foods, a dietary staple for most Americans, occupy the opposite end of the spectrum, with a lot of "total calories" relative to "caloric cost" and thus not much of a thermogenic effect. Take white bread, for example. It has been so extensively degraded by processing that your body's work has been done for it by the manufacturer of the food. Your body does not have to work (i.e., pay a caloric cost), because the food is already broken down.

One way to estimate the thermogenic value of a particular food is to assess how much work you must do from the time you put the food in your mouth until you swallow it (I call this the "chew test"). This parallels the amount of energy that will be expended during the balance of the digestive process. When comparing the thermogenic effect of different foods, be sure to compare quantities of equal caloric value.

Bearing this instruction in mind, let's compare 100 calories worth of white bread with 100 calories worth of steak. The steak requires a lot of chewing, whereas the white bread practically dissolves in your saliva with very little chewing required – similarly to cotton candy. What about steak vs. ground beef? Steak wins - know why? Because ground beef has been processed and, as noted a moment ago, processing diminishes the thermogenic value of food. What about apple vs. banana? This one is a closer call, but the apple wins –know why? Because an apple has almost twice as much fiber per ounce.

Thermogenic Foods

Fruits and Vegetables

Fruits and vegetables exert a substantial thermogenic effect because carbohydrate in general is moderately thermogenic, and fiber is highly thermogenic. However, some fruits and vegetables are more carbohydrate-dense than others. For example, potatoes are thermogenic and so are bananas, but they also contain more active carbohydrate than do apples or strawberries. Stated differently, apples and strawberries are more **thermogenic per unit of carbohydrate**. Cruciferous vegetables like broccoli and cauliflower are so thermogenic per unit of carbohydrate that they do not count toward your daily carbohydrate limit after the 7-day metabolic shift period (see below). Everyone knows that broccoli has relatively few total calories, but, in view of its strong thermogenic effect, broccoli has even fewer actual calories.

Because you will be restricting carbohydrate intake during the downcycle, you will want to economize carbohydrate consumption. Eating carbohydrate foods that are thermogenic per unit of carbohydrate allows you to consume a greater volume of food than if you were eating foods of a higher carbohydrate density. A greater volume of food is positively correlated not only with metabolic rate but also with satiety.[10,11] Food volume is important in appetite regulation, because gastric distention and intestinal stimulation send satiety signals to the brain.[12,13,14,15,16,17] Many breakfast cereals, for example, are high in fiber, but have a low thermogenic/carbohydrate ratio. You are limited in how much of such foods you can eat, and bird-like portions are neither satisfying nor significantly increase metabolic rate.

High-fiber/high-water-content (HIFWAC) fruits and non-starchy vegetables are ideal for optimizing thermogenesis. Conversely, consuming carbohydrate foods low in water and fiber forces you to miniaturize portion sizes to stay within carb limits. HIFWAC fruits are less carbohydrate-dense, and thus have greater thermogenic value per unit of carbohydrate than do other fruits.

HIFWAC Fruits (Excellent Thermogenic/Carbohydrate Ratio)	Non-HIFWAC Fruits (Inferior Thermogenic/Carbohydrate Ratio)
Apples, Apricots, Blueberries, Cherries, Grapes, Peaches, Pears, Raspberries, Strawberries	Bananas, Dates, Dried Fruit, Figs, Raisins, Watermelon

An easy way to identify which carbohydrate foods have high thermogenic value per unit of carbohydrate is to assess "active carbs" (see Chapter 14). The lower the active carb rating of a particular carbohydrate food, the more thermogenic that food is per unit of carbohydrate. The reason for this correspondence is that, when calculating active carbs, you subtract fiber (the non-caloric thermogenic element) from total carbohydrate. Accordingly, active carbs can be viewed as a measure of how "unthermogenic" a food is per unit of carbohydrate.

Lower Active Carb Content = More Thermogenic Per Unit of Carbohydrate = Greater Volume Per Unit of Carbohydrate

To illustrate how widely foods vary in volume and thermogenic potency per unit of carbohydrate, consider that in terms of active carbohydrate:

3 cups of broccoli = 3 french fries = 7 jellybeans = 7 cups of mushrooms = 1 marshmallow = 14 cups of lettuce.

As you can see, there is a vast difference between how much calorie-costly work your metabolism must undertake to digest an equivalent amount of active carbohydrate derived from different sources. Suffice to say, eating and digesting 14 cups of lettuce entails much greater thermogenesis than eating and digesting one marshmallow.

Note also from the carbohydrate exchanges above that carbohydrate-dense foods tend to be nutrient-sparse, and carbohydrate-sparse foods tend to be nutrient-dense. Therefore, even a modest increase in your daily intake of carbohydrate-sparse foods will substantially increase your nutrient intake. A *substantial* increase in your daily intake of these foods may even put you on par nutritionally with the ancient warriors (See "You Can Learn a Lot from an Ancient Warrior," in Chapter 5.) The NHE Eating Plan encourages consumption of carbohydrate-sparse foods – and this is one of the many ways in which the NHE Eating Plan promotes optimal health.

The emphasis on the thermogenic/carbohydrate ratio is not meant to imply that you should never eat fruits in the non-HIFWAC category; nor must you completely abstain from other foods with an inferior thermogenic/carbohydrate ratio (like bagels, English muffins, or pasta) during the downcycle. It is important to be comfortable and to adapt the Eating Plan to your tastes. However, with regard to starchy foods, if you are one of those people who "can't eat just one" and finds it more difficult to eat starchy foods in small quantities than not at all, then I recommend eliminating them entirely from your standard fat-burning meals, sticking instead to HIFWAC fruits and non-starchy vegetables. When the carb-load rolls around, you can (and should) eat as much starchy food as you want.

Below, you will find a list of vegetables with exceptionally high thermogenic/carbohydrate ratio - so high, in fact, that they do not count toward your daily carbohydrate limit after the 7-day metabolic shift period. In other words, you can eat them in unlimited quantity. You are encouraged to eat these foods, but watch your toppings/dressings – you must account for them. If you are experiencing difficulty meeting your carb-load minimum (see p. 125), go easy on these bulky vegetables when carb-loading. If you are not having such a problem, then feel free to increase thermogenesis by adding these vegetables to your carb-load meals.

152

Vegetables with the Highest Thermogenic/Carbohydrate Ratio*
(and which can be eaten in unlimited quantity after the first 7 days)

Asparagus	Lettuce
Broccoli	Mushroom
Cabbage	Radicchio
Cauliflower	Radish
Celery	Spinach

If these vegetables don't strike you as being among the most appetizing foods you've ever eaten, remember, as noted in Chapter 13, melted butter or melted cheese can do wonders for the taste. And both of these toppings are permissible in moderate quantities. Furthermore, you will notice from the list that you have the makings of a tasty salad; and since you are allowed to consume fat in moderation, feta cheese, sunflower seeds, and rich dressings are all possibilities. One word of caution, though: many dressings contain more carbohydrate than you might imagine. Be sure to account for the carbohydrate content of the dressing and the croutons if there are any.

Protein Foods

Now that you appreciate how thermogenesis assists your fat loss efforts, you will be happy to know that the NHE Eating Plan has a built-in thermogenic effect deriving from the plentiful protein it prescribes. As mentioned earlier, protein foods are generally the most highly thermogenic. Therefore, *by switching from a carbohydrate-based diet to a protein-based diet, you automatically increase thermogenesis.*

There are two exceptions to the rule that protein foods are the most highly thermogenic: 1) protein foods that are high in fat (fat has low thermogenic value) and 2) protein foods that have been processed. A classic example of a highly processed protein food is protein powder (however, protein powder has compensating virtues that we'll discuss in Chapter 21). Lunch meats, too, are processed; and have lower thermogenic value than fresh, cooked meat (and they are inferior to fresh meat in all other nutritional respects as well; so don't rely on lunch meats as your primary protein source.)

In addition to being powerfully thermogenic, meat is an excellent food in terms of its nutritional content. If you are a vegetarian, tofu and other soy-based products are fine substitutes for meat. Soy protein, having been found to improve cholesterol

---

* There are many vegetables, besides the ones listed, that have an excellent thermogenic/carbohydrate ratio and superb nutrient profile (like tomatoes, peppers, and carrots, for instance). If your favorite vegetable did not make the "all-star team," it means only that they are not freebees and you must account for them in your daily carbohydrate allowance, like you would for any other carbohydrate food. (Technically, tomatoes and peppers are fruits because they contain seeds.)

levels[18,19,20,21] and help prevent cancer,[22,23,24,25] is rapidly attaining nutritional superstar status. Tofu, a soy product, is an outstanding food. In addition to protein, tofu contains "good fat" (see Chapter 18) and is thermogenic (although not to the extent of lean meat, which is the king of thermogenic foods). Soy-based products are crucial for vegetarians on the NHE Eating Plan and can add tasty variety, and health benefits, to the meat-eater's diet. All soy products, however, are not created equal in terms of carbohydrate content; so read the label carefully, and do the appropriate calculation to determine "active carbs."

When preparing meat, take reasonable measures, like draining grease, to avoid excess fat. It is not necessary, however, to surgically remove all visible fat, a practice common among low-fat devotees. Along the same line, make sure that most of the meat you consume contains more protein than fat. Sausage and bacon are fine every once in a while, but stick to lean meat most of the time.

References

1. Segal KR, et al. Thermic Effect of Food at Rest, during Exercise, and after Exercise in Lean and Obese Men of Similar Body Weight. *J Clin Invest* 1985;76:1107.

2. D'Alessio DA. Thermic Effect of Food in Lean and Obese Men. *J Clin Invest* 1988;81:1781.

3. Carlson GL. Nutrient Induced Thermogenesis. *Baillieres Clin Endocrinol Metab* 1997;11:603.

4. Garrow JS, Hawes SF. The Role of Amino Acid Oxidation in Causing Specific Dynamic Action in Man. *Br J Nutr* 1972;27:211.

5. Schwartz RS, et al. The Thermic Effect of Carbohydrate Versus Fat Feeding in Man. *Metabolism* 1985;34:285.

6. Jequier E. Carbohydrate-Induced Thermogenesis in Man. *Int J Vitam Nutr Res* 1986;56:193.

7. Karst H, et al. Diet-Induced Thermogenesis in Man: Thermic Effects of Single Proteins, Carbohydrates and Fats Depending on their Energy Amount. *Ann Nutr Metab* 1984;28:245.

8. Nair KS, Halliday D, Garrow JS. Thermic Response to Isoenergetic Protein, Carbohydrate or Fat Meals in Lean and Obese Subjects. *Clin Sci* 1983;65:307.

9. Zed C, James WP. Dietary Thermogenesis in Obesity. Response to Carbohydrate and Protein Meals: The Effect of Beta-Adrenergic Blockade and Semistarvation. *Int J Obes* 1986;10:391.

10. Crovetti R, et al. The Influence of Thermic Effect of Food on Satiety. *Eur J Clin Nutr* 1998;52:482.

11. Westerterp-Plantenga MS, et al. Satiety Related to 24 H Diet-Induced Thermogenesis during High Protein/Carbohydrate vs High Fat Diets Measured in a Respiration Chamber. *Eur J Clin Nutr* 1999;53:495.

12. Davis JD, Collins BJ. Distention of the Small Intestine, Satiety, and the Control of Food Intake. *Am J Clin Nutr* 1978;31(Suppl):S255.

13. Read N, French S, Cunningham K. The Role of the Gut in Regulating Food Intake in Man. *Nutr Rev* 1994;52:1.

14. Pappas TN, Melendez RL, Debas HT. Gastric Distension is a Physiologic Satiety Signal in the Dog. *Dig Dis Sci* 1989;34:1489.

15. Schick RR, et al. Effect of Intraduodenal or Intragastric Nutrient Infusion on Food Intake in Man. *Z Gastroenterol* 1991;29:637.

16. Wirth JB, McHugh PR. Gastric Distension and Short-Term Satiety in the Rhesus Monkey. *Am J Physiol* 1983;245:R174.

154

17. Rolls BJ, et al. Volume of Food Consumed Affects Satiety in Men. *Am J Clin Nutr* 1998;67:1170.

18. Baum JA, et al. Long-Term Intake of Soy Protein Improves Blood Lipid Profiles and Increases Mononuclear Cell Low-Density-Lipoprotein Receptor Messenger RNA in Hypercholesterolemic, Postmenopausal Women. *Am J Clin Nutr* 1998;68:545.

19. Nagata C, et al. Decreased Serum Total Cholesterol Concentration is Associated with High Intake of Soy Products in Japanese Men and Women. *J Nutr* 1998;128:209.

20. Carroll KK. Review of Clinical Studies on Cholesterol-Lowering Response to Soy Protein. *J Am Diet Assoc* 1991;91:820.

21. Wong WW, et al. Cholesterol-Lowering Effect of Soy Protein in Normocholesterolemic and Hypercholesterolemic Men. *Am J Clin Nutr* 1998;68(Suppl):1385S.

22. Messina MJ, et al. Soy Intake and Cancer Risk: In Vitro and In Vivo Data. *Nutr Cancer* 1994;21:113.

23. Constantinou AI, AE Krygier, RR Mehta. Genistein Induces Maturation of Cultured Human Breast Cancer Cells and Prevents Tumor Growth in Nude Mice. *Am J Clin Nutr* 1998;68(Suppl):1426S

24. Stephens FO. Phytoestrogens and Prostate Cancer: Possible Preventive Role. *Med J Aust* 1997;167:138.

25. Schleicher RL, et al. The Inhibitory Effect of Genistein on the Growth and Metastasis of a Transplantable Rat Accessory Sex Gland Carcinoma. *Cancer Lett* 1999;136:195.

Chapter 17

Protein Optimization
and
Meal Frequency

Health nuts are going to feel stupid someday, dying of nothing.
Redd Foxx

The more the "experts" preach, the fatter we get; and the fatter we get, the more the "experts" preach.
Rob Faigin

Nothing illustrates more clearly the bankruptcy of the conventional wisdom on diet than the way in which protein has been relegated to second-class status, and meat, a major source of protein and many other nutrients, condemned. Amid the misguided fat-phobia frenzy, protein has been found guilty by association because many protein sources, like red meat and dairy products, contain a substantial amount of fat. Because both fat and protein, when utilized properly, are our allies and not our enemies, this has been a double-blunder. It is one of the many reasons why the more the "experts" preach, the fatter we get.

Protein, made-up of amino acids, has an extremely impressive resume. Except for water, it is more plentiful in our bodies than any other substance. Protein is derived from the Greek word *protos*, "first" – a fitting description given that it is the main constituent of all living cells. Our immune system is chiefly composed of protein, and so are the thousands of enzymes that catalyze every bodily function from the blink of an eye to the burning of fat. The vital anabolic processes by which the body renews and rebuilds itself require protein. Protein deficiency is marked by wholesale deterioration of the body that mirrors the aging process, including impaired immunity, loss of lean body mass, and diminished mental function and physical vigor. While some amino acids can be synthesized by the body, others must be supplied by diet and are termed "essential amino acids." Specifically, absent regular dietary intake of the following amino acids, human life cannot be sustained: leucine, isoleucine, valine, lysine, methionine, phenylalanine, threonine, tryptophan.

These and other amino acids not only sustain life but also afford metabolic and hormonal advantages integral to physique enhancement. Protein elevates metabolic rate by means of the thermogenic effect discussed in the previous chapter. Hormonally, protein intake is positively correlated with growth hormone,[1,2] IGF-1,[3,4,5] and glucagon.[6,7] These hormones, collectively, exert an anabolic and lipolytic effect.

Notwithstanding protein's many virtues, more is not necessarily better. In the ongoing controversy between the low-fat crowd and the Atkins dieters, the low-fatties hurl accusations that a high-protein diet damages kidneys. This charge is a stretch, but not completely unfounded.[8] Excessive protein intake over a long period of time can adversely affect kidney health; but a protein-rich diet that is not excessive does not present a problem.[9,10] If you adhere to the 50-gram-per-meal limit on protein intake and you do not have existing kidney problems, protein overconsumption will not be an issue on the NHE Eating Plan.

Another beneficial function of the NHE Eating Plan's per-meal limit on protein intake is prevention of fat storage. This brings us to the second reason why more protein is not necessarily better. In Chapter 10, "The Hormonal Response to Food," you learned that, while carbohydrate is the primary stimulus for insulin secretion, protein too can propel insulin levels into the fat-storage zone when too much of it is eaten at one sitting. This is why the Eating Plan emphasizes protein optimization, not maximization.

Protein *consumption* does not equate precisely with protein *absorption*. This subtle point is widely missed, rarely discussed, and very important. Maximizing protein absorption is advantageous because it allows you to consume less protein than would otherwise be necessary to derive the same benefits, thus avoiding the fattening hormonal response that results from consuming too much protein. Hence, with protein optimization you maximize the benefits of dietary protein while avoiding its potential drawbacks.

Consumption ≠ Absorption

Optimization: A Recurring Theme of Natural Hormonal Enhancement

Optimization means maximizing the good while minimizing the bad. It is a recurring theme of Natural Hormonal Enhancement because hormonal effects are rarely a black-and-white matter. Most factors that affect your hormones are to some extent a double-edged sword.

In Chapter 11, you saw how this phenomenon plays-out in respect to carbohydrate - restrict carbs too tightly and IGF-1 is suppressed; eat too many carbs and growth hormone is suppressed. In addition, individual hormones sometimes have both "good" and "bad" functions (see, for example, the discussion in Chapter 10 concerning insulin and glucagon). This is why the simplistic good-food/bad-food dichotomy that dominates current dietary philosophy is fatally flawed. **The key to building a great body is subtler than eliminating "bad" foods from your diet or exercising "more"; it involves successfully navigating the course between good hormonal effects and bad ones.**

This double-edged-hormonal-effects phenomenon applies to exercise, too. Exercise often stimulates both good and bad hormones, simultaneously. However, by knowing how properly to manipulate exercise variables (i.e., volume, frequency, intensity, duration, load, and exercise selection) you can maximize the good, while minimizing the bad, hormonal effects. This can translate to a tremendous difference in the results you achieve from exercise (see Chapter 21).

How Much to Consume?

There is a distinct lack of consensus on this topic in the scientific community, and it has long been one of the more divisive issues among nutritionists and health writers. I wish I had the definitive answer that would still the waters of dissension and bring closure to this contentious issue - but I don't. Nor do I think such an answer is possible.

The answer to how much protein to consume cannot be generalized; it depends on several factors that vary from individual to individual. In theory, there is an optimal protein level for each person, influenced by activity level (particularly whether you exercise and the volume and type of exercise), percentage of lean body mass, caloric intake, age, and overall nutritional status. Several health writers have thrown their hat into this ring of controversy by advancing sophisticated formulas for determining how much protein one should consume each day. *The Zone*, by Dr. Barry Sears, is a prime example of this worthy but doomed effort. While I admire the intellectual energy that goes into developing such an elaborate system, I believe that protein consumption formulas are more likely to mislead than enlighten because they do not account for all of the relevant variables. Any formula that did account for all the variables would probably necessitate that you enlist the services of a Wall Street accounting firm to figure-out what to eat.

Even more misleading than protein consumption formulas is the RDA, which ignores all of the variables enumerated in the foregoing paragraph. In any case, when discussing the RDA, it is important to bear in mind that the RDA reflects the amount of a nutrient necessary to stave-off deficiency. When I hear defenders of the RDA point to these paltry allowances and say, "that's all you need," I just shake my head in dismay. By the same reasoning, we all might as well settle for earning minimum wage since "that's all we need" - to eke-out an impoverished existence.

In addition, the RDA has not kept pace with research in sports nutrition that has established that protein needs increase with intensive exercise,[11,12,13,14,15,16,17,18] thereby rendering the RDA irrelevant for athletes and bodybuilders. Furthermore, the NHE Eating Plan uses protein as a dietary instrument to elicit advantageous hormonal and metabolic responses; the RDA certainly does not envision this aspect of protein consumption. In short, the RDA should not be cast idly aside - rather it should be thrown with great force.

Most health authorities maintain that the American diet contains more than enough protein and that we should crank-up the carbs rather than concerning ourselves with protein. I suspect that this position is colored by the prevailing pro-carbohydrate/anti-protein bias. When you get past fashionable statements paying homage to conventional wisdom and look at the evidence, a different picture emerges.

Setting aside the issue of "enough for what?" (averting deficiency or promoting optimal health?), a recent USDA food intake study[19] suggests that the reigning notion that Americans get all the protein they need is untrue for older individuals, and especially women, even if "enough" is defined in the scantiest terms. This study found that approximately 25% of men and 30% of women over 50 years of age fall below the RDA for protein, with this figure rising to 36% for men over 70 years of age, and 43% for women in that age group. The study shows, moreover, that approximately 13% of all women (20 years of age and older) are below 75% of the RDA for protein. Among the over-70-years-of-age group, 15% of men and 17% of women fall below 75% of the RDA for protein. I would suggest to the "experts" that they review this data before casually dismissing the idea that there is reason to be concerned about getting enough protein.

Given the importance of protein for maintaining muscle mass and immune function, it is clear, by negative implication, that sub-optimal protein intake can accelerate the age-related decline in muscle mass and immune function. While the importance of adequate protein for maintaining a strong, healthy body is old news, these particular facts bear repeating to those people whose approach to combating the degenerative effects of aging includes avoiding protein in order to pack-in the carbs. Interestingly, the long-lived, rice-eating Japanese, with an average lifespan of 80+ years, who are frequently held out as an example of the benefits of a high-carbohydrate diet, consume more protein than do Americans on a percentage-of-total-calories basis.[20] *

Having noted above that excessive protein intake over a long period of time is unhealthy, let us also observe that excessive anything isn't usually good for you. Those authorities who warn against too much protein are often referring to unbalanced liquid protein crash diets, which were responsible for several deaths in the 1970's due to electrolyte imbalance and consequent heart arrhythmia caused by this extreme approach. Stay away from these diets - weight loss doesn't do you any good when it occurs in the cemetery.

While the recommendation to avoid extreme protein diets is sound, the general proposition that a protein-rich diet is unhealthy also has gained currency. And this notion is fundamentally ridiculous in view of the evidence presented in Chapter 5 showing that human beings evolved on a protein-rich diet. As noted earlier, anti-protein is typically an offshoot of anti-fat. In addition, anti-protein is a byproduct of the pro-carbohydrate movement inasmuch as protein gets displaced from the diet in the misled effort to elevate carbohydrate to the recommended 60%-70% of total caloric intake. It is interesting how the high-carb crowd advances vague, unfounded warnings that protein is bad for you while ignoring the fact that refined-carbohydrate-based diets have been linked to virtually every major degenerative disease that afflicts the Western world (see Chapter 8).

While more is not necessarily better, too little protein is unhealthy because, unlike carbohydrate, the human body requires a certain amount of protein to function properly. The NHE Eating Plan, by making protein the centerpiece of your diet, effectively precludes deficiency. But this is an incidental benefit given that our objective is to build an excellent body, not merely to keep from becoming afflicted with deficiency disorders.

* The Japanese lifespan, which places them among the longest living people on Earth, is truly remarkable when one considers that they live on a cramped, overcrowded, heavily air-polluted island. Moreover, their diet is significantly higher in carbohydrate than other healthy, long-lived populations like the French and the Eskimos, discussed in Chapter 8. There are three plausible explanations for this: vegetables, soy, and fish (green tea probably contributes, too). Fish and soy are the principal protein sources of the Japanese, and, as noted above, the Japanese diet is considerably higher in protein than commonly believed.

Soy, fish, and vegetables each possess potent disease-fighting attributes. In addition, recall from Chapter 8 that high carbohydrate *plus* high fat is considerably more destructive than high carbohydrate alone. The Japanese diet is relatively low in fat, which would tend to mitigate the harm caused by their higher-than-ideal carbohydrate intake. In any event, I suspect that a lifetime of high-vegetable, high-soy, and high-fish intake collectively confers a very powerful cardiovascular-/cancer-protective effect that more than compensates for any transgressions committed in the area of carbohydrate consumption. All in all, in terms of diet, the Japanese do much more right than wrong - and that is probably a major reason why they live so long.

Maximizing Absorption

You learned in Chapter 10 that carbohydrate can be stored as glycogen or bodyfat and used later for energy. Dietary fat too can be stored, as bodyfat, for later usage. Protein is the only macronutrient that cannot be stored in a readily accessible form. When sufficient dietary protein is not forthcoming, protein that has been incorporated into your body structure, as muscle, is broken down under the direction of catabolic hormones (see Chapter 11). Therefore, protein consumption pattern is pivotal to combating catabolism. And as we know, minimizing catabolism is one of the keys to building a strong body and counteracting the physical deterioration of aging.

To prevent muscle from being degraded, while simultaneously promoting muscular enhancement/growth, you must maintain a supply of readily available amino acids in your bloodstream. Compounding the fact that you cannot store protein is the fact that you are limited in how much protein you can absorb at one sitting to between 30-50 grams.[21] Accordingly, **spread-out protein consumption by consuming less protein more frequently, rather than more protein less frequently**.

Spreading-out protein consumption allows for greater absorption and more efficient use of ingested protein.[22] Furthermore, frequent protein feedings keep your blood amino acid pool "topped-off" so your muscles always have a ready supply of amino acids to use as building blocks in the construction of a better body. In addition, frequent protein intake increases amino acid availability to the brain for conversion to neurotransmitters to enhance emotional well-being and mental productivity.*

Gorging oneself with protein is antagonistic to fat loss because at high intake levels, protein provokes an aggressive insulin response. And since you cannot absorb more than approximately 50 grams of protein at one sitting anyway, you are not getting any redeeming benefit from the extra protein. Protein is the least apt of the macronutrients to be turned into fat, but it can happen if you consume too much protein at one sitting.

There are several reasons why protein is less likely than either fat or carbohydrate to be stored as bodyfat. In addition to the fact that protein stimulates far less insulin per gram than does carbohydrate (see Chapter 10), converting protein to fat is a

---

* In Chapter 11, in our discussion of serotonin, I stated that "you can increase baseline serotonin levels, but if you send it soaring - look-out below." By providing a steady incoming supply of tryptophan, you support serotonin production. By contrast, a high-carbohydrate/low-protein meal, by causing a temporary hormonal imbalance, precipitates a flood of tryptophan into the brain thereby inducing an unnatural serotonin spike, without furnishing the raw material (tryptophan) to finance the spike. In addition to serotonin, other amino acids, too, support the production of other neurotransmitters pertinent to mental performance and emotional well-being (see Chapters 10, 11). And utilization of these amino acids, as well, can be maximized by frequent protein feedings (but remember to keep the feedings small- to medium-sized).

metabolically inefficient process (meaning it requires a lot of energy relative to the energy provided by protein). Besides, your body would rather use protein for the many constructive purposes that protein serves. Nevertheless, if you consume too much protein at one sitting, your body has no choice. Insulin gets called forth to clear the excess amino acids from the bloodstream, and amid high insulin everything you eat - protein, carbohydrate, and fat – is more prone to be converted to bodyfat (this is the "conveyor-belt problem" described in Chapter 10). **Stay below 50 grams of protein per meal**, especially a mixed meal in which carbohydrate is present, and you will avoid this pitfall.

Meal Frequency

In the same way that a regimen of more frequent, smaller meals maximizes absorption and utilization of protein, it also maximizes absorption and utilization of other nutrients. But the advantages of this powerful dietary technique go further. It also neutralizes cravings, and promotes fat loss and muscle maintenance/development.

In both animal[23,24,25] and human studies,[26,27,28,29,30] more frequent eating is associated with less fat storage at a given level of caloric intake. I suspect that this fact is partly attributable to a greater cumulative thermogenic effect resulting from this pattern of eating. The primary explanation, though, is hormonal. Specifically, a regimen entailing more frequent, smaller feedings stabilizes and lowers insulin levels.[31,32,33,34] Consequently, you tend to eat less food overall (see p. 100); and of the food you do eat, less gets stored as bodyfat.

Remember, insulin is fat-producing only when it reaches high levels. Hence, by keeping insulin levels out of the "fat-storage zone," you defuse its lipogenic properties. Stated differently, more frequent insulin secretions of lesser magnitude is preferable to less frequent insulin secretions of greater magnitude. This explains why the "starve and stuff" eating pattern, common among dieters, is hormonally incorrect. The "starve and stuff" format results from resisting the urge to eat until overcome by it, and it is the most effective form of eating for propelling insulin into the fat-storage zone. Conversely, distributing caloric intake among more, smaller, feedings achieves the twin objectives of lowering insulin and narrowing its range of fluctuation. In so doing, you avoid triggering insulin's fat-promoting capability while enjoying its anabolic benefits.

Speaking of anabolic benefits, a recently published study indicates that, in addition to facilitating fat loss, more frequent eating helps preserve muscle mass against the ravages of calorie restriction.[35] * The subjects of this study were two groups of boxers on a calorie-restricted diet. While both groups consumed 1,200 calories a day, the two-meal-a-day group lost significantly more lean body mass than did the six-meal-a-day group.

---

* It is not uncommon for trial and error, although a highly inefficient way of learning, to get ahead of science. This is one such case, as bodybuilders have been devoutly practicing meal frequency for decades based on the belief, now found to be true, that more frequent, smaller meals facilitate muscular development.

This finding harmonizes with a study published in the *New England Journal of Medicine*, which found that, in addition to lowering insulin levels, more frequent, smaller feedings lowers cortisol levels.[36]*

While "three squares" a day may seem more natural than frequent nibbling, don't make the mistake of confusing "conventional" with "natural." In fact, there is no evidence that the "ancient warriors," whose eating habits we explored in Chapter 5, partitioned their food intake into three equally spaced feedings as do modern day *Homo sapiens*. The more plausible view is that the three-meal-a-day convention emerged contemporaneously with the Industrial Revolution, prompted by the need to conform eating patterns to factory life. Studies of nonindustrialized societies, showing an absence of the "three square" custom, reinforce the idea that "meals" as we know them are artificial constructs.

If you are not yet sold on the benefits of more frequent, smaller meals, consider the fact that gorging (eating one or two large meals per day) has been linked to an increased risk of heart disease.[37] Conversely, increasing meal frequency alone, with no alteration in the kind or amount of food consumed, can improve blood lipid profile.[38,39,40,41,42,43] This benefit is likely owed to the insulin-lowering effect of smaller, more frequent meals (recall from Chapter 8 that insulin regulates cholesterol and triglyceride production). Clearly, a little nibbling can go a long way toward better health and improved body composition, whereas "three squares a day" is more likely to make you round. So remember, it's better to graze than to gorge.

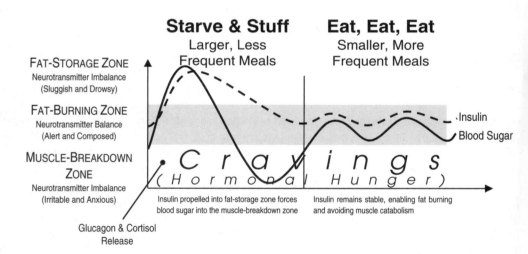

---

* It makes perfect sense that stabilizing insulin would lower cortisol. Recall from the discussion of the "sugar-burner-deprived-of-sugar" scenario, in Chapter 11, that when blood sugar levels become depressed as a result of an insulin surge, muscle-eating catabolic hormones like cortisol are released. Therefore, the "muscle-breakdown zone" for blood sugar is the opposite side of the coin of the "fat-storage zone" for insulin.

References

1. Suminski RR, et al. Acute Effect of Amino Acid Ingestion and Resistance Exercise on Plasma Growth Hormone Concentration in Young Men. *Int J Sport Nutr* 1997;7:48.

2. Isidori A, LoMonaco A, Cappa M. A Study of Growth Hormone Release in Man After Oral Administration of Amino Acids. *Curr Med Res Opin* 1981;7:475.

3. Isley WL, Underwood LE, Clemmons DR. Dietary Components that Regulate Serum Somatomedin-C Concentrations in Humans. *J Clin Invest* 1983;71:175.

4. Clemmons DR, Seek MM, Underwood LE. Supplemental Essential Amino Acids Augment the Somatomedin-C/Insulin-Like Growth Factor I Response to Refeeding after Fasting. *Metabolism* 1985;34:391.

5. Schurch MA, et al. Protein Supplements Increase Insulin-like Growth Factor-I Levels and Attenuate Proximal Femur Bone Loss in Patients with Recent Hip Fracture. A Randomized, Double-Blind, Placebo-Controlled Trial. *Ann Int Med* 1998;128:801.

6. Schmid R, et al. Circulating Amino Acids and Pancreatic Endocrine Function after Ingestion of a Protein-Rich Meal in Obese Subjects. *J Clin Endocrinol Metab* 1989;68:1106.

7. Schmid R, et al. Contribution of Postprandial Amino Acid Levels to Stimulation of Insulin, Glucagon, and Pancreatic Polypeptide in Humans. *Pancreas* 1992;7:698.

8. Dunger A, et al. Functional Alterations in the Rat Kidney Induced Either by Diabetes or High Protein Diet. *Exp Clin Endocrinol Diabetes* 1997;105(Suppl):48S.

9. Skov AR, et al. Changes in Renal Function during Weight Loss Induced by High vs Low-Protein Low-Fat Diets in Overweight Subjects. *Int J Obes Relat Metab Disord* 1999;23:1170.

10. Blum M, et al. Protein Intake and Kidney Function in Humans: Its Effect on 'Normal Aging'. *Arch Intern Med* 1989;149:211.

11. Tarnopolsky MA, MacDougall JD, Atkinson SA. Influence of Protein Intake and Training Status on Nitrogen Balance and Lean Body Mass. *J Appl Physiol* 1988;64:187.

12. Lemon PW. Do Athletes Need More Dietary Protein and Amino Acids? *Int J Sport Nutr* 1995;(5 Suppl):S39.

13. Friedman JE, Lemon PW. Effect of Chronic Endurance Exercise on Retention of Dietary Protein. *Int J Sports Med* 1989;10:118.

14. Tarnopolsky MA, et al. Evaluation of Protein Requirements for Trained Strength Athletes. *J Appl Physiol* 1992;73:1986.

15. Lemon PW. Effects of Exercise on Dietary Protein Requirements. *Int J Sport Nutr* 1998;8:426.

16. Lemon PW, Dolny DG, Yarasheski KE. Moderate Physical Activity Can Increase Dietary Protein Needs. *Can J Appl Physiol* 1997;22:494.

17. Lemon PW, et al. Protein Requirements and Muscle Mass/Strength Changes during Intensive Training in Novice Bodybuilders. *J Appl Physiol* 1992;73:767.

18. Meredith CN, et al. Dietary Protein Requirements and Body Protein Metabolism in Endurance Trained Men. *J Appl Physiol* 1989;66:2850.

19. *USDA Continuing Survey of Food Intakes by Individuals, 1994-1995;* ARS, Beltsville Human Nutrition Center, Food Surveys Research Group.

20. McArdle WD, Katch FI, Katch VL. *Exercise Physiology.* Baltimore, MD: Williams and Wilkins 1996, p. 26.

21. Colgan M. *Optimum Sports Nutrition.* NY: Advanced Research Press 1993, p. 165.

22. Bujko J, et al. Benefit of More But Smaller Meals at a Fixed Daily Protein Intake. *Z Ernahrungswiss* 1997;36:347.

23. Armstrong MK, Romsos DR, Leveille GA. Time Sequence of Lipogenic Changes in Adipose Tissue of Rats when Converted from Ad Libitum Feeding to Meal-Eating. *J Nutr* 1976;106:884.

24. Ticca M, Tomassi G. Effect of Age and Duration of Meal-Eating on Body Composition and on Lipogenesis and Cellularity of Adipose Tissue in Male Rats. *S TA NU* 1975;5:23.

25. Palmquist DL, Learn DB, Baker N. Re-Evaluation of Effects of Meal Feeding on Lipogenic Activation by Glucose in Rats. *J Nutr* 1977;107:502.

26. LeBlanc J, Mercier I, Nadeau A. Components of Postprandial Thermogenesis in Relation to Meal Frequency in Humans. *Can J Physiol Pharmacol* 1993;71:879.

27. Fabry P, et al. Effect of Meal Frequency in School Children, Changes in Weight-Height Proportion and Skinfold Thickness. *Am J Clin Nutr* 1966;18:358.

28. Metzner HL, et al. The Relationship between Frequency of Eating and Adiposity in Adult Men and Women in the Tecumseh Community Health Study. *Am J Clin Nutr* 1977;30:712.

29. Bray GA. Lipogenesis in Human Adipose Tissue: Some Effects of Nibbling and Gorging. *J Clin Invest* 1972;51:537.

30. Ortega RM, et al. [Relationship between the Number of Daily Meals and the Energy and Nutrient Intake in the Elderly. Effect on Various Cardiovascular Risk Factors]. *Nutr Hosp* 1998;13:186. Spanish.

31. Jones PJ, Namchuk GL, Pederson RA. Meal Frequency Influences Circulating Hormone Levels but Not Lipogenesis Rates in Humans. *Metabolism* 1995;44:218-23

32. Bertelsen J, et al. Effect of Meal Frequency on Blood Glucose, Insulin, and Free Fatty Acids in NIDDM Subjects. *Diabetes Care* 1993;16:4.

33. Jones PJ, Leitch CA, Pederson RA. Meal-Frequency Effects on Plasma Hormone Concentrations and Cholesterol Synthesis in Humans. *Am J Clin Nutr* 1993;57:868.

34. Jenkins DJ, et al. Nibbling Versus Gorging: Metabolic Advantages of Increased Meal Frequency. *N Engl J Med* 1989;321:929.

35. Iwao S, Mori K, Sato Y. Effects of Meal Frequency on Body Composition during Weight Control in Boxers. *Scand J Med Sci Sports* 1996;6:265.

36. See, supra, note 34.

37. Fabry P, Tepperman J. Meal Frequency - A Possible Factor in Human Pathology. *Am J Clin Nutr* 1970;23:1059.

38. Arnold LM, et al. Effect of Isoenergetic Intake of Three or Nine Meals on Plasma Lipoproteins and Glucose Metabolism. *Am J Clin Nutr* 1993;57:446.

39. McGrath SA, Gibney MJ. The Effects of Altered Frequency of Eating on Plasma Lipids in Free-Living Healthy Males on Normal Self-Selected Diets. *Eur J Clin Nutr* 1994;48:402.

40. Edelstein SL, et al. Increased Meal Frequency Associated with Decreased Cholesterol Concentrations; Rancho Bernardo, CA, 1984-1987. *Am J Clin Nutr* 1992;55:664.

41. See, supra, note 30.

42. See, supra, note 33.

43. See, supra, note 34.

Using Dietary Fat to Burn Bodyfat

The important message is not to eliminate fat, but to replace the bad fat with the good.
Dr. Walter Willet, Professor of Epidemiology and Nutrition, Harvard University

Essential fats may be the savior of twentieth-century disease conditions and immune disorders.
Ann Gittleman, *Beyond Pritikin*

In trying to eliminate fat from our diets, we may wind up tossing out our health - and our fitness - as well.
Living Fit magazine, Aug. 1997

There is no longer any doubt in science that inadequate intake of [essential fats] means
higher bodyfat no matter what diet, fat-loss drugs, or other attack on fat you may adopt.
Dr. Michael Colgan, *Natural Muscular Development,* Oct. 1997

Eating a fat-restricted diet won't make you live longer, it'll just make your life seem longer.
Rob Faigin

The idea that eating fat can help you shed bodyfat may be a bit disorienting in view of the prevailing negativity about this most maligned of macronutrients. But without dietary fat, your fat loss efforts will surely come to failure so you had better banish the fat phantoms from your head before you begin the NHE Eating Plan. If you have not read Chapter 8, please do so now as this chapter is a sequel to that chapter.

First, I cannot overemphasize the following fact, which I have stressed repeatedly throughout this book: WHETHER OR NOT DIETARY FAT IS FATTENING DEPENDS ON YOUR HORMONAL STATE. If you are a sugar-burner, your metabolism is geared toward carbohydrate utilization and incoming dietary fat gets channeled to adipose tissue to be added to your fat stockpile. By contrast, as a fat-burner, the sugar-burning (glycolytic) pathway is suppressed and the fat-burning (lipolytic) pathway is activated. Consequently, incoming dietary fat gets burned at a high rate along with its biochemical sibling - bodyfat. This does not mean that a fat-burner does not use both glucose and fat, but that the relative reliance on each of these fuel sources is skewed toward fat and away from sugar.

The NHE Eating Plan calls for moderate fat intake and an emphasis on good fat. I will elaborate on what is meant by "moderate" and "good" in a moment. But first, let's examine the relationship between dietary fat and fat burning. For one, fat helps you get into, and stay in, a fat-burning mode. In other words, dietary fat facilitates the metabolic shift from sugar burning to fat burning. Additionally, fat is essential to defeating cravings, which, otherwise, will likely defeat you.

It's fascinating to observe how nutrition myths get propagated to the point where they become, supposedly, common knowledge. One such myth is that we need carbohydrate for energy. The perpetuation of this myth is partly attributable to commercial considerations. High-carbo drinks and bars, which bring-in a fortune each year for the companies that manufacture and sell them, are comprised mainly of high fructose corn syrup, one of the cheapest food ingredients known to man. Alternatively, many of these ingeniously marketed "performance" foods contain maltodextrin or glucose polymers which, despite the impressive, high-tech-sounding names are basically dirt-cheap, nutrient-deplete, laboratory-manipulated starches.

The most insidious aspect of the myth that you need carbohydrate for energy is that it is somewhat of a self-fulfilling prophecy. When you regularly consume a high quantity of carbohydrate, you become a sugar-burner; and as a sugar-burner, your body relies heavily on sugar and is inefficient at burning fat for energy. So, in a twisted way, you *do* need carbohydrate for energy - *if* you buy into the concept that you need carbohydrate for energy!

This is not to say that carbohydrate cannot be beneficial. It can be, especially for athletes, and this is why the carb-load is a feature of the NHE Eating Plan. But the importance of carbohydrate as a fuel source has been grossly overblown by mistaken "experts" and clever marketing folks.

Recall from Chapter 8 that the traditional Eskimo diet is virtually devoid of carbohydrate, particularly in winter, and yet their metabolism continues humming along just fine. There are "essential amino acids," discussed in the previous chapter; and there are "essential fats," discussed below; but there are no "essential carbohydrates" (if you ever hear that term, check your pockets, because someone is trying to get your money).

The actual amount of carbohydrate required by human beings is *zero*. By contrast, a certain amount of protein and fat is required; without it, your health unravels like a ball of yarn and you die. Above these minimums (and, of course, a certain amount of vitamins, minerals, and water), you must provide your body with energy. As a strict matter of survival, it does not matter whether energy enters your system in the form of protein, carbohydrate, or fat. Your body is capable of utilizing any of these macronutrients for fuel.

The adenosine triphosphate (ATP) molecule is the fundamental energy unit for all living things from single-celled algae to human beings. Your body needs ATP to execute the functions necessary for survival, as well as any other activities in which you choose to engage. The notion that glucose (derived from dietary carbohydrate) is necessary for energy fails to appreciate the fact that free fatty acids (derived from bodyfat and dietary fat) can, like glucose, be broken down to ATP. And as we discussed in Chapter 10, free fatty acids are the superior of the two fuel sources for 95% of your daily activity. In terms of our current discussion, free fatty acids yield more ATP than does glucose. Thus, the million-dollar question becomes: from what will you derive your ATP, glucose or free fatty acids? The answer is simple: if you are a sugar-burner, then primarily from glucose; if you are a fat-burner, then primarily from free fatty acids.

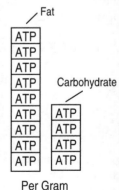

Your metabolism adapts to the most available energy source by becoming more efficient at converting that energy source into ATP.[1,2] Accordingly, when fat becomes more available than carbohydrate, your body becomes more efficient at using fat for energy. The lipolytic effect of dietary fat has been observed in both human[3,4] and animal[5,6] studies. Specifically, dietary fat activates fat-metabolizing enzymes, called *lipases*;[7,8,9,10] and suppresses the lipogenic enzymes, *malic* and *fatty acid synthase*.[11,12,13] Carbohydrate ingestion has the opposite effect on lipogenic enzymes,[14,15] and activates enzymes that increase glucose utilization.[16] Hormonally, it has been demonstrated in studies comparing isocaloric high-fat/low-carbohydrate and low-fat/high-carbohydrate diets that the former decreases the insulin/glucagon ratio.[17]

Hence, dietary fat helps you become a fat-burner by means of the hormonal and enzymatic adaptations it induces. In less technical terms, dietary fat revs-up the fat-burning machinery inside your body. Either way you express it, carbohydrate consumption is a crucial qualifier: if carbohydrate intake is not restricted, these fat-burning adaptations will either be muted or will not occur at all.

Like every other feature of metabolism, this mechanism was shaped by evolution. Survival through the ages favored those individuals whose metabolism was capable of shifting to accommodate different fuel sources. Those unfortunate folks who could not make the necessary metabolic adjustments in response to the vicissitudes of the hunter-gatherer lifestyle died out hundreds-of-thousands of years ago, and so did their genetic legacy.

Fat consumption is particularly important in connection with the NHE Eating Plan because with carbohydrate restricted most of the time, if you restrict fat too, you would wind-up eating either too much protein or too few calories or both. Too few calories is bad because it slows your metabolism, stimulates catabolic hormones, and causes hunger (see Chapters 9, 11). Too much protein is bad because it raises insulin levels, which keeps you in a sugar-burning mode (see Chapter 17). Therefore, if you restrict fat and carbohydrate and eat only protein, you invite hunger, catabolism, metabolic depression, and sugar burning - none of which is a condition favorable to physique improvement.

Another reason why moderate fat consumption is key is because it quells cravings. The primary way that fat accomplishes this helpful task is by stimulating the release of *cholecystokinin* (CCK),[18,19] a hormone/neurotransmitter that sends a satiety signal to the brain[20,21,22] and delays gastric emptying.[23,24] * Slower emptying of the contents of the stomach into the bloodstream blunts the resultant rise in blood sugar and postpones hunger.[25]

* Interestingly, when CCK was discovered it was hailed as a breakthrough when researchers discovered that, when administered to rats, it drastically reduced appetite.[25a] But later studies showed that it did not work so well in humans, because the pancreas adapts to exogenous CCK by producing neutralizing enzymes. Consequently, the satiating effect of exogenous CCK dwindles to nil within a few weeks. The story of CCK is instructive: it illustrates, once again, the problems inherent in administering substances into the body that are naturally produced within the body. When possible, natural enhancement is the better course to pursue. By consuming fat in moderation, you can naturally stimulate CCK.

Natural Hormonal Enhancement

Cravings are the undoing of anyone trying to adhere to a dietary plan, so keeping them in check is imperative. The general framework of the NHE Eating Plan, by shifting the insulin/glucagon axis away from insulin predominance, knocks-out the main source of cravings: hormonal hunger. However, cravings are like the villain in a low-budget horror movie - they have a tendency to keep creeping back from the dead. But fear not, the satiating power of fat, along with subdued insulin levels, and stable blood sugar, should keep cravings in the grave.

It is one of the more basic, but overlooked, facts of human metabolism that the body strives to store that which is in short supply. This is another example of the innate "intelligence" of the human body, which we discussed in Chapter 9. For example, you may have heard that the more water you drink, the less water you retain, and vice versa. This may seem counter-intuitive, but it makes perfect sense from the standpoint of survival. Many a bodybuilder has wound-up "holding water" on competition day because he began water restriction too early in the week and consequently gave his body a signal to cling to every molecule of water contained in the foods he ate in the days leading-up to the contest.

This counterregulatory dynamic is a central feature of human metabolism. In Chapter 11, we examined this phenomenon in connection with carbohydrate and how to use it to your advantage. In Chapter 9, we explored the counterregulatory mechanism in relation to calories and how it renders calorie restriction futile. The same principle applies to protein: when abundance prevails, the body uses some protein for "optional" processes (like building muscle) and wastes, or excretes, the remainder.[26] But when protein scarcity prevails, the body becomes much more conservative with the precious little it receives. In this scenario, no protein is excreted and muscle growth ceases and then is rolled-back as the body breaks down muscle to get the amino acids not forthcoming in the diet.[27]

The same feedback phenomenon that applies to carbohydrate, protein, water, and calories also applies to fat. Tightly restricting fat consumption induces aggressive retention coupled with fat cravings to get more of it into the body. Conversely, when fat is abundantly available, the body is more liberal in burning it for energy.[28,29] Once again, we see that human physiology does not conform precisely to the laws of logic which, in this case, would suggest that the less of something you consume, the less of it you store. Rather, the human body has its own agenda, governed by the drive to survive not logic, and this dynamic must be accounted for if your fat loss efforts are to be successful.

How Much is Moderate?

I could, like so many other health writers, tell you how much fat you should be consuming each day - but I am not going to do so. Experience counsels that to be effective, a dietary program must be practical and convenient. Many health writers get so lost in trying to craft the ultimate formula for fat loss that they forget this golden rule. The fact of the matter is that few people will go through life calculating macronutrient percentages and apportioning their food intake into perfect ratios. The NHE Eating Plan is designed, not as an intellectual exercise, but to help real-life people improve their health and physique. I am already asking you to count carbohydrate grams. To ask you to do more counting would risk causing you to lose your patience instead of your bodyfat.

Having said that, here are some easy-to-follow guidelines regarding how much fat to eat. For one, try to eat mostly lean meat. Bacon and sausage are okay occasionally, but most of the meat you consume should contain significantly more protein than fat. Recall from Chapter 5 that the "ancient warriors" ate plenty of meat. It bears noting, however, that meat from wild game is considerably leaner than the meat sold in supermarkets. Domesticated animals are always fatter, both in terms of subcutaneous fat and marbling within the muscle, than their wild counterparts due to their greater food supply and reduced level of physical activity. Additionally, breeders have undertaken efforts, through genetics management and feeding techniques, to increase the proportion of fat in order to satisfy the public demand for tender meat.[30]

Furthermore, fat from wild animals has a healthier composition. It contains less saturated fat[31] (but approximately the same amount of cholesterol since the cholesterol content of fat does not differ greatly from that of lean tissue[32]). The fat of wild animals also contains a significant amount of eicosapentaenoic acid (omega 3), whereas domestic beef does not.[33] The point here is not to suggest that you hunt your own dinner, but rather to point-out the shortcomings of domesticated meat. To counter these deficiencies, supply the missing omega 3 fat and select lean cuts of meat.

It is best to keep fat moderate throughout the day for maximum craving-control. However, should you find halfway through the day that your fat consumption for that day is front-loaded, reduce fat on the back-end, keeping dinner lean. For example, if you ate ground beef for lunch, and snacked on almonds in the afternoon, it would be preferable to eat chicken breast for dinner rather than spare ribs. I call this "common-sense compensation." Another common sense guideline is that you should take reasonable measures to avoid excess fat. Drain-away the extra fat from cooked meat and put just enough dressing on your salad, or melted butter on your vegetables, to enhance the taste. I call this the "No Floating Vegetables Rule."

Most people possess a fairly accurate sense of what the word "moderate" means, and I am confident in your ability to gauge where "low" ends and "high" begins. My confidence is reinforced by the fact that fat tends to be self-regulating on the NHE Eating Plan (see Chapter 9). It is highly possible, in fact, that you will wind-up eating less fat than you do currently, especially since "hidden fat," which is ubiquitous in the refined carbohydrate foods that comprise the bulk of the American diet, will be essentially eliminated from your diet.

169

On the NHE Eating Plan, you will be eating fat in a readily identifiable form, which is the form in which fat has its highest satiety value. With the standard American diet, by contrast, fat sneaks into your body piggy-backed onto carbohydrate-laden foods. What is worse, most of the fat in processed carbohydrate foods is trans fat (a.k.a., "partially hydrogenated" oil). As the research unfolds, trans fat is emerging as the next dietary villain. But this time, the bad rap is well-deserved (more about this later).

Good Fat

Fat serves many vital functions in the body. In particular, fat is necessary for absorption of fat-soluble vitamins: A,D,E, and K.[34] Extremely low-fat diets compromise absorption of these vitamins.[35] As is the case with amino acids, there are "essential" fatty acids which cannot be synthesized by the body and, therefore, must be derived from food.

Dietary fat plays an important role in immune function.[36,37] To illustrate, a recent study found that highly trained runners on a medium-fat diet (32%) had superior immune status as compared with their low-fat counterparts (17%).[38] The relationship between dietary fat and immunity bears particular significance for athletes, given that they are the group most likely to practice dietary fat restriction and tax their immune system via high-volume exercise. Notwithstanding the importance of adequate dietary fat, all fats are not created equal. Some fats are greatly beneficial, some are not so great, and some are roadblocks on the path to a better body.

In the last few years, certain types of fat have captured the attention of the scientific community - this time in a positive light. The recent explosion of interest in this area is attributable to two convergent avenues of research. For one, we have come to appreciate that, not only is it true that not all types of fat are bad for serum cholesterol and triglyceride levels, but some types of fat are actually good for blood lipid levels. With heart disease the leading cause of death in the United States, and unfavorable blood lipid profile a significant risk factor for heart disease, you would think that every health authority in the U.S. would be shouting this information from the highest rooftop. But that is not happening. Rather, this potentially lifesaving information is being drowned-out by the insistent admonition to restrict fat altogether.

The other line of research into fats relates to eicosanoids. The outstanding work of Dr. Barry Sears, author of *The Zone*, has shed light on the sweeping importance of these hormone-like substances. Eicosanoids have been found to regulate a wide range of functions critical to health, including: immune response, cholesterol production, inflammation, blood clotting, blood pressure, and tumor growth.[39,40,41] As the building blocks of eicosanoids,[42] essential fatty acids have ridden the coattails of these findings to newfound appreciation.

Eicosanoids: The Master Key to Disease - and its Prevention

If you are wondering whether you have any control over eicosanoids, you do. In fact, although eicosanoid research is ultra-cutting-edge, controlling eicosanoid production is easy. Eicosanoids are regulated by insulin/glucagon, the focal point of the NHE Eating Plan. Insulin predominance stimulates "bad" eicosanoids by activating the enzyme, *delta 5 desaturase*, which shifts eicosanoid synthesis toward production of "bad" eicosanoids.[43,44,45] As you might expect, glucagon, the hormonal antagonist of insulin, inhibits this enzyme, thereby stimulating production of "good" eicosanoids. The direct impact of the hormones insulin and glucagon on the all-important eicosanoids demonstrates that the insulin/glucagon axis is the pivot-point not only for fat loss, but for overall health and well-being as well.

In addition to its role in growth and development and as an energy source and eicosanoid precursor, scintillating new research shows that dietary fat influences gene expression.[46,47,48,49] This finding reveals that the quantity and type of fat we eat impacts upon our well-being more profoundly than previously imagined; and it has made fatty acid metabolism one of the hottest areas of research in nutritional science. But despite their fundamental role in the body, fats have been shrouded in misunderstanding and prejudice for so long that misconceptions about fat have become deeply rooted in public consciousness. For this reason, it will likely be a long time before the prevailing anti-fat mentality is extinguished, given the persistence of hare-brained pronouncements from health authorities equating healthy eating with low-fat eating. Much remains to be discovered regarding the physiological effects of the various types of dietary fat. But what we have learned indicates, unequivocally, that consumption of the right kinds of fat, rather than fat restriction, is conducive to optimal health.

You should aim to fulfill your moderate fat allowance with fats that afford health and fat loss benefits. By enabling you to enjoy the advantages of "good fat," the NHE Eating Plan is superior to a low-fat diet which, by its nature, restricts your ability to do so. The principal good fats are monounsaturated fat and omega 3 fat. Both have been found to protect against cardiovascular disease, among many other benefits that they confer.

Monounsaturated Fat and the Oil Controversy

Both olive oil and canola oil have become increasingly popular in recent years. While health commentators uniformly agree that these two oils are healthful substitutes for saturated fat, controversy exists as to which is better. Olive oil contains more monounsaturated fat, while canola oil contains more essential fatty acids. Specifically, canola oil provides more omega 6 than does olive oil and, more significantly, provides a modest amount of the scarcer omega 3s, which olive oil does not.

Olive oil, due to its high monounsaturated content, is more resistant than canola oil to unhealthy free-radical formation caused by heat-induced oxidation.[50] Therefore, olive oil is preferable for cooking. (Incidentally, saturated fat, predominant in butter, too, is relatively resistant to heat-induced oxidation, in contrast to polyunsaturated fat, predominant in most vegetable oils.[51]) Oxidized fats are pro-oxidative, meaning they exert the opposite action of antioxidants. In addition to its suitability for cooking, olive oil's taste and culinary versatility are big pluses.

171

Olive oil boasts an unsurpassed health record. In particular, the acclaimed Mediterranean diet, which corresponds with exceptionally low rates of cardiovascular disease and cancer, features olive oil as its centerpiece.[52,53,54] Since the 1960's, when the remarkable low incidence of atherosclerosis in Greece and Southern Italy was first documented, researchers and public health specialists have been scrutinizing this epidemiological phenomenon. In particular, the fact that approximately 30% of caloric intake in these countries derives from monounsaturated fat has focused attention on this type of fat as a possible coronary risk reducer.[55]

The Mediterranean island of Crete presents the most compelling case study. Inhabitants of this island have the lowest rate of cardiovascular disease in the world,[56] despite the fact that fat comprises 40-45% of their total caloric intake.[57] Notably, olive oil represents the chief source of fat in the Cretan diet, and their per capita olive oil consumption is among the highest in the world. In fact, Cretan field laborers are reputed to drink olive oil by the glassful to provide energy for their physically demanding work (unless you intend to toil like a Cretan laborer, I wouldn't recommend this practice).

The monounsaturated fat in olive oil has been shown to lower both LDL/HDL cholesterol ratio and serum triglyceride levels.[58,59,60,61,62] * Moreover, recent research suggests that the beneficial effect of monounsaturated fat on blood lipids is accompanied by an anti-oxidative effect exerted by the polyphenols (also found in red wine) present in olive oil.[63,64,65] These twin advantages amount to a formidable cardioprotective force, and suggest that a causal relationship exists between high olive oil consumption and low incidence of cardiovascular disease in Mediterranean countries. Furthermore, studies comparing a diet high in monounsaturated fat with a high-carbohydrate/low-fat diet consistently find that a high-monounsaturated-fat/reduced-carbohydrate diet is more effective at improving blood lipid profile[66,67,68] and, in diabetics, stabilizing blood sugar.[69,70,71] Sadly, despite this evidence, a high-carb/low-fat diet is still widely prescribed to coronary patients and diabetics.

Virgin olive oil is the only widely available, mass-marketed, unprocessed oil. All other oils sold in grocery stores have undergone a makeover consisting of some combination of degumming, bleaching, refining, and/or deodorizing.[72] Because virgin olive oil is unprocessed, all of its minor components are intact. More than 100 discrete compounds, all with names you wouldn't want to try to pronounce, have been identified in olive oil.[73]** Because many of these substances have not been studied, their physiological effects remain a mystery. But it is clear that the overall effect of olive oil on health is positive.

---

* When olive oil was compared head-to-head with canola oil at the Lipid Metabolism Laboratory at Tufts University, canola oil lowered total cholesterol to a greater degree than did olive oil (12% vs. 7%). But canola oil also dropped HDL by 7% (a commonly observed shortcoming of polyunsaturated fat). Since olive oil, characteristically, only lowered LDL, the contest was basically a draw.[73a]

** Here are a few of the minor components of olive oil: *beta sitosterol, oleic acid, triterpenic acids, 2-phenylethanol, hydroxytyrosol, p-tyrosol, cycloartenol.* People lose sight of the fact that some of the most potent, healthful substances are found naturally in food. I would not be surprised if a supplement manufacturer came out with olive oil gelcaps but listed all those big, impressive words on the label and charged you $30 per bottle.

172

All factors considered, olive oil is the best oil and an outstanding food overall. Buy "extra virgin" olive oil to ensure the highest quality. Olive oil that does not say "virgin" has been "de-virginized" through a process that diminishes its healthful properties.[74,75] Canola oil is the second-best oil, and it can be used to add variety and provide both omega 3 fat and monounsaturated fat.

Additional sources of monounsaturated fat include avocados, nuts, and seeds. Nuts and seeds also contain omega 6 fat. Walnuts, soybeans, and pumpkin seeds each contain small amounts of omega 3 fat in the form of alpha-linolenic acid, along with omega 6 and monounsaturated fat.

Saturated Fat vs. Polyunsaturated Fat: A Critical Reassessment

Vegetable oil is held in high esteem by the American public due to oil company advertising campaigns that trumpet the fact that it is cholesterol-free; and also due to the advice of health authorities to reduce saturated fat in favor of polyunsaturated fat contained in vegetable oil. Given that dietary cholesterol is of minimal import to heart disease and saturated fat is not the villain it has been made out to be (see Chapter 8), I believe the time has come to reevaluate the wisdom of emphasizing polyunsaturated fat intake. At the very least, health organizations should replace the questionable recommendation to substitute polyunsaturated fat for saturated fat with the more meaningful and helpful distinction between "good fat" and "bad fat."

Health authorities have argued for many years that changing our diet to include more polyunsaturated fat and less saturated fat will reduce cardiovascular disease. However, the benefit, in terms of serum cholesterol, of substituting polyunsaturated fat for saturated fat is not evident. Rather, studies show that this approach decreases both HDL and LDL cholesterol,[76,77,78,79] thus not reducing coronary risk. Furthermore, a study published in the *Journal of the American Medical Association* found that overall fat, monounsaturated fat, and saturated fat consumption correlated with a reduced risk of stroke; but polyunsaturated fat correlated with an increased risk of stroke.[80] Until such time as this finding is corroborated by further studies, you should regard it as preliminary but worth noting. It is yet another indication that fat is not the enemy, and polyunsaturated fat is not the savior, that it has been made out to be.

Another feature of this developing picture is the effect of fat on testosterone levels. Again, polyunsaturated fat is "odd man out," with both monounsaturated fat and saturated fat, but not polyunsaturated fat, having been shown to increase testosterone levels (see Chapter 22). The upshot is that the experts' recommendations to reduce fat intake and replace saturated fat with polyunsaturated fat appears to be the perfect dietary prescription for lowering mens' testosterone levels!

So, polyunsaturated fat is not a panacea - but might it actually be bad for you? Polyunsaturated fat, because of its chemical structure, is more susceptible to oxidation by exposure to light, heat, and oxygen than either monounsaturated fat or saturated fat.

Oxidation of lipids in the body generates highly reactive, "renegade" molecules called free radicals.[81,82] In the early 1980's, Durk Pearson and Sandy Shaw, in their 800-page bestseller, *Life Extension*, sounded an alarm about polyunsaturated fat, asserting that it promotes free radical generation.[83] Unfortunately, their message never established traction because health authorities had already determined, incorrectly, that saturated fat was the enemy. Since then, the laws of biochemistry have not changed - polyunsaturated fat remains a potentially disease-promoting prooxidant.

Compelling evidence exists indicating that free radicals are responsible for much of the damage and corrosion associated with aging, cardiovascular disease, and cancer[84,85,86,87,88,89] (and as noted in Chapter 4, growth hormone and IGF-1 combat free radical damage). There is also evidence specifically implicating polyunsaturated fat in disease.[90,91,92,93,94] Furthermore, although there are surely other factors at play, it is noteworthy that the sharp rise in cancer incidence during the twentieth century correlates with the sharp rise in consumption of polyunsaturated vegetable oil. Since 1900, when cancer was not nearly the force it is today, saturated fat consumption has not increased but consumption of polyunsaturated fat and its mutant cousin, trans fat, has increased dramatically.[95,96]

Trans Fatty Acids: Mutant Child of Technology

While the recommendation to shun saturated fat in favor of polyunsaturated fat is of questionable soundness, the movement toward trans fatty acids is undoubtedly an ominous development. Trans fat is like a criminal in disguise, showing up in our food but not on the package label.* While trans fat has not officially been charged with wrongdoing, the incriminating evidence is mounting rapidly.

The presence of trans fat can be detected by the words "partially hydrogenated" on the label. Production of partially hydrogenated fat began early in the 20th century, and it rose steadily throughout the 1900's. The hydrogenation process is designed to increase the shelf-life of polyunsaturated fat by making it more resistant to oxidation. In effect, hydrogenation involves artificially saturating fat by adding hydrogen atoms to its structure. Whereas butter is naturally saturated, solid margarine is unnaturally partially saturated. While the artificial saturation process helps avoid the health problems caused by oxidized fat, it introduces new problems by creating trans fat.

The process of chemically manipulating fat to increase hydrogen content alters its structure from the natural *cis* configuration to the aberrant *trans* configuration, thereby giving these fats their name and giving those who consume them exposure to mutant fat

---

* As this book goes to press, the Food and Drug Administration has announced plans to include the trans-fatty-acid content of foods on product labels. This comes after years of rebuffing the entreaties of public health advocates brandishing highly persuasive evidence of the pathogenic effects of trans fat. Ascherio and Willett of the Harvard School of Public Health estimate that 30,000 premature deaths per year in the United States are attributable to consumption of trans fat.[96a] How many of those deaths would have been avoided had the FDA been more responsive to the manifest risks of trans fat consumption rather than expending resources trying to regulate or outlaw dietary supplements that can help prevent the same diseases that trans fat causes?

molecules. In the words of G.J. Brisson, Professor of Nutrition at Laval University in Quebec, "between the parent oil. . . and the partially hydrogenated product. . . there is a world of chemistry that alters profoundly the composition and physiochemical properties of natural oils."[97] Trans fat promotes cardiovascular disease (see below) and interferes with essential fatty acid metabolism and eicosanoid formation.[98,99,100,101] In other words, trans fat is the quintessential "bad fat": it not only inflicts harm directly but also impairs the body's ability to utilize "good" fats.

With respect to the trans fat/heart disease connection, a recent study that tracked 85,095 women found that a high intake of trans-fat-laden foods such as margarine raised the risk of heart disease by as much as 50%.[102] Viewed in conjunction with similar studies in the U.S.,[103] U.K.,[104,105,106] and Finland,[107] the association between trans fat consumption and cardiovascular disease appears striking. But, as Chapter 8 underscores, association does not equate with causation. Hence, the higher incidence of heart disease among populations that consume a high quantity of trans fat does not prove causation any more than being present at the scene of a crime proves guilt.

But before we dismiss the charges for lack of evidence, a smoking gun can be found in the fact that trans fatty acids have been shown to exert an across-the-board adverse effect on cholesterol levels by raising total cholesterol, lowering HDL, and raising LDL.[108,109,110,111,112] Compare this with saturated fat, which has never been shown to lower HDL cholesterol (but has been shown to increase it[113,114]). In two studies in which trans fat was compared head-to-head with saturated fat, trans fat had a substantially worse effect on coronary risk factors.[115,116] Moreover, as demonstrated in Chapter 8, whether or not saturated fat is unhealthy depends upon one's hormonal state. Trans fat is unhealthy regardless of hormonal state.

In my view, any study that purports to show a causal connection between overall fat intake or saturated fat intake and disease is invalid if it does not control for the variables of trans fat consumption, polyunsaturated fat consumption, and hormonal state (given that each of these factors is capable of contributing to, or independently causing, every health problem blamed on saturated fat). Shockingly, if my view were to prevail, not one shred of evidence would exist to show that fat in general or saturated fat in particular causes disease. Instead, we would be left with the French, the Eskimos, the Mediterraneans, our *Homo sapien* ancestors, and all the other evidence reviewed in this book showing that neither fat in general nor saturated fat in particular causes anything, except tasty flavor and perhaps increased testosterone levels in men.

Whereas humans have consumed saturated fat since the beginning of time, trans fat is essentially a twentieth-century invention. In addition to the evidence that trans fatty acids cause disease, the fact that they are a recent addition to the human diet and that their effects on the body are not fully understood is unsettling. As the research unfolds, it is unlikely that we will discover anything good about trans fat. Rather, it is probable that more damning evidence will emerge. Preliminary evidence suggests that trans fatty acids may adversely affect infant and fetal development,[117,118] may lower testosterone levels in men,[119] and may heighten breast cancer risk.[120]

175

Movements are afoot in several countries to eliminate or regulate trans fat. Canada and Germany have taken steps in this direction. Most countries, though, blindly follow the U.S. government on matters of diet and nutrition, not realizing the extent to which food lobbies and bureaucratic incompetence impact governmental recommendations on these issues. Even so, the greater portion of the blame for the presence of trans fat in the food supply rests not with sheep-like governments but with a food processing industry devoid of social responsibility, which, instead of fixing the problem, spends millions of dollars propping-up the ailing cholesterol bogeyman and advertising the health benefits of products unfit for consumption by anyone desiring to be healthy.

The NHE Eating Plan affords considerable protection from trans fat by virtue of minimizing consumption of processed carbohydrate foods, which generally contain the highest concentrations of them. Aside from that, if you steer clear of margarine that is solid at room temperature and check the mayonnaise label, you will be consuming far less trans fat than the vast majority of Americans.

Butter vs. Margarine:
Making Sound Health Choices in the Sound-Byte Era

The butter vs. margarine debate continues to rage, dividing health authorities into opposing camps. I have observed that health commentators, especially in magazines and on TV, tend to exaggerate the hazards of suspect foods. This is because overstated representations of the risks, or benefits, of foods attract attention and make good copy. People are more likely to purchase a magazine or tune-in to a TV program when the headline or teaser is couched in life-altering terms.

In the fast-paced, sound-byte era in which we live, the enormous surplus of information makes it exceedingly difficult to capture the attention of a jaded public. When it comes to health information, people want to know what is going to kill them or restore youth and vitality overnight - they have no time for a balanced analysis leading to an equivocal conclusion. The result is that health information is skewed toward sensationalism.

Some health authorities would have you believe that the trans fatty acids in margarine are the most hazardous substance not labeled with a skull and crossbones. Other health authorities are equally vehement in asserting that butter will plug-up your arteries like industrial putty. The truth usually lies somewhere in the middle. In this case, upon close examination of the evidence on both sides, the anti-trans-fat argument is far more persuasive than the anti-saturated-fat argument.

The so-called information age is not an unqualified positive from the standpoint of health. The average American is becoming increasingly dismayed and frustrated by the overwhelming volume of conflicting health information that he/she encounters on a regular basis. This sometimes results in a "who knows, who cares" attitude which, in turn, results in wholesale disengagement from any effort to eat healthy. This mindset is exemplified in a poem by James Kavanaugh in which he says that after listening to all the contradictory advice from numerous medical and nutrition experts, he decided it was easier to just live on Fritos and Jack Daniels. It is my sincere hope that this book will dispel your confusion and impart the knowledge and direction you need to achieve your health and fitness objectives (so hold-off on the Fritos and Jack at least until you finish reading this book).

Chapters 6 and 7 provide answers to the question of why health information, as a whole, is largely inaccurate. In terms of practical advice about how to navigate the information ocean without drowning in exasperation, **don't believe every sound-byte you hear on the subject of health and fitness**. The "experts" have an annoying tendency to generalize from the isolated to the infinite. Keep all information in context, and take it with a grain of salt. **Make your health choices based on the weight of the evidence**.

176

Scrutinize the motives and allegiances of any person dispensing health and fitness information. Is the commentator an independent thinker or a follow-the-leader type who still believes that dietary cholesterol causes heart disease and the RDA is all the nutrition a person needs? Does he or she have a vested interest? *Vested interest, or bias resulting from a follow-the-leader mentality, negates credibility even when the so-called expert has a wall full of unpronounceable degrees from the world's foremost academic institutions.*

In addition, ask yourself this: from what source(s) is the commentator getting his or her information? I believe that anyone making statements concerning health is obligated to cite his/her sources. Information that is rigorously researched and meticulously cited should be accorded more weight than bald assertions reflecting nothing more than the opinion of the commentator (as obvious as this may seem, many people miss this point and automatically give equal credence to everything they see in print). The fact is that some experts are wise, and some are otherwise. **A health "expert" who fails to relate the basis of his or her statements by providing specific scientific citations is owed little deference.** Always remember that, in the words of Dr. Michael Colgan:

Science is a system of evidence that owes no allegiance to title or position.

Be an independent thinker and be confident in your own common sense reasoning and your ability to discern the truth amid the volumes of information that you encounter every day as a beneficiary, or victim, of the information age.

Omega 3

Human beings evolved on a diet that contained roughly equal amounts of omega 3 and omega 6 fatty acids.[121] During the past 150 years, consumption of omega 6 fatty acids has increased in Western nations due to an increase in vegetable oil consumption. During this same period, consumption of omega 3 fatty acids has declined due to livestock domestication (see p. 169) and food processing that disproportionately destroys the more fragile omega 3's.[122] As a result, the ratio of omega 6 to omega 3 consumption has altered radically.[123] Studies indicate that fatty acid imbalance has far-reaching adverse physiological effects mediated via eicosanoids; and it is likely a contributory factor in the upsurge of degenerative disease that has occurred during the latter part of the twentieth century.

The prevalence of omega 3 deficiency coupled with the substantial health and fat loss benefits of omega 3 consumption, warrants taking deliberate measures to incorporate it into your diet. There are three sources of omega 3 fatty acids: alpha-linolenic acid (ALA), eicosapentaenoic acid (EPA), and docosahexaenoic acid (DHA). Omega 3 fatty acids have earned a spot at the forefront of nutritional research, showing promise in connection with both degenerative conditions and sports performance. Many more discoveries regarding the benefits of omega 3 fat are, I believe, yet to come.

In Chapter 8, you learned that traditional Eskimos remain largely unscathed by degenerative diseases running rampant in the U.S. and other industrialized countries. Omega 3 fat, abundant in the Eskimo diet, has been credited as central to this phenomenon;[124,125] and is associated with reduced coronary mortality in other populations, as well.[126,127,128,129,130] The mechanism by which omega 3 fatty acids protect against cardiovascular disease is a potent triglyceride-lowering effect,[131,132,133,134] and possibly an anticoagulant (blood-thinning) effect.[135,136] By comparison to its effect on serum triglyceride levels, the effect of omega 3 fat on cholesterol levels is minor – which reinforces the significance of triglyceride as a coronary risk factor. In addition to its well-established cardioprotective influence, mounting evidence suggests that omega 3 fatty acids protect against cancer.[137,138,139,140]

Omega 3 fat is also emerging as an important factor in fat loss. For one, omega 3 fat improves insulin sensitivity[141,142,143,144,145] (which sheds light on how it reduces serum triglyceride levels given that excess insulin promotes accumulation of triglyceride in the blood, see p. 48). Heightened insulin sensitivity facilitates fat loss by making insulin work more efficiently. The more sensitive cells are to insulin, the less of it the pancreas must emit in response to a given amount of blood sugar. This helps keep insulin levels out of the fat-storage zone (see p. 162). (Other nutrients and exercise also affect insulin sensitivity.) Consistent with its favorable effect on insulin function, omega 3 fatty acids have been shown to reduce abdominal fat storage in laboratory animals.[146,147]

Of particular interest to bodybuilders and athletes, preliminary studies indicate that omega 3 fatty acids can help maintain nitrogen balance under catabolic conditions.[148,149] This anti-catabolic effect translates to less muscle-breakdown consequent to intense training and other forms of stress. The research into the effects of omega 3 fat on athletic performance and body composition is at an early stage - but is very promising.

Newly acquired insights into the functions of eicosanoids suggest that the diverse benefits of omega 3 fatty acids stem from a common source. The unifying factor appears to be that omega 3 fat increases production of "good" eicosanoids, by inhibiting the delta 5 desaturase enzyme in much the same way, but less powerfully, as does glucagon[150,151,152] (see p. 171). Unquestionably, omega 3 fat is your ally in the quest for optimal health and physique.

The best food source of omega 3 fat is cold-water fish. Salmon, herring, trout, mackerel, halibut, and sardines are rich in EPA and DHA. Low-fat fish such as sole, swordfish, snapper, and flounder are comparatively low in omega 3 content. Sources of alpha-linolenic acid, which is converted in the body to EPA and DHA, include dark green leafy vegetables, walnuts, pumpkin seeds, soybeans, and canola oil. Flaxseed oil, one of the more highly touted supplements in recent years, is the richest source of alpha-linolenic acid and has earned special treatment below, for reasons not entirely positive.

Healthy Bacon?

The problem of the relative scarcity of omega 3 fat was tackled recently by food technologists who fed fish oil to pigs so that the quality of their bacon would be higher. This seems like a clever idea, doesn't it? Most people like the taste of bacon but they avoid it because of its high-fat content; so you turn this negative into a positive by creating bacon that contains omega 3 fat. Healthy bacon is a marketer's dream. Unfortunately, though, not all bright ideas are right ideas: they succeeded in producing healthier bacon, but it smelled so much like fish that it was deemed inedible.

178

Fish oil supplements are available at health food stores, but eating fish is a better and more economical way to get omega 3 fat. Eight ounces of Atlantic salmon contains as much omega 3 fat as a handful of fish oil pills. And if you like the taste of fish, you will derive considerably more pleasure from a fish dinner than from swallowing a small pile of pills. In addition to the pleasure factor, fish, but not fish oil, is a rich source of protein. Remember, when selecting fish, the fattier the fish, the more omega 3. Stated differently: fat is where it's at.

All Fats Aren't Created Equal

Maximize your "good fat" intake within your moderate fat quota.

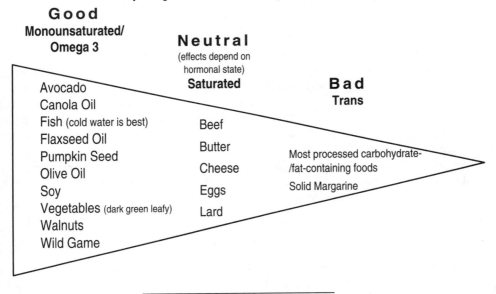

To Flax or Not to Flax

Flaxseed oil's star status among the constellation of highly publicized dietary supplements is owed to recent discoveries of the benefits of omega 3 fatty acids. As a rich source of omega 3, flaxseed oil is worthy of much of the favorable attention it has received. There are, however, drawbacks to flaxseed oil, as well.

For one, the chemical structure of flaxseed oil, a "superunsaturated" fat, renders it exceptionally susceptible to oxidation.[153] What is worse, unsaturated fats oxidize without smelling or tasting rancid.[154] The fragility of flaxseed oil accounts for why it is packaged in a black container. Light, heat, and air can each ruin flaxseed oil; and at a pricey 15 dollars a bottle, its temperamental nature doesn't please me as the consumer. To counter the oxidation problem, keep your flaxseed oil refrigerated when you are not using it, buy smaller containers so you can finish it sooner after opening it, and never cook with it.

Another shortcoming of flaxseed oil is it contains alpha-linolenic acid (ALA), which must be converted to EPA/DHA in the body. This imperfect conversion process becomes even less efficient with advancing age due to a decline in the enzyme that makes EPA/DHA from ALA.[155,156] In addition, the vast majority of studies demonstrating the benefits of omega 3 fat use EPA and DHA, not alpha-linolenic acid (remember, too, the heart-healthy Eskimos consume fish, not flaxseed oil).

Furthermore, Dr. Barry Sears cautioned in The Zone of an adverse impact of ALA on eicosanoid synthesis by means of inhibiting the delta 6 desaturase enzyme (not to be confused with the delta 5 desaturase enzyme that we discussed earlier - delta 6 desaturase "activates" dietary fatty acids into

Natural Hormonal Enhancement

gamma-linolenic acid (GLA), whereas delta 5 desaturase directs metabolism of activated fatty acids toward "bad" eicosanoids as opposed to "good" eicosanoids). More recently, Michael and Mary Dan Eades, in *Protein Power*, stepped-up the attack on alpha-linolenic acid, recommending avoidance of flaxseed (57% ALA) and canola oil (10% ALA). [157] I disagree.

I believe that the importance of consuming a substantial amount of omega 3 fat outweighs the negatives of flaxseed oil, especially given that the delta-6-inhibitory-problem that the authors of *Protein Power* find so troubling can be readily circumvented by supplementing GLA. Evening primrose oil and borage seed oil are good sources of GLA. Human breast milk is a richer, though less conveniently available, source of GLA.

If you like fish, or at least don't dislike it, stick with that and save yourself the money and annoyance of dealing with flaxseed oil. If, however, you find fish unpalatable or wish to avoid it for other reasons, then I recommend flaxseed oil and GLA. One way or another, omega 3 fat is too beneficial to do without.

I recommend eating high-fat fish at least twice per week. Or, if you are relying on low-fat fish like tuna to supply omega 3, then I recommend at least four servings per week. Unfortunately, the purity of our waterways leaves much to be desired, and the Great Lakes are notoriously bad.[158] To minimize exposure to heavy metals (particularly, PCBs, lead, and mercury) and bacterial contaminants, here are two recommendations: avoid shellfish and eat low on the food chain (i.e., small fish). Remember, "you are what you eat" applies to all creatures. When a big fish eats a small fish, the big fish retains in its body the metallic pollutants resident in the small fish. And don't forget about the non-fish sources of omega 3 fat. By incorporating "good fat" into your diet, you will be doing a service to your heart, your waistline, and your muscles.

References

1.   Flatt J-P. Use and Storage of Carbohydrate and Fat. *Am J Clin Nutr* 1995;61:952S.

2.   Thomas CD, et al. Nutrient Balance and Energy Expenditure During Ad Libitum Feeding of High Fat and High Carbohydrate Diets in Humans. *Am J Clin Nutr* 1992;55:934.

3.   Kather H, et al. Influences of Variation in Total Energy Intake and Dietary Composition on Regulation of Fat Cell Lipolysis in Ideal-Weight Subjects. *J Clin Invest* 1987;80:566.

4.   Kasper H, et al. Response of Body Weight to a Low Carbohydrate, High Fat Diet in Normal and Obese Subjects. *Am J Clin Nutr* 1973;26:197.

5.   Kelwick A, Pawan GLS. The Effect of High-Fat and High-Carbohydrate Diets on Rates of Weight Loss in Mice. *Metabolism* 1964;13:87.

6.   Lester T, Czarnecki-Maulden G, Lewis D. Cats Increase Fatty Acid Oxidation when Isocalorically Fed Meat-Based Diets with Increasing Fat Content. *Am J Physiol* 1999;277:R878.

7.   Armand M, et al. Dietary Fat Modulates Gastric Lipase Activity in Healthy Humans. *Am J Clin Nutr* 1995;62:74.

8.   Borel P, et al. Gastric Lipase: Evidence of an Adaptive Response to Dietary Fat in the Rabbit. *Gastroenterology* 1991;100:1582.

9.   Gidez LI. Effect of Dietary Fat on Pancreatic Lipase Levels in the Rat. *J Lipid Res* 1973;14:169.

10. Sabb JE, Godfrey PM, Brannon PM. Adaptive Response of Rat Pancreatic Lipase to Dietary Fat: Effects of Amount and Type of Fat. *J Nutr* 1986;116:892.

11. Shillabeer G, et al. Hepatic and Adipose Tissue Lipogenic Enzyme mRNA Levels are Suppressed by High Fat Diets in the Rat. *J Lipid Res* 1990;31:623.

Chapter 18 - Using Dietary Fat to Burn Bodyfat

12. Sandretto AM, Tsai AC. Effects of Fat Intake on Body Composition and Hepatic Lipogenic Enzyme Activities of Hamsters Shortly After Exercise Cessation. *Am J Clin Nutr* 1988;47:175.

13. Tsai AC, Gong T-W. Modulation of the Exercise and Retirement Effects by Dietary Fat Intake in Hamsters. *J Nutr* 1987;117:1149.

14. M'Zali H, et al. Time-Dependent Effects of Insulin on Lipid Synthesis in Cultured Fetal Rat Hepatocytes: A Comparison between Lipogenesis and Glycogenesis. *Metabolism* 1997;46:345.

15. Sadur CN, Eckel RH. Insulin Stimulation of Adipose Tissue Lipoprotein Lipase. Use of the Euglycemic Clamp Technique. *J Clin Invest* 1982;69:1119.

16. Suzuki M, et al. In Vitro Stimulation of Glucose Utilization by Insulin in Primary Cultures of Rat Hepatocytes. *Diabetes Res Clin Pract* 1991;13:163.

17. Lewis SB, et al. Effect of Diet Composition on Metabolic Adaptations to Hypocaloric Nutrition: Comparison of High Carbohydrate and High Fat Isocaloric Diets. *Am J Clin Nutr* 1977;30:160.

18. Hildebrand P, et al. Hydrolysis of Dietary Fat by Pancreatic Lipase Stimulates Cholecystokinin Release. *Gastroenterology* 1998;114:123.

19. Hildebrand P, Beglinger C. [The Role of Cholecystokinin as a Regulator of Gastrointestinal Functions]. *Schweiz Rundsch Med Prax* 1998;87:1821. German.

20. Dourish CT, Rycroft W, Iversen SD. Postponement of Satiety by Blockade of Brain Cholecystokinin (CCK-B) Receptors. *Science* 1989;245:1509.

21. Rehfeld JF. Cholecystokinin as Satiety Signal. *Int J Obes* 1981;5:465.

22. Schick RR, et al. Brain Regions Where Cholecystokinin Exerts its Effect on Satiety. *Ann N Y Acad Sci* 1994;713:242.

23. Liddle RA, et al. Regulation of Gastric Emptying in Humans by Cholecystokinin. *J Clin Invest* 1986;77:992.

24. Konturek JW, et al. Role of Cholecystokinin in the Control of Gastric Emptying and Secretory Response to a Fatty Meal in Normal Subjects and Duodenal Ulcer Patients. *Scand J Gastroenterol* 1994;29:583.

25. Cunningham KM, Read NW. The Effect of Incorporating Fat into Different Components of a Meal on Gastric Emptying and Postprandial Blood Glucose and Insulin Responses. *Br J Nutr* 1989;61:285.

25a. Antin J, et al. Cholecystokinin Elicits Complete Behavioural Sequence of Satiety in Rats. *J Comp Physiol Psychol* 1975;89:784.

26. Moundras C, et al. Dietary Protein Paradox: Decrease of Amino Acid Availability Induced by High-Protein Diets. *Am J Physiol* 1993;264:1057.

27. Tawa NE, Goldberg AL. Suppression of Muscle Protein Turnover and Amino Acid Degradation by Dietary Protein Deficiency. *Am J Physiol* 1992;263:317.

28. Verboeket-van de Venne WP, Westerterp KR, ten Hoor F. Substrate Utilization in Man: Effects of Dietary Fat and Carbohydrate. *Metabolism* 1994;43:152.

29. Schrauwen P, et al. Changes in Fat Oxidation in Response to a High-Fat Diet. *Am J Clin Nutr* 1997;66:276.

30. Wittwer SH. Altering Fat Content of Animal Products through Genetics, Nutrition, and Management. In: National Research Council. *Fat Content and Composition of Animal Products.* Washington DC: National Academy of Sciences 1976:80-84.

31. Crawford MA. Fatty-Acid Ratios in Free Living and Domestic Animals. *Lancet* 1968;1:1329.

32. Feeley RM, Criner PE, Watt BK. Cholesterol Content of Foods. *J Am Diet Assoc* 1972;61:134.

33. Simopoulos AP. New Products from the Agri-Food Industry: The Return of N-3 Fatty Acids into the Food Supply. *Lipids* 1999;34(Suppl):S297.

34. Erasmus U. *Fats that Heal Fats that Kill.* BC, Canada: Alive Books 1993, p. 161.

35. Jequier E. Response to and Range of Acceptable Fat Intake in Adults. *Eur J Clin Nutr* 1999;53(Suppl):S84.

36. Perez RV, Alexander JW. Immune Regulation by Lipids. *Transplant Proc* 1988;20:1162.

37. Kinsella JE, Lokesh B. Dietary Lipids, Eicosanoids, and the Immune System. *Crit Care Med* 1990;18:S94.

38. Venkatraman JT, et al. Influence of the Level of Dietary Lipid Intake and Maximal Exercise on the Immune Status in Runners. *Med Sci Sports Exer* 1997;29:333.

39. Fletcher JR. Eicosanoids. Critical Agents in the Physiological Process and Cellular Injury. *Arch Surg* 1993;128:1192.

40. Reilly MP, Lawson JA, FitzGerald GA. Eicosanoids and Isoeicosanoids: Indices of Cellular Function and Oxidant Stress. *J Nutr* 1998;128(Suppl):434S.

41. Booyens J, van der Merwe CF, Katzeff IE. Chronic Arachidonic Acid Eicosanoid Imbalance: A Common Feature in Coronary Artery Disease, Hypercholesterolemia, Cancer and other Important Diseases. Significance of Desaturase Enzyme Inhibition and of the Arachidonic Acid Desaturase-Independent Pathway. *Med Hypotheses* 1985;18:53.

42. Das UN. Interaction(s) between Essential Fatty Acids, Eicosanoids, Cytokines, Growth Factors and Free Radicals: Relevance to New Therapeutic Strategies in Rheumatoid Arthritis and Other Collagen Vascular Diseases. *Prostaglandins Leukot Essent Fatty Acids* 1991;44:201.

43. Medeiros LC, et al. Insulin, But Not Estrogen, Correlated with Indexes of Desaturase Function in Obese Women. *Horm Metab Res* 1995;27:235.

44. el Boustani S, et al. Direct In Vivo Characterization of Delta 5 Desaturase Activity in Humans by Deuterium Labeling: Effect of Insulin. *Metabolism* 1989;38:315.

45. Sears B. *The Zone*. NY: Harper Collins 1995.

46. Jump DB, Clarke SD. Regulation of Gene Expression by Dietary Fat. *Annu Rev Nutr* 1999;19:63.

47. Pegorier JP. Regulation of Gene Expression by Fatty Acids. *Curr Opin Clin Nutr Metab Care* 1998;1:329.

48. Vanden Heuvel JP. Peroxisome Proliferator-Activated Receptors: A Critical Link Among Fatty Acids, Gene Expression and Carcinogenesis. *J Nutr* 1999;129:575

49. Grimaldi PA, et al. Long Chain Fatty Acids as Modulators of Gene Transcription in Preadipose Cells. *Mol Cell Biochem* 1999;192:63.

50. Erasmus U. *Fats that Heal Fats that Kill*. BC, Canada: Alive Books 1993, p. 40, 126.

51. Id. at p. 16-17, 126.

52. Helsing E. Traditional Diets and Disease Patterns of the Mediterranean, Circa 1960. *Am J Clin Nutr* 1995;61:1329S.

53. Keys A, et al. The Diet and 15-Year Death Rate in the Seven Countries Study. *Am J Epidemiol* 1986;124:903.

54. Buzina R, Suboticanec K, Saric M. Diet Patterns and Health Problems: Diet in Southern Europe. *Ann Nutr Metab* 1991;35(Suppl):32.

55. Massaro M, Carluccio MA, De Caterina R. Direct Vascular Antiatherogenic Effects of Oleic Acid: A Clue to the Cardioprotective Effects of the Mediterranean Diet. *Cardiologia* 1999;44:507.

56. Menotti A, et al. Food Intake Patterns and 25-Year Mortality from Coronary Heart Disease: Cross-Cultural Correlations in the Seven Countries Study. The Seven Countries Study Research Group. *Eur J Epidemiol* 1999;15:507.

57. Kafatos A, et al. Nutrition Status of the Elderly in Anogia, Crete, Greece. *J Am Coll Nutr* 1993;12:685.

58. Mata P, et al. Effects of Long-Term Monounsaturated- vs Polyunsaturated-Enriched Diets on Lipoproteins in Healthy Men and Women. *Am J Clin Nutr* 1992;55:846.

59. Sirtori CR, et al. Olive Oil, Corn Oil, and N-3 Fatty Acids Differently Affect Lipids, Lipoproteins, Platelets, and Superoxide Formation in Type II Hypercholesterolemia. *Am J Clin Nutr* 1992;56:113.

60. Mata P, et al. Effect of Dietary Monounsaturated Fatty Acids on Plasma Lipoproteins and Apolipoproteins in Women. *Am J Clin Nutr* 1992;56:77.

61. Mensink RP, Katan MB. Effect of a Diet Enriched with Monounsaturated Fatty or Polyunsaturated Fatty Acids on Levels of Low-Density and High-Density Lipoprotein Cholesterol in Healthy Men and Women. *N Engl J Med* 1989;321:436.

62. Kris-Etherton PM, et al. High-Monounsaturated Fatty Acid Diets Lower Both Plasma Cholesterol and Triacylglycerol Concentrations. *Am J Clin Nutr* 1999;70:1009.

63. Manna C, et al. The Protective Effect of the Olive Oil Polyphenol (3,4-Dihydroxyphenyl)-Ethanol Counteracts Reactive Oxygen Metabolite-Induced Cytotoxicity in Caco-2 Cells. *J Nutr* 1997;127:286.

Chapter 18 - Using Dietary Fat to Burn Bodyfat

64. Caruso D, et al. Effect of Virgin Olive Oil Phenolic Compounds on In Vitro Oxidation of Human Low Density Lipoproteins. *Nutr Metab Cardiovasc Dis* 1999;9:102.

65. Baroni SS, et al. Solid Monounsaturated Diet Lowers LDL Unsaturation Trait and Oxidisability in Hypercholesterolemic (Type IIb) Patients. *Free Radic Res* 1999;30:275.

66. Baggio G, et al. Olive-Oil-Enriched Diet: Effect on Serum Lipoprotein Levels and Biliary Cholesterol Saturation. *Am J Clin Nutr* 1988;47:960.

67. Grundy SM, et al. Comparison of Monounsaturated Fatty Acids and Carbohydrates for Reducing Raised Levels of Plasma Cholesterol in Man. *Am J Clin Nutr* 1988;47:965.

68. Grundy SM. Comparison of Monounsaturated Fatty Acids and Carbohydrates for Lowering Plasma Cholesterol. *N Engl J Med* 1986;314:745.

69. Rasmussen OW, et al. Effects on Blood Pressure, Glucose, and Lipid Levels of a High-Monounsaturated Fat Diet Compared with a High-Carbohydrate Diet in NIDDM Subjects. *Diabetes Care* 1993;16:1565.

70. Campbell LV, et al. The High-Monounsaturated Fat Diet as a Practical Alternative for NIDDM. *Diabetes Care* 1994;17:177.

71. Rasmussen OW, et al. [Favourable Effect of Olive Oil in Patients with Non-Insulin-Dependent Diabetes. The Effect on Blood Pressure, Blood Glucose and Lipid Levels of a High-Fat Diet Rich in Monounsaturated Fat Compared with a Carbohydrate-Rich Diet]. *Ugeskr Laeger* 1995;157:1028. Danish.

72. Erasmus U. *Fats that Heal Fats that Kill.* BC, Canada: Alive Books 1993, p. 255.

73. Id. at 256.

73a. Lichtenstein AH, et al. Effects of Canola, Corn, and Olive Oils on Fasting and Postprandial Plasma Lipoproteins in Humans as Part of a National Cholesterol Education Program Step 2 Diet. *Arterioscler Thromb* 1993;13:1533.

74. Wiseman SA, et al. Dietary Non-Tocopherol Antioxidants Present in Extra Virgin Olive Oil Increase the Resistance of Low Density Lipoproteins to Oxidation in Rabbits. *Atherosclerosis* 1996;120:15.

75. Ramirez-Tortosa MC, et al. Extra-Virgin Olive Oil Increases the Resistance of LDL to Oxidation More than Refined Olive Oil in Free-Living Men with Peripheral Vascular Disease. *J Nutr* 1999;129:2177.

76. Fumeron F, et al. Lowering of HDL2-Cholesterol and Lipoprotein A-I Particle Levels by Increasing the Ratio of Polyunsaturated to Saturated Fatty Acids. *Am J Clin Nutr* 1991;53:655.

77. Jackson RL, et al. Influence of Polyunsaturated and Saturated Fats on Plasma Lipids and Lipoproteins in Man. *Am J Clin Nutr* 1984;39:589.

78. Rudel LL, Haines JL, Sawyer JK. Effects on Plasma Lipoproteins of Monounsaturated, Saturated, and Polyunsaturated Fatty Acids in the Diet of African Green Monkeys. *J Lipid Res* 1990;31:1873

79. Vessby B, Lithell H, Boberg J. Reduction of Low Density and High Density Lipoprotein Cholesterol by Fat-Modified Diets. A Survey of Recent Findings. *Hum Nutr Clin Nutr* 1982;36:203.

80. Brunner R. Dietary Fat and Ischemic Stroke. *JAMA* 1998;279:1171.

81. Mylonas C, Kouretas D. Lipid Peroxidation and Tissue Damage. *In Vivo* 1999;13:295.

82. Kanner J, German JB, Kinsella JE. Initiation of Lipid Peroxidation in Biological Systems. *Crit Rev Food Sci Nutr* 1987;25:317.

83. Shaw S, Pearson D. *Life Extension.* NY: Warner Books 1982.

84. Vendemiale G, Grattagliano I, Altomare E. An Update on the Role of Free Radicals and Antioxidant Defense in Human Disease. *Int J Clin Lab Res* 1999;29:49.

85. Casaril M, Corso F, Corrocher R. [Free Radicals in Human Pathology]. *Recenti Prog Med* 1991;82:39. Italian.

86. Bunker VW. Free Radicals, Antioxidants and Ageing. *Med Lab Sci* 1992;49:299.

87. Ames BN. Dietary Carcinogens and Anticarcinogens. Oxygen Radicals and Degenerative Diseases. *Science* 1983;221:1256.

88. Proctor PH, Reynolds ES. Free Radicals and Disease in Man. *Physiol Chem Phys* 1984;16:175.

89. Cross CE, et al. Oxygen Radicals and Human Disease. *Ann Int Med* 1987;107:526.

Natural Hormonal Enhancement

90. Gower JD. A Role for Dietary Lipids and Antioxidants in the Activation of Carcinogens. *Free Radic Biol Med* 1988;5:95.

91. Jenkinson A, et al. Dietary Intakes of Polyunsaturated Fatty Acids and Indices of Oxidative Stress in Human Volunteers. *Eur J Clin Nutr* 1999;53:523.

92. Durak I, et al. High-Temperature Effects on Antioxidant Systems and Toxic Product Formation in Nutritional Oils. *J Toxicol Environ Health* 1999;57:585.

93. Eritsland J. Safety Considerations of Polyunsaturated Fatty Acids. *Am J Clin Nutr* 2000;71:197.

94. Braden LM, Carroll KK. Dietary Polyunsaturated Fat in Relation to Mammary Carcinogenesis in Rats. *Lipids* 1986;21:285.

95. Enig MG, Munn RJ, Keeney M. Dietary Fat and Cancer Trends--A Critique. *Fed Proc* 1978;37:2215.

96. Keeney M. Comments on the Effects of Dietary Trans-Fatty Acids in Humans. *Cancer Res* 1981;41:3743.

96a. Ascherio A, Willett WC. Health Effects of Trans Fatty Acids. *Am J Clin Nutr* 1997;66(Suppl):1006S.

97. Brisson GJ. *Lipids in Human Nutrition.* NJ: Burgess 1981, p. 39.

98. Sugano M, Ikeda I. Metabolic Interactions between Essential and Trans-Fatty Acids. *Curr Opin Lipidol* 1996;7:38.

99. Kinsella JE, et al. Metabolism of Trans Fatty Acids with Emphasis on the Effects of Trans, Trans-Octadecadienoate on Lipid Composition, Essential Fatty Acid, and Prostaglandins: An Overview. *Am J Clin Nutr* 1981;34:2307.

100. Mahfouz M. Effect of Dietary Trans Fatty Acids on the Delta 5, Delta 6 and Delta 9 Desaturases of Rat Liver Microsomes In Vivo. *Acta Biol Med Ger* 1981;40:1699.

101. Mahfouz MM, Smith TL, Kummerow FA. Effect of Dietary Fats on Desaturase Activities and the Biosynthesis of Fatty Acids in Rat-Liver Microsomes. *Lipids* 1984;19:214.

102. Willett WC, et al. Intake of Trans Fatty Acids and Risk of Coronary Heart Disease among Women. *Lancet* 1993;341:581.

103. Ascherio A, et al. Trans Fatty Intake and Risk of Myocardial Infarction. *Circulation* 1994;89:94.

104. Thomas LH. Ischaemic Heart Disease and Consumption of Hydrogenated Marine Oils in England and Wales. *J Epidemiol Community Health* 1992;46:78.

105. Thomas LH, Winter JA, Scott RG. Concentration of 18:1 and 16:1 Transunsaturated Fatty Acids in the Adipose Body Tissue of Decedents Dying of Ischaemic Heart Disease Compared with Controls: Analysis by Gas Liquid Chromatography. *J Epidemiol Community Health* 1983;37:16.

106. Thomas L. Mortality from Arteriosclerotic Disease and Consumption of Hydrogenated Oils and Fats. *Brit J Preven Soc Med* 1975;29:82.

107. Pietinen P, et al. Intake of Fatty Acids and Risk of Coronary Heart Disease in a Cohort of Finnish Men. The Alpha-Tocopherol, Beta-Carotene Cancer Prevention Study. *Am J Epidemiol* 1997;145:876.

108. Mensink RP, Katan MB. Effect of Dietary Trans Fatty Acids on High Density and Low Density Cholesterol Levels in Healthy Subjects. *N Engl J Med* 1990;323:439.

109. Katan MB, Zock PL, Mensink RP. Trans Fatty Acids and their Effects on Lipoproteins in Humans. *Annu Rev Nutr* 1995;15:473.

110. Judd JT, et al. Dietary Trans Fatty Acids: Effects on Plasma Lipids and Lipoproteins of Healthy Men and Women. *Am J Clin Nutr* 1994;59:861.

111. Zock PL, Mensink RP. Dietary Trans-Fatty Acids and Serum Lipoproteins in Humans. *Curr Opin Lipidol* 1996;7:34.

112. Zock PL, Katan MB. Trans Fatty Acids, Lipoproteins, and Coronary Risk. *Can J Physiol Pharmacol* 1997;75:211.

113. Mensink RP, Katan MB. Effect of Dietary Fatty Acids on Serum Lipids and Lipoproteins: A Meta-Analysis of 27 Trials. *Arterioscler Thromb* 1992;12:911.

114. Berglund L, et al. HDL-Subpopulation Patterns in Response to Reductions in Dietary Total nd Saturated Fat Intakes in Healthy Subjects. *Am J Clin Nutr* 1999;70:992.

115. Aro A, et al. Stearic Acid, Trans Fatty Acids, and Dairy Fat: Effects on Serum and Lipoprotein Lipids, Apolipoproteins, Lipoprotein(A), and Lipid Transfer Proteins in Healthy Subjects. *Am J Clin Nutr* 1997;65:1419.

184

116. Sundram K, et al. Trans (Elaidic) Fatty Acids Adversely Affect the Lipoprotein Profile Relative to Specific Saturated Fatty Acids in Humans. *J Nutr* 1997;127:514S.

117. Carlson SE, et al. Trans Fatty Acids: Infant and Fetal Development. *Am J Clin Nutr* 1997;66(Suppl):715S.

118. Koletzko B. [Supply, Metabolism and Biological Effects of Trans-Isomeric Fatty Acids in Infants]. *Nahrung* 1991;35:229. German.

119. Hanis T, et al. Effects of Dietary Trans-Fatty Acids on Reproductive Performance of Wistar Rats. *Br J Nutr* 1989;61:519.

120. Kohlmeier L, et al. Adipose Tissue Trans Fatty Acids and Breast Cancer in the European Community Multicenter Study on Antioxidants, Myocardial Infarction, and Breast Cancer. *Cancer Epidemiol Biomarkers Prev* 1997;6:705.

121. Simopoulos AP, et al. Overview of Evolutionary Aspects of Omega 3 Fatty Acids in the Diet. *World Rev Nutr Diet* 1998;83:1.

122. Erasmus U. *Fats that Heal Fats that Kill*. BC, Canada: Alive Books 1993, p. 52.

123. Simopoulos AP. Essential Fatty Acids in Health and Chronic Disease. *Am J Clin Nutr* 1999;70(Suppl):560S.

124. Parkinson AJ, et al. Elevated Concentrations of Plasma Omega-3 Polyunsaturated Fatty Acids among Alaskan Eskimos. *Am J Clin Nutr* 1994;59:384.

125. Feskens EJ, Kromhout D. Epidemiologic Studies on Eskimos and Fish Intake. *Ann N Y Acad Sci* 1993;683:9.

126. Daviglus ML, et al. Fish Consumption and the 30-Year Risk of Fatal Myocardial Infarction. *N Engl J Med* 1997;336:1046.

127. Albert CM, et al. Fish Consumption and Risk of Sudden Cardiac Death. *JAMA* 1998;279:23.

128. Guallar Castillon E, et al. [Fish Consumption and Coronary Mortality in the General Population: A Meta-Analysis of Cohort Studies]. *Gac Sanit* 1993;7:228. Spanish.

129. Kromhout D, Bosschieter EB, de Lezenne Coulander C. The Inverse Relation between Fish Consumption and 20-Year Mortality from Coronary Heart Disease. *N Engl J Med* 1985;312:1205.

130. Siscovick DS, et al. Dietary Intake and Cell Membrane Levels of Long-Chain N-3 Polyunsaturated Fatty Acids and the Risk of Primary Cardiac Arrest. *JAMA* 1995;274:1363.

131. Phillipson BE, et al. Reduction of Plasma Lipids, Lipoproteins, and Apoproteins by Dietary Fish Oils in Patients with Hypertriglyceridemia. *N Engl J Med* 1985;312:1210.

132. Harris WS. Dietary Fish Oil and Blood Lipids. *Curr Opin Lipidol* 1996;7:3.

133. Roche HM, Gibney MJ. Long-Chain N-3 Polyunsaturated Fatty Acids and Triacylglycerol Metabolism in the Postprandial State. *Lipids* 1999;34(Suppl):S259.

134. Harris WS. Nonpharmacologic Treatment of Hypertriglyceridemia: Focus on Fish Oils. *Clin Cardiol* 1999;22(Suppl):II40.

135. Nieuwenhuys CM, et al. Hypocoagulant and Lipid-Lowering Effects of Dietary N-3 Polyunsaturated Fatty Acids with Unchanged Platelet Activation in Rats. *Arterioscler Thromb Vasc Biol* 1998;18:1480.

136. McIntosh GH, et al. The Influence of Dietary Fats on Plasma Lipids, Blood Pressure and Coagulation Indices in the Rat. *Atherosclerosis* 1985;55:125.

137. Kromhout D. The Importance of N-6 and N-3 Fatty Acids in Carcinogenesis. *Med Oncol Tumor Pharmacother* 1990;7:173.

138. Cave WT Jr. Dietary n-3 (omega-3) Polyunsaturated Fatty Acid Effects on Animal Tumorigenesis. *FASEB J* 1991;5:2160.

139. de Deckere EA. Possible Beneficial Effect of Fish and Fish N-3 Polyunsaturated Fatty Acids in Breast and Colorectal Cancer. *Eur J Cancer Prev* 1999;8:213.

140. Latham P, Lund EK, Johnson IT. Dietary n-3 PUFA Increases the Apoptotic Response to 1,2-Dimethylhydrazine, Reduces Mitosis and Suppresses the Induction of Carcinogenesis in the Rat Colon. *Carcinogenesis* 1999;20:645.

141. Raheja BS, et al. Significance of the N-6/N-3 Ratio for Insulin Action in Diabetes. *Ann N Y Acad Sci* 1993;683:258.

142. Behme MT. Dietary Fish Oil Enhances Insulin Sensitivity in Miniature Pigs. *J Nutr* 1996;126:1549.

143. Luo J, et al. Dietary (n-3) Polyunsaturated Fatty Acids Improve Adipocyte Insulin Action and Glucose Metabolism in Insulin-Resistant Rats: Relation to Membrane Fatty Acids. *J Nutr* 1996;126:1951.

144. Chicco A, et al. Effect of Moderate Levels of Dietary Fish Oil on Insulin Secretion and Sensitivity, and Pancreas Insulin Content in Normal Rats. *Ann Nutr Metab* 1996;40:61.

145. Liu S, et al. Dietary Omega-3 and Polyunsaturated Fatty Acids Modify Fatty Acyl Composition and Insulin Binding in Skeletal-Muscle Sarcolemma. *Biochem J* 1994 1;299:831.

146. Belzung F, Raclot T, Groscolas R. Fish Oils N-3 Fatty Acids Selectively Limit the Hypertrophy of Abdominal Fat Depots in Growing Rats Fed High Fat Diets. *Am J Physiol* 1993;264:R1111.

147. Parrish CC, Pathy DA, Angel A. Dietary Fish Oils Limit Adipose Tissue Hypertrophy in Rats. *Metabolism* 1990;39:217.

148. Ross JA, Moses AG, Fearon KC. The Anti-Catabolic Effects of N-3 Fatty Acids. *Curr Opin Clin Nutr Metab Care* 1999;2:219.

149. Hayashi N, et al. Effect of Intravenous Omega-6 and Omega-3 Fat Emulsions on Nitrogen Retention and Protein Kinetics in Burned Rats. *Nutrition* 1999;15:135.

150. Gronn M, et al. Effects of Dietary Purified Eicosapentaenoic Acid (20:5 (N-3)) and Docosahexaenoic Acid (22:6(N-3)) on Fatty Acid Desaturation and Oxidation in Isolated Rat Liver Cells. *Biochim Biophys Acta* 1992;1125:35.

151. Fischer MA, Black HS. Modification of Membrane Composition, Eicosanoid Metabolism, and Immunoresponsiveness by Dietary Omega-3 and Omega-6 Fatty Acid Sources, Modulators of Ultraviolet-Carcinogenesis. *Photochem Photobiol* 1991;54:381.

152. Garg ML, Thomson AB, Clandinin MT. Effect of Dietary Cholesterol and/or Omega 3 Fatty Acids on Lipid Composition and Delta 5-Desaturase Activity of Rat Liver Microsomes. *J Nutr* 1988;118:661.

153. Erasmus U. *Fats that Heal Fats that Kill*. BC, Canada: Alive Books 1993.

154. Sandy S, Pearson D. *Life Extension*. NY: Warner Books 1982, p. 368.

155. Dinh TK, Bourre JM, Durand G. Effect of Age and Alpha-Linolenic Acid Deficiency on Delta 6 Desaturase Activity and Liver Lipids in Rats. *Lipids* 1993;28:517.

156. Bordoni A, et al. Dual Influence of Aging and Vitamin B6 Deficiency on Delta-6-Desaturation of Essential Fatty Acids in Rat Liver Microsomes. *Prostaglandins Leukot Essent Fatty Acids* 1998;58:417.

157. Eades M, Eades MD. *Protein Power*. NY: Bantam Books 1996, p. 80-81.

158. Foran JA, Cox M, Croxton D. Sport Fish Consumption Advisories and Projected Cancer Risks in the Great Lakes Basin. *Am J Public Health* 1989;79:322.

186

Chapter 19

Common Mistakes
and
How to Avoid Them

Fools never learn;
Intelligent men learn from their own mistakes;
Wise men learn from the mistakes of others.
Unknown

Failure is an opportunity to begin again more intelligently.
Henry Ford

Better to prepare and prevent than to repair and repent.
Unknown

The less you leave to chance, the better chance you'll have.
Ross Perot

Based on my experience coaching people on the NHE Eating Plan, as well as my own experience on the Eating Plan, I have isolated a few of the lurking pitfalls to which the unwary often fall victim. As I have said before, if you follow the Eating Plan, *you cannot fail*. It's like going into a Chinese restaurant and ordering bagels and lox - failure is simply not on the menu.

Unless you are among the rare exceptions, you will lose bodyfat steadily and predictably if you follow the Eating Plan. The key words are, "if you follow the Eating Plan." The NHE Eating Plan puts subtle but powerful fat-burning forces into action in your body; and it is easy to make subtle but powerful mistakes that negate these forces and deny you the fabulous results the Eating Plan is capable of producing.

I hope that you will resolve, at the outset, to avoid these mistakes. If, however, after a few weeks, you find that you are not seeing the results you expect from the Eating Plan, you should revisit this chapter and try to identify the source of your difficulties. The majority of the time, the resolution to your fat loss shortcoming can be found on the pages of this chapter. Once you identify the problem and make the appropriate changes, you will be back on the fast track to permanent fat loss.

For further assistance, go to www.extique.com and click on "Ask Rob." There you will find my answers to frequently asked questions.

Witch's Brew, Misplaced Loyalty, and the Felt Need to Conform

One mistake is mixing diets, combining aspects of currently popular diets with the NHE Eating Plan and putting them together into your own personal dietary witch's brew. Don't. Should you feel a need to make modifications, do so within the framework of the Eating

Plan, as discussed in Chapter 15. If, instead, you make self-invented modifications, you may wind-up modifying your way out of the Eating Plan and into the nether world of conventional dieting. Failure and frustration are the standard penalties for such false ingenuity.

While eating too much fat is a mistake, it is less common than you might suppose. In the absence of hormonal hunger and with "hidden fat" eliminated from your diet, it is unlikely that you will consume too much fat. A more common mistake is eating too little fat in an effort to remain faithful to the misled forces in society that have labeled dietary fat as some kind of monster.

I have gone to considerable lengths in this book to dispel the "fat makes you fat" myth in an effort to protect you from falling into the trap of undue fat restriction. Even so, some people will still feel the need to remain loyal to their low-fat master. The high-carb/low-fat paradigm is quickly falling from grace as its profound ineffectiveness gains belated recognition. But its ultimate collapse will not come soon enough for those people who cannot resist the pervasive anti-fat hysteria that has gripped our society. Low-fat is the in-thing; it's accepted, and it's fashionable. But having a low-fat body is even more fashionable than eating low fat, so keep your sights set on your ultimate objective and don't be diverted by the same felt need to conform that has led so many people down a blind alley.

Don't Get Nickeled and Dimed to Death by Hidden Carbs

The NHE Eating Plan does not require a great deal of willpower because self-deprivation, the outstanding element of conventional diets, is not part of the program. Vigilance, however, is required. Without it, hidden carbohydrates infiltrate your diet and undercut your efforts to lose fat. The problem here is that carbohydrate is hidden in many foods that are not typically associated with carbohydrate.

It is common knowledge that potatoes, pasta, bread, and dessert foods contain carbohydrate. But what about ketchup, salad dressing, barbecue sauce, breaded or processed meats, and gourmet coffee? All of these foods contain "hidden carbs." Hidden carbs are ubiquitous in today's processed-food, sweet-tooth, food culture. In fact, your best bet is to assume that everything (except eggs and unprocessed meat) contains hidden carbs, then proceed to figure-out just how many grams of carbohydrate are hiding in your food. The smoke and mirrors of hidden carbs can be very tricky; some salad dressings (like Italian or blue cheese) contain virtually zero grams of carbohydrate while other dressings (like French) are loaded with them.

This is not to suggest that hidden carbs should be avoided altogether, merely that you must be aware at all times of how much carbohydrate you are consuming and make the proper adjustments respecting carb limits. Otherwise, carbs add-up, little by little, bit by bit, and can wind-up pushing you over your daily carb-intake allocation. You think you are following the NHE Eating Plan to a tee, but, unwittingly, you are exceeding your carbohydrate limit every day. When the fat doesn't come off like it's supposed to, you are befuddled - "what happened?" you ask. Answer: you got nickeled and dimed to death by hidden carbs.

I've seen it happen many times and it's a back-breaker on the NHE Eating Plan, because everything is predicated on your being in a fat-burning state. When carbohydrate intake is too high, you never fully make the metabolic shift. Instead, you wind-up in metabolic no-man's land, and this can be the worst of all worlds. In this state (somewhere between heaven and hell), you never completely shake hormonal hunger and you are continually at risk of storing dietary fat as bodyfat since fat is fattening when you are not in a fat-burning state.

Metabolic Purgatory

Be Proactive, Not Reactive

On the NHE Eating Plan, if you fail to plan - you plan to fail. Another popular saying also applies to the Eating Plan: the five Ps - proper preparation prevents poor procedure. More directly, if you begin the day with no idea of what you are going to eat that day, you're in trouble. Market forces favor processed, carbohydrate-laden foods. These foods are everywhere and eating them on a regular basis is incompatible with fat loss. If you don't bring food to work and you are constantly forced to improvise, you will experience difficulty adhering to the Eating Plan.

When suitable food is not readily available, and time and convenience are pressing factors, fast-food beckons. Most fast-foods are loaded with refined carbohydrate. Ordering a cheeseburger "hold the bread" is fine occasionally, but you can't do that every day. The fast-food environment presents you with a very narrow selection of acceptable options, and tempts you to partake of the unacceptable options.

In addition, when you do not have suitable food on hand, you are more likely to put-off eating until you are hungry rather than eating to prevent hunger. And under the influence of hunger, you are more likely to make poor food choices. You must plan ahead. If you are constantly rolling with the punches, you will eventually get knocked-out.

The solution is simple: prepare food in advance and have suitable snacks available at all times, particularly in the beginning when you are becoming accustomed to a new way of eating and battling cravings into submission. If you do not own airtight food containers, that should be your first investment. If you are on the road a lot, a cooler for your car would also be a good investment. As the American Civil War illustrated more than a century ago, no matter how brilliant the battleplan, and no matter how strong the will of those carrying it out, an undertaking cannot succeed without adequate support and supplies. With this in mind, I offer the following suggestion to you in your war against bodyfat: whatever paraphernalia you need in order to ensure that you have Eating-Plan-friendly food available at all times, get it.

189

Snacking: When and Why

Eat every few hours irrespective of whether you are hungry. Each between-meal interval does not have to be the exact same duration, *but no interval should be longer than 4 hours.* Whether you designate a particular feeding a "meal" or a "snack" is mere semantics. What matters is that you **eat to prevent hunger rather than eating in response to hunger**. Should you find that you have no desire to eat within 4 hours after your last meal/snack, fine - simply eat a small snack like a handful of nuts, or a tablespoon of peanut butter, or a few slices of cheese or turkey, or a protein shake. In other words, *desire to eat influences the size of the feeding NOT whether or not you feed.*

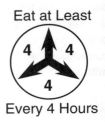

Eat at Least

Every 4 Hours

Animals are wholly influenced by primal drives and appetites, but humans typically give consideration to other factors like, for instance: how long they wish to live, how good they wish to feel, and what they wish their body to look like. For NHE adherents, in particular, decisions regarding nutrient intake are based on a systematic strategy of self-betterment that preempts mindless impulses like hunger. By eating when you are *not* hungry, you are being proactive and guaranteeing that hunger will stay away for another few hours. If you do this perpetually, you'll never be hungry.

If, however, you allow more than 4 hours to elapse without eating, you relinquish control. In this scenario, you are, in effect, sitting back and waiting for hunger to strike - *you are letting the enemy in the door.* Under the influence of an appetite surge, your eating decisions are likely to become distorted. Don't make matters unnecessarily difficult for yourself - get with the program.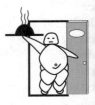

If you are doing things right, after you have settled into the NHE Eating Plan you will rarely, if ever, have an urge to gorge yourself. Ravenous hunger and intense cravings are abnormal appetite manifestations resulting from any or a combination of the following: 1) a "starve and stuff" pattern of eating, 2) chronic high-carbohydrate consumption, 3) excessive restriction of fat or calories. The Eating Plan stamps-out all three of these practices.

If appetite flare-ups do occur, they should be interpreted as an indication that you have made a mistake somewhere. Are you eating too little fat? Is your carb-load comprised mainly of sugary carbs rather than starchy carbs? Are you allowing more than 4 hours to elapse between feedings? With both hormonal hunger and real hunger nullified, you will be left with a normal, healthy appetite (see Chapters 10 and 11). Feel free to eat more or less sizable meals as your appetite dictates - but "more sizable" should never amount to gorging (see Chapter 17 for a discussion of meal size).

Snacking: What and How

Nuts (cashews, almonds, walnuts, pecans, etc. - take your pick) are portable and convenient. Raw nuts and seeds, sold at health food stores, are craving-killing dynamos, containing protein (particularly rich in the superstar amino acid, arginine), "good fat," fiber, potassium and magnesium, more naturally occurring vitamin E than any other food, and conferring a strong thermogenic effect. What else could you ask for in a snack? Less carbohydrate perhaps, but as long as you eat nuts in moderation this relatively-low-active-carb food is not a threat to carb limits.

Based on the superb nutrient profile of nuts, and the fact that nut trees grow **Nuts** abundantly in the heart-healthy Mediterranean region where they are a dietary tradition, it has long been suspected that this relatively high-fat food helps prevent heart disease. Even so, recent research confirming this hypothesis has surpassed expectations. To quote an article in the September 1999 issue of the *American Journal of Clinical Nutrition*,[1] "one of the most unexpected and novel findings in nutritional epidemiology in the past 5 yrs. has been that nut consumption seems to protect against ischemic heart disease." The same article, after reviewing the remarkably strong inverse correlations observed not only for nut consumption/heart disease but also for nut consumption/all-cause mortality, concluded that "nut consumption may not only offer protection against [heart disease], but also increase longevity."

The epidemiological studies finding that nuts protect against heart disease[2,3,4] are consistent with clinical trials finding that nut consumption lowers LDL and triglyceride levels.[5,6,7] Based on the evidence to date, frequent nut consumption may decrease coronary risk by up to 40%.[8] In one study published in the *Archives of Internal Medicine*, eating nuts 5 times per week was associated with a lower risk of heart disease than exercising 3 times per week.[9] (Incidentally, this same study found donut consumption to be hazardous, correlating with high risk of both coronary mortality and all-cause mortality – we may have identified a new cop killer.)

Based on the apparent potency of its cardioprotective effect, it is likely that a synergism exists among the various nutritive elements of nuts. Not coincidentally, humans and our genetic predecessors have been snacking on nuts for millions of years. By contrast, potato chips and pretzels have been around for only as long as widespread obesity and degenerative disease have plagued humankind, approximately 100 years.

If nuts are the best snacks, which are the best nuts? Recall from Chapter 18 that walnuts, pumpkin seeds, and soybeans each contain omega 3 fat in addition to other good fats. Also recall from Chapter 18 that omega 3 fat facilitates fat loss in addition to conveying other health benefits. Raw nuts are better than roasted, processed ones because raw nuts generally contain less fat, less sodium, and superior essential fatty acid content (the heat of roasting deactivates essential fatty acids). In either event, be sure to account for nuts' modest carbohydrate content in your daily and per-meal carb calculation. And remember to subtract dietary fiber to get "active carbs" (see Chapter 14); otherwise, you are cheating yourself out of permissible carbohydrate. Bottom line: go nuts.

191

Nut butter is a tasty and spreadable variation on the nut theme. Don't limit yourself to peanut butter. At your local natural food store you should find any or all of the following: almond butter, cashew butter, hazelnut butter, and tahini (sesame seed butter). Nut butter is more calorie-dense than raw nuts, with more fat due to added oil. Thus, a little bit goes a long way toward preventing cravings. In fact, nut butter does such a good job of neutralizing cravings that if you eat too much of it at one sitting, you are likely to "ruin your appetite" (just what your mother always warned you about) for many hours afterwards - so use it sparingly. *Remember, your mindset should always be:* "I don't want to eat too much now, because I'll be eating again in just a few hours" - and then live-up to your word by eating again in a few hours. Before you know it, eating smaller more frequent meals will become a habit.

Be sure to buy only natural nut butters. Those are the ones that do not bear the words "partially hydrogenated" or "hydrogenated" on the label. The basis of this recommendation is that unnatural oils contain trans fatty acids which, as you learned in Chapter 18, represent roadblocks on the path to a better body. Because they are not hydrogenated, natural nut butters tend to be less creamy, with a grainier texture, and the oil tends to separate from the nutmush.* As a general rule, the more wholesome the food, the more quickly it spoils (especially if it contains fat). Accordingly, foods containing natural oils should be stored in the refrigerator.

Fruit

Fruit, too, is a suitable snack (see Chapter 15 for recommended fruits). Fruit is not as good of a snack as nuts and seeds, however, because fruit contains only carbohydrate and fiber - scant protein and negligible fat (both of which augment the satiety value of a food). But if you are creative, you can circumvent this shortcoming. For example, an apple combined with peanut butter contains carbohydrate, protein, and fat. Similarly, strawberries and cream contains carbohydrate and fat (not quite as good as apple and peanut butter). Fruit is an excellent food, containing vitamins, minerals, antioxidants, and fiber; but it must be eaten in measured moderation if you are to stay within carb limits.

Lean Meat

Lean meat is a terrific snack in terms of its substance, but it does not rank highly in the categories of convenience and portability since it must be cooked and refrigerated; and even then, it does not have nearly the edible lifespan of nuts. If you opt to snack on meat, I recommend cooking steak or chicken/turkey and keeping it in your cooler or refrigerator for easy access. Recall from Chapter 16 that lean meat is "the king of thermogenic foods," which means it cranks-up your metabolism. But be careful, the more convenient and portable meat snacks are usually the processed ones which often contain hidden carbs. For example, lunch meats and beef jerky each can vary widely in carbohydrate content from zero to as much as a piece of candy.

* Don't look for it in the dictionary.

Cheese is another worthy snack. Unlike meat, it does not require cooking, **Cheese**
but it too requires refrigeration, which limits portability. As with meat, be
judicious in your cheese consumption so as not to go overboard with saturated fat, which
cheese contains in abundance. Real cheese is very low in carbohydrate, but beware of
"cheese food," which looks exactly like real cheese and tastes similar but usually
contains corn syrup or other carb-garbage. Based on my observations, up to 70% of the
sliced cheese sold in the dairy section of grocery stores is "cheese food." Apparently
cheese food sells well, probably because it costs less to buy (and much less to produce)
and most people do not imagine that there is a difference between cheese (a food) and
"cheese food."

Cottage cheese is an outstanding snack, containing less fat and **Cottage Cheese**
substantially more protein than cheese. I prefer 4% lowfat cottage
cheese, which contains approximately 5 grams of fat (3 grams saturated) per ½ cup, just
enough to counteract cravings and confer a rich taste, and 13 grams of protein. By
adding cottage cheese (or ricotta cheese which has essentially the same nutritional
profile, but a different taste and texture) to salad or fruit, you transform a low-protein
meal into a moderate-/high-protein meal. In this way, cottage cheese can help you
achieve your "protein optimization" objectives (see Chapter 17).

Better Living Through Better Brain Chemistry:
Using Food to Enhance Mental Performance and Emotional Well-Being

Cheese and cottage cheese have another virtuous attribute. The relatively unknown fact is that
cheese and cottage cheese are powerful brain boosters. They achieve this effect by means of their
impact on brain chemicals called neurotransmitters, which we've discussed in other parts of this
book. Neurotransmitters convey impulses across neuronal synapses in the brain. Collectively, these
impulses comprise the symphony of thoughts and emotions that you experience as an intelligent,
self-aware being.

Each protein food has a unique amino acid profile. For instance, egg white protein and whey
protein are high in branched chain amino acids (leucine, isoleucine, and valine). Cheese and
cottage cheese are high in the amino acids phenylalanine and tyrosine, which are precursors to the
neurotransmitters norepinephrine and dopamine. Recall from Chapter 10 that these
neurotransmitters increase the rate of activity (i.e., neurotransmission) in the brain, thereby
increasing mental productivity and mental clarity. Norepinephrine, also called noradrenaline, is very
similar to the hormone adrenaline. In fact, noradrenaline is sometimes referred to as "the brain's
adrenaline."

Eating cheese, cottage cheese, or soy before an exam or business meeting can work to your
advantage by enhancing mental clarity and literally making you think quicker. If, on the other hand,
you are nervous or anxious about your meeting, exam, etc. to the point where it may impair your
performance, increase the carbohydrate content of this meal - the resulting serotonin boost will
produce a calming effect. You should determine the optimal mental state for the task ahead, and
then structure your meal accordingly. (Vitamins C and B-6 facilitate conversion of phenylalanine
and tyrosine to norepinephrine and thus can heighten the potency of a brain-boosting meal.)

Caffeine and, to a much greater degree, cocaine, exert their stimulatory effect by means of
inducing the release of stored norepinephrine in the brain. Hence, the characterization of caffeine
as a mind-accelerating mood booster is not just hype brewed-up by the coffee industry. However,
there are important differences between the neurochemical dynamics of a drug-induced brain
boost and a protein-induced brain boost.

For one, you develop a tolerance to stimulant drugs, which renders a given dosage decreasingly potent over time. Furthermore, where an unaccustomed dose is ingested, you "crash" from the drugs because they deplete the neurotransmitters that they stimulate. By contrast, when you eat foods containing phenylalanine and tyrosine, you supply the raw materials to support production of norepinephrine and dopamine; hence, there is no crash suffered nor tolerance acquired. (Other protein foods, too, like chicken, fish, and eggs, contain phenylalanine and tyrosine but in lower concentrations than cheese, cottage cheese, and tofu.) Protein foods also contain tryptophan, the amino acid precursor to serotonin. Whereas a protein meal supports production of serotonin, a carbohydrate meal provokes a sharp, unnatural serotonin spike (see Chapters 9 and 16).

In general, stress increases nutritional needs. In particular, stress depletes norepinephrine, resulting in mental fatigue, loss of concentration, and heightened susceptibility to depression. Often when you feel mentally "drained" you are, in fact, suffering from a drain on your norepinephrine stores that has outstripped your brain's ability to replace. Low norepinephrine, like low serotonin, manifests itself emotionally and behaviorally. For example, deficits in either of these neurotransmitters can cause depression. However, because of the fundamentally different effects of these two neurotransmitters, the type of depression is different in each case. Whereas low-norepinephrine depression is characterized by lethargy and lack of motivation, low-serotonin depression is characterized by anxiety, irritability, and insomnia. In addition to emotional well-being and mental performance, neurotransmitters (particularly their decline with advancing age) play a key role in senility, the great dehumanizer that turns alert, sensitive, self-sufficient persons into apathetic, shuffling zombies. (Evidence discussed in the next chapter suggests that Alzheimer's disease, the most dementing form of senility, is hormonally rooted.)

Don't hold your breath waiting for the medicine men or the legal drug dealers in this country to acknowledge (or become aware of) the link between nutrition and mental health. Although this connection is firmly grounded in scientific fact and bears important implications for everyone (especially the millions whose lives are darkened by depression), it presents no profit potential to the health establishment and runs counter to the institutional bias against natural approaches to health.

References

1. Sabate J. Nut Consumption, Vegetarian Diets, Ischemic Heart Disease Risk, and All-Cause Mortality: Evidence from Epidemiologic Studies. *Am J Clin Nutr* 1999;70(Suppl):500S.

2. Fraser GE, Shavlik DJ. Risk Factors for All-Cause and Coronary Heart Disease Mortality in the Oldest-Old. The Adventist Health Study. *Arch Intern Med* 1997;157:2249.

3. Fraser GE, et al. A Possible Protective Effect of Nut Consumption on Risk of Coronary Heart Disease. The Adventist Health Study. *Arch Intern Med* 1992;152:1416.

4. Hu FB, et al. Frequent Nut Consumption and Risk of Coronary Heart Disease in Women: Prospective Cohort Study. *BMJ* 1998;317:1341.

5. Spiller GA, et al. Nuts and Plasma Lipids: An Almond-Based Diet Lowers LDL-C while Preserving HDL-C. *J Am Coll Nutr* 1998;17:285.

6. Abbey M, et al. Partial Replacement of Saturated Fatty Acids with Almonds or Walnuts Lowers Total Plasma Cholesterol and Low-Density-Lipoprotein Cholesterol. *Am J Clin Nutr* 1994;59:995.

7. Chisholm A, et al. A Diet Rich in Walnuts Favourably Influences Plasma Fatty Acid Profile in Moderately Hyperlipidaemic Subjects. *Eur J Clin Nutr* 1998;52:12.

8. Fraser GE. Nut Consumption, Lipids, and Risk of a Coronary Event. *Clin Cardiol* 1999;22(Suppl):III11.

9. See, supra, note 2.

Chapter 20

Lifestyle Factors:
Small Modifications Can Make a Major Difference in Your Hormonal Status

Stress and Mental Outlook

He who fears suffering is already suffering from what he fears.
Michel de Montaigne

Hardening of the heart can kill you faster than hardening of the arteries.
Unknown

The emptier the pot, the quicker the boil –
an angry person is seldom reasonable; a reasonable person is seldom angry.
Unknown

All that we are is a result of what we have thought. What we think we become.
Buddha

Thoughts that uplift the mind, cleanse the body; thoughts that degrade the mind, foul the body.
Rob Faigin

Hatred does more damage to the container in which it is stored than to the object on which it is poured.
Unknown

Half the things we worry about never happen, and the other half happen anyway. So one good reason for not worrying is so you won't feel like a fool when everything turns-out all right, and another good reason is so you don't foolishly upset yourself brooding over the inevitable.
Rob Faigin

Stress is detrimental to health generally and to body composition in particular. For one, stress triggers food cravings in many people. Specifically, as discussed in Chapter 1, stressed individuals crave the serotonin fix that a carbohydrate-rich food confers. What does "stressed" spell backwards?) **The principal consequence of stress is that it stimulates a rise in cortisol, the catabolic, pro-aging, anti-immunity, anti-testosterone, anti-growth hormone, insulin-raising, hormone**. Cortisol directly destroys muscle tissue (see Chapter 11); and it indirectly (via its antagonistic effect on other hormones) promotes central fat deposition (i.e., potbelly).[1,2,3,4]

The central nervous system is closely linked with the endocrine system. The stress response begins at the hypothalamus in the brain, which secretes *corticotropin-releasing hormone*.[5,6] Corticotropin-releasing hormone travels a short distance to the pituitary gland (also in your head), where it prompts release of *adrenocorticotropic hormone* (ACTH).[7,8] ACTH, in turn, activates the outer part of the adrenal glands, called the *adrenal cortex*.[9,10] The adrenals, positioned directly above the kidneys, weigh only a fraction of an ounce. Although tiny, the adrenals pack a wallop in terms of their ability to affect human biochemistry. Cortisol is produced via the process outlined in Chapter 22; and in response to ACTH, the adrenal cortex releases cortisol into the bloodstream.

One type of stress, exercise-related physical stress, can be applied constructively to improve the testosterone/cortisol ratio and to generate other advantageous hormonal shifts (see Chapter 21). However, many people who exercise, because they do not understand the relationship between frequency/intensity/duration/load/volume and hormones, are systematically raising cortisol and lowering testosterone and growth hormone levels. Other physical stressors, like illness and injury, also stimulate cortisol release, but, unlike exercise, without the redeeming potential of testosterone enhancement or any other hormonal benefit. The drastic muscle wastage that attends severe illness graphically illustrates cortisol's catabolic dynamism.

The catabolic specter also rises in response to mental stress. Accordingly, you should strive to minimize mental stress, although achieving this objective is increasingly challenging in today's fast-paced and complex society. Anxiety, fear, and anger, each can, within minutes, raise cortisol levels.[11] Hence, being all wound-up can be as bad for your health as being all run-down, and a negative outlook can negatively affect your physical well-being.

The mind/body connection is an exciting and promising frontier in health and human performance. Both the average lay person and the average medical doctor scoff at the notion that thoughts can influence health. The prevailing textbook view envisions immunity as a discrete system separate and apart from the brain and hormones. This compartmentalized mode of conception impedes progress toward a greater understanding of the human condition and perpetuates the burn, cut, and poison approach of conventional medicine.

The rapidly growing field of *neuroendocrinimmunology* - a discipline that combines research on the brain, nervous system, hormones, and immune system – presents convincing evidence of the intimate interrelationship among these systems.[12,13,14,15] The human body is not an organic machine consisting of distinct independent components, as the medicine men would have you believe. Rather, the human body is an integrated biological entity comprised of various parts working interdependently in fluid cooperation.

The immune system responds to physical and mental stress similarly to how it responds to an infection.[16,17,18,19] And like an infection, stress compromises the body's ability to defend against other immune challenges.[20,21,22,23,24] This fact is demonstrated by a 1998 study published in the *Proceedings of the National Academy of Sciences* in which monkeys were injected with the simian equivalent of the human immunodeficiency virus (HIV), and subjected to differing degrees of social stress. In monkeys assigned to more stressful conditions, the virus manifested itself more aggressively and post-infection survival rates among this group were lower.[25] Two other simian AIDS studies, using social separation and housing relocations as stress markers, also found an association

196

between disease progression and stressful experiences.[26,27] Studies of homosexual HIV-infected men are in accord, finding that stress can triple[28] or quadruple[29] the likelihood of progression of HIV to AIDS in the first few years after infection.

Depression acts as a stressor, and patients with depression exhibit impaired immune function.[30,31,32,33,34,35,36] This applies not only to clinical depression, but also to situational depression resulting from major adverse life events.[37,38,39,40,41] The immunosuppressive impact of a melancholy mindset likely explains the higher rates of mortality and morbidity among the surviving spouse of a recently deceased person[42,43,44,45,46,47] (especially when the husband is the survivor[48,49,50]).* Conversely, optimism and positive mood mitigate stress-induced immune suppression (see below). This shows that thoughts are not, as many people believe, confined to your head. Rather, your thoughts can make you physically sick. This negative mind/body effect is mediated by - you guessed it - cortisol.

In addition to chewing up muscle tissue and weakening immunity, excess cortisol damages the brain, by degrading the *hippocampus*.[51,52,53] The hippocampus is an area of the brain involved in memory and intelligence. Rich in glucocorticoid receptors, the hippocampus is exceptionally vulnerable to cortisol's catabolic effects.[54,55] Because of its neurotoxicity and its role in accelerating age-related brain degeneration, cortisol has become suspect in the rising tide of Alzheimer's disease.[56,57,58,59] Depression, too, has burgeoned in recent years into a major health problem, and elevated cortisol levels are common among depressives.[60,61,62,63,64,65] To what extent hypercortisolism is a cause of depression and to what extent it is a result of depression is not clear; this is one of the many questions confronting researchers in this fascinating field.

Stress reduction is central to enhancing hormonal status naturally. The resultant reduction in cortisol levels will bolster testosterone levels in men;** and it will facilitate growth hormone release[66,67,68,69] and improve insulin sensitivity in both sexes (see p. 92). The benefits to health and physique of these across-the-board hormonal improvements can be profound, especially in the long run.

The immunosuppressive effect of excess cortisol is well-established (see p. 92), and it stands to reason that long-term immune suppression resulting from chronically elevated cortisol levels increases susceptibility to all kinds of sickness and disease. The totality of the evidence points unmistakably to one fact: your thoughts can destroy you. That's a drastic statement so let me clarify that I'm not talking about occasional or fleeting negative

---

* Poignant accounts of an aggrieved hero "dying of a broken heart" in the wake of his lover's death may have more scientific credibility than storytellers and poets realize.

** Chapter 22 explains how cortisol competitively reduces testosterone production and opposes testosterone's anabolic action. There is also evidence that stress impacts testosterone status by suppressing luteinizing hormone (LH), the hormone that directs the testes to produce testosterone.[69a,69b,69c,69d,69e] Studies further show that stress can reduce the sensitivity of testicular LH receptors;[69f,69g,69h,69i,69j,69k] thereby rendering the testes "deaf" to messages coming down from the hypothalamus-pituitary command center, via luteinizing hormone, to pump-out testosterone. This does not mean that you should eliminate *all* stress. In fact, stress can be applied strategically to *increase* testosterone levels (see "Strategic Stress," in Chapter 21). Chronic stress, though, physical or mental, will retard testosterone production - no doubt about it.

thoughts. Rather, I am referring to the kind of chronic negative mental imagery and stress that can be caused by a tension-drenched job, a rotten personal relationship, or a pessimistic or angry outlook on life. The fact is that, while sound nutrition is essential to good health, many people suffer poor health not because of what they are eating, but because of what is eating them.

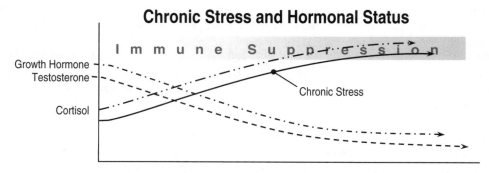

Chronic Stress and Hormonal Status

Stress has many sources. The form of stress easiest to monitor and control is physical stress. In Chapter 21, we'll discuss how to harness advantageously this type of stress. By contrast, psychosocial and emotional stress are more difficult to regulate and they lack the constructive potential of physical stress.

Cortisol's evolutionary function as an activator of the fight or flight response[70] is of minimal utility in the post-industrial age, in which we do less fighting and fleeing and more fretting and fussing. Modern-day humans are confronted with far fewer life-threatening situations than were our ancient ancestors. But in our increasingly complex society, we are buffeted by a myriad of less dire but more persistent stressors related to work, finances, and personal relationships. These stressors, while they do not cause immediate bodily harm, foster gradual bodily degeneration.

Unlike the fight-or-flight stressors that we are evolutionarily equipped to handle, modern-day stressors lack a physical outlet for dissipating stress. You can't physically run away from a work deadline. And if you pummel your boss with a blunt object like Paleolithic man did to creatures that made his cortisol levels rise, you are likely to wind-up in handcuffs, which will make your cortisol levels rise even higher. Physical activity serves to neutralize stress by providing both a sense of control and a means of discharging energy. Taking action under stressful conditions, as opposed to remaining passive, is a powerful coping tool.[71] But the stressful conditions of modern society are generally not susceptible to resolution by physical exertion.

Although stress management is a greater challenge today than it was thousands of years ago, conquering stress is an achievable objective. First, it is important to understand that the physiological impact of a particular stressor is determined by how you perceive it and deal with it.[72,73,74] Optimism and positive mood buffer the physiological response to stress, whereas pessimism exacerbates it.[75,76,77,78] Using the example above, a work deadline can be perceived in various ways: as a threat, as a challenge, or as a date-certain after which you will no longer have to concern yourself with a given task. Similarly, you can view a negative comment as an insult, as constructive criticism, or as completely inconsequential. The key point is that: external circumstances are inherently incapable of affecting hormone levels within your body; your cognitive perception and evaluation of events determines whether and to what extent they physiologically impact upon you.

Because we are not strictly rational beings, even our best efforts at self-mastery are subject to being undercut by passion and emotion. Even so, the stress response, and by extension cortisol levels, are largely controllable. Bear in mind the powerful effect that thoughts can have on hormone levels. Fear, anger, jealously, and hatred serve little constructive purpose and can diminish your health and quality of life. Bottom line: if you want to be the picture of health, you'd better have a positive frame of mind.

Sleep

The amount of sleep required by the average person is just five minutes more.
Unknown

The best sleep aid is a clear conscience - a few extra dollars in the bank doesn't hurt either.
Unknown

Oversleeping allows more time for dreaming but prevents you from making your dreams come true.
Unknown

From the earliest times, scientists and philosophers have wondered why we spend one-third of our existence in an unconscious state. You may be surprised to learn that scientists in the 21st century are not much closer than Aristotle was to resolving this vexing question. An article published in *Medical Hypotheses* offered the following explanation for sleep: the vegetative state is primary and the waking state is a periodic departure superimposed upon vegetative life.[79] (I could have used this theory in my own defense as a high school student when I got caught snoozing in class.) The profound restorative role of sleep has long been appreciated on a general level, but the physiological events that occur during sleep and their specific functions remain elusive. Until we fully understand what goes on inside our body and brain during sleep, we will not be able to answer the question of why 30% of our existence is spent in a state of suspended animation. One fact is clear, however. Sleep is much more than a time of repose.

Contrary to the popular conception of sleep as an idle and inert state, it is, in fact, a physiologically eventful period. Within the outwardly motionless body, electro-neurological oscillations and cascading hormones define the biologic turbulence of sleep. Furthermore, the complex hormonal and brainwave activities that occur during sleep are crucial to immune system operation, cognitive function, emotional well-being, and physical development. The overarching importance of nighttime sleep stems from the fact that circadian hormonal rhythms, which orchestrate all biological processes, are dependent upon the sleep-wake cycle.[80,81,82,83] Thus, it is not surprising that experimental animals deprived of sleep for extended periods exhibit severe metabolic and neuroendocrine abnormalities.[84,85,86] In humans, too, sleep deprivation is inimical to health.

199

Sleep is particularly important for athletes and others engaged in physical training because it helps stave-off overtraining syndrome, marked by elevated cortisol levels. The same volume of exercise that will produce an overtrained state in a sleep-deprived athlete might not in a well-rested athlete. Athlete or not, **adequate nighttime sleep is vital to optimizing hormone levels**.

The emphasis on *nighttime* sleep bears elaboration. Nocturnalism defies human adaptability, as demonstrated by studies of night shift workers showing persistently distorted hormonal rhythms and greater incidence of health problems.[87,88,89,90,91] These findings have prompted research into endocrine phase-shifting techniques, including appropriately timed full-spectrum light exposure and administration of melatonin, designed to ameliorate the woes of night shift work. The bottom line is that, while daytime naps can be beneficial on an adjunctive basis (see below), no amount of daytime sleep can substitute for a good night's sleep.

Daily life imposes assorted physical, mental, and emotional stressors that conspire to disrupt the biological homeostasis of the body. Nighttime sleep is a time of restorative reorganization, in which the chaotic influence of stress is turned back. Hence, sleep is a bulwark against stress and a cortisol neutralizer. Conversely, sleep deprivation amplifies the impact of stress and is, itself, a stressor capable of raising cortisol levels.[92,93,94,95,96,97,98] Other hormonal effects of sleep deprivation include: impaired insulin function,[99,100,101] alterations in thyroid hormones,[102,103,104,105] decreased growth hormone output (see below), and in men, decreased testosterone levels.[106,107,108,109] The hormonal effects of sleep deficiency are remarkably similar to the hormonal changes associated with aging. And these two conditions are mutually reinforcing insofar as reduced sleep quality in older individuals is both a cause and a result of hormonal decline.[110,111,112,113]

Growth hormone status is especially dependent on sleep, because a major growth hormone surge occurs during the first episode of slow-wave sleep, approximately 30-70 minutes after sleep on set. Disturbed or interrupted sleep can cause growth hormone output to be reduced or aborted. Therefore, not merely sleep, but sound sleep, is essential to maximizing growth hormone release.[114,115,116,117,118,119,120]

The major episodes of slow-wave sleep occur during the first half of the night, at which time surging growth hormone coincides with the lowest cortisol levels of the day. Conversely, the second half of the night is marked by diminished growth hormone output, and cortisol levels rising toward a morning peak.[121,122,123,124,125] Sleep researchers postulate that the early period, during which growth hormone levels and cortisol levels are maximally disassociated in favor of growth hormone, is a time of uniquely

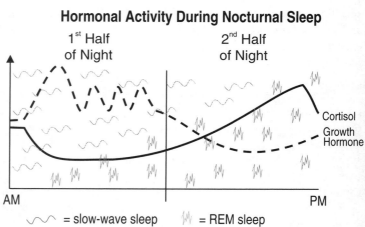

Hormonal Activity During Nocturnal Sleep

1st Half of Night

2nd Half of Night

AM — PM

Cortisol
Growth Hormone

~~~ = slow-wave sleep   ⋀⋀ = REM sleep

200

significant anabolic activity. With advancing age, the nighttime sleep-induced growth hormone peak falls and the cortisol nadir rises,[126] consonant with the general age-related reduction in the anabolic/catabolic ratio.[127,128] The hormonal shift toward catabolism is largely responsible for the physical deterioration of aging (see Chapter 4); and the closing of the nocturnal "anabolic window" may play a central role in this connection.

Growth hormone release is influenced not only by aging, but also by diet. Recall from Chapter 11 that insulin (more precisely, high blood sugar) is antagonistic to growth hormone. Chapter 21 addresses the blood sugar/growth hormone relationship, and explores its implications for the pre-workout and post-workout meals. The issue here is whether consuming carbohydrate before bed, by causing a rise in blood sugar, will blunt the nocturnal growth hormone surge.

Interestingly, there is some evidence indicating that the sleep-related growth hormone spurt is not suppressed by hyperglycemia.[129] This suggests that repeated observations of the suppressive effect of high blood sugar levels on growth hormone release in the waking state (see Chapter 21) may not apply equally to the sleeping state - but more studies are needed to clarify this. In any event, other studies show that fasting prior to sleep can heighten sleep-related growth hormone output.[130,131] Therefore, based on all the evidence in both the sleeping and waking state, going to bed with a belly-full of carbs is hormonally unwise and may diminish, if not nullify, nocturnal growth hormone release. Conversely, allowing ample time after consuming carbohydrate before retiring to bed will help maximize nighttime growth hormone release. Therefore, **to enhance growth hormone output, refrain from consuming carbohydrate within 90 minutes of going to bed**. (On the NHE Eating Plan, this will not be much of an issue except on carb-load days.)

Seven hours of sleep per day is a good target for the average person. Athletes and bodybuilders should aim for between 7 and 9 hours of sleep (including naps, which are optional but recommended for this group), to combat overtraining syndrome and to maximize performance and recovery. Don't worry about occasional sleep deficiency, the body responds to acute shortfalls in sleep by increasing sleep efficiency on the following night (specifically, the recovery night is characterized by shorter sleep onset latency, more R.E.M. sleep, and more stage-IV sleep).[132,133,134,135,136] Chronic sleep deprivation, however, is another matter.

A continuum of biological individuality exists in relation to how much sleep is needed, but this range is not as wide as commonly believed - at least as far as hormones are concerned. While you may be able to "get by" on reduced sleep, eventually you will pay the price. Before the consequences of sleep deficiency become symptomatically evident, consistently getting less than six hours of sleep is likely to exact a toll by raising cortisol levels. Even modestly elevated cortisol levels, over time, can create subtle but significant mischief. Chronic sleep deficiency is prevalent in modern society,[137] and people who average less than six hours of sleep per night have an approximately 150% higher death rate than their longer-sleeping counterparts.[138,139] Bottom line: if you don't snooze, you lose.

Natural Hormonal Enhancement

Daytime naps, while not a substitute for adequate nighttime sleep, can "pinch-hit" for nighttime sleep on a limited basis and offset sleep deprivation. As to growth hormone release, sleep trumps circadian rhythm making daytime naps a viable growth hormone stimulus.[140,141] (There is evidence suggesting that more growth hormone is secreted during naps occurring after 4 PM as opposed to earlier.[142]) By contrast, cortisol suppression is chiefly controlled by circadian rhythm, not sleep.[143,144] This does not mean that napping cannot help counter cortisol. It can, but only indirectly via its relaxing or "de-stressing" effect, not by directly inhibiting the pituitary-adrenal axis – the latter effect is circadian-dependent and exclusively associated with the first half of nocturnal sleep.

The circadian rhythmicity of hormonal secretions is a hot area of research. We are learning that not only baseline hormone levels, but also the synchronicity of hormonal rhythms determines health and rate of biological aging. Increasing circadian misalignment and hormonal disorderliness with advancing age promote degeneration and disease.[145,146,147,148,149,150] Similarly, regular disruption of circadian rhythm by night-shift work, jetlag, or partying 'till dawn can accelerate aging. This research bodes ill for individuals partaking of the current growth hormone and testosterone injection craze because, as explained in Chapter 3, exogenous hormones override the body's natural daily rhythms.

Hours of sleep that begin earlier and end earlier are more in harmony with hormonal rhythms and are more valuable than an equivalent amount of sleep that begins later and ends later.[151,152,153] This is one of the many instances in which scientific research validates ancient wisdom; the proverb "one hour's sleep before midnight is worth two after" is correct in essence. Accordingly, **to optimize hormonal status, maximize darkness hours spent sleeping and maximize daylight hours spent awake**. This is another way of expressing the "early to bed, early to rise" adage. If you balk at this recommendation because you consider yourself a "night person," you will probably find that once you change your sleeping pattern you become a "morning person."

Additionally, going to bed at approximately the same time each night facilitates more restful sleep as compared with an irregular sleeping pattern.[154,155,156] Accordingly, if you are forced to curtail sleep due to a demanding work schedule or other lifestyle imperatives, you can maximize the value of the sleep you do get by going to bed early and at the same time each night. It is probably no coincidence that the vast majority of long-lived individuals go to bed early, are "early risers," and have routinized sleep habits. A 1989 study published in the *International Journal of Aging and Human Development* found that nuns are exceptionally good sleepers. This may offer further proof of the benefit of a strict sleep schedule, or it may bespeak the benefits of spiritualism and inner peace. Then again, it may simply be a result of not being subjected to a bedmate stealing the covers.[157]

Sunlight

The best protection against skin cancer is a good tan.
George Hamilton

Keep your face to the sunshine and you'll never see the shadows.
Helen Keller

The sun not only makes life possible, but it is the central organizing force in the living world exerting both daily and seasonal influences. In animals, the sun governs reproductive, activity-rest, and feeding patterns. Even the animals imprisoned in our homes for our amusement and protection will establish a resting spot near a window and will bask in the sun when let out.* In the human world, the development of artificial light has reduced dependence on sunlight. Biologically, however, we are still creatures of the sun.

Until the late twentieth century, scientists believed that activity, sleep, and social interactions controlled circadian rhythms. In the last twenty years, new research has come to light. We now know that in organisms as diverse as single-celled algae and humans, light is the primary stimulus regulating the circadian biological clock.[158] The mammalian circadian pacemaker, located in the suprachiasmatic nucleus (SCN) of the hypothalamus, generates 24-hour rhythms for many physiologic functions including body temperature and hormonal secretion.[159,160,161]

Light enters the body via the retino-hypothalmic pathway: through the eyes, converted to nerve impulses, and transmitted to the SCN.[162] The SCN conveys this information to the pineal gland, a key interface between environmental lighting and hormonal output. The pineal produces melatonin which, in turn, signals activities throughout the endocrine system via its influence on the pituitary gland and hypothalamus.[163,164] Pineal melatonin, in effect, "feeds back" on the SCN, thereby influencing the SCN's activities.[165,166] Based on the interdependent cooperation between the pineal and the SCN, they can be aptly described as coequal regulators of our biological clock, sharing a position atop the hormonal chain of command.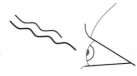

Both the light-sensitive SCN and the light-sensitive pineal are centrally involved in sex drive and reproductive function,[167,168,169,170,171] and marked differences in the size and morphology of the SCN exist among women, heterosexual men, and homosexual men.[172,173,174] In male rodents, experimental light deprivation causes profound testicular

---

* Being the egotistical species that we are, we assume that those creatures we have taught to "speak," beg, roll-over, and excrete waste on command want nothing more than our love. In reality, I suspect that the animals we have adopted as "pets" would choose physical activity, freedom to roam in the open air, and sunlight over human affection any day. Animals don't need our doting approval, and if they could express themselves collectively they'd surely ask to be left alone to prosper in their natural habitat as they have for millions of years. Like most people, I am strongly in favor of animal rights – and I also support our right as superior beings to cut animals into pieces and examine their innards in the name of scientific advancement.

shrinkage and a reduction in testosterone levels to near-castrate levels.[175,176,177,178] In a wide range of other animals, summer to winter light changes induce decrements in reproductive hormones, copulatory performance, and gonadal mass.[179,180,181,182,183,184,185,186,187,188,189] Furthermore, breeding season in animals can be delayed or advanced by altering light availability;[190,191] and in humans, circadian (daily) hormonal rhythms can be delayed or advanced by the same means.[192,193] Without wishing to crassly disillusion anyone, hot summer nights of love and romance may not be entirely unrelated to animalistic seasonal breeding influences.

Humans are not seasonal breeders in the sense of some animals that mate only during a particular time of the year. Even so, a light-related seasonal influence on human libido cannot be discounted in view of studies showing that in both males[194,195,196] and females[197,198] sex hormone levels are highest during the time of the year when the sun shines the longest. The fact that light is testosterone-enhancing is illuminating news for men. And it suggests that men who report an increased sex drive after spending a day at the beach seeing women in swimsuits basking in the sun may be as much aroused by the sunlight as by the women. To enhance testosterone levels in men, and to increase sex drive in both sexes, maximize daylight hours by retiring early and rising early; and get outside as much as possible.

In addition to synchronizing biorhythms, sensational new research demonstrates that the sun acts as a hormonal catalyst-precursor. When solar ultraviolet radiation in the wavelength range of 290-320 nanometers (UVB) strikes exposed areas of the body, it chemically reacts with a type of cholesterol present in the skin called *epidermal 7-dehydrocholesterol*, converting it to vitamin D.[199] This much we knew since the early 1920's. But here's where it gets exciting.

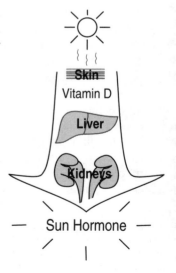

Vitamin D then undergoes an assembly-line chemical makeover first in the liver then in the kidneys.[200] Through this process, mild-mannered vitamin D turns into a "super hormone" inelegantly named *1,25-dihydroxyvitamin D3* (I prefer to call it "sun hormone"). Early reports on sun hormone showed that it regulated intestinal, bone, and kidney function. These findings shed light on the mechanisms by which vitamin D exerts its classical effects on skeletal health, given that all three of these organs are involved in calcium metabolism (via absorption, mobilization, and reabsorption, respectively).[201] Recent research has revealed that the biologic effect of sun hormone is more comprehensive than originally believed, with positive implications for many disease states including osteoporosis, cancer, psoriasis, multiple sclerosis, and arthritis.[202,203,204,205,206]

The sun hormone/cancer connection is particularly provocative when considered in the context of the prevailing twin messages from health authorities that we should 1) void the sun, and 2) wear sunscreen, to protect ourselves from skin cancer. I dissent from this consensus; and I further maintain that the combined effect of these two recommendations is an increase in cancer and other forms of pathology and woe, including osteoporosis and depression. Before we discuss the role of sun hormone in cancer prevention, let's address the role of sunlight in cancer causation. As you will see, the relationship between sunlight and skin cancer is at variance with popularly accepted notions.

The incidence of all types of skin cancer has risen dramatically in the U.S. and around the world since the 1970's.[207,208,209] However, because this has occurred concurrently with an increase in many types of cancer (see Chapter 6), it is more accurate to say that we have a cancer problem including skin, rather than a skin cancer problem per se. This is an important clarification because it is likely that all types of cancer are caused by the same or related factors. (For example, ultraviolet radiation depletes epidermal and dermal antioxidants;[210,211,212] and antioxidant supplementation has been shown to protect against skin cancer and many other types of cancer, as well.[213,214,215]) DNA resides in every cell of our body, and every cell is intimately interconnected with every other cell (this dynamic integration of parts distinguishes a living organism from a machine). DNA is constantly damaged by oxidative stress, and repaired (see Chapter 4). Unrepaired damage to DNA can cause abnormal cell growth leading to cancer. Therefore, cancer reflects a critical interruption in the biologic harmony of life resulting in aberrant cellular behavior. This is the larger picture.

The causative role of ultraviolet radiation in skin cancer varies with the type of skin cancer. The deeper in the skin cancer occurs, the more complex is the inducing influence of the sun. Highly common, easily treatable, non-aggressive, and rarely life-threatening, squamous and basal cell carcinoma occur superficially on the skin and directly correlate with cumulative sunlight exposure. Melanoma, by contrast, occurs deeper in the skin and although treatable early, spreads quickly and kills many. Unlike squamous and basal cell carcinoma, melanoma is not related to total sunlight exposure.[216,217,218]

In a nutshell, here's what the research tells us about melanoma risk: a suntan is protective whereas intermittent intense sunlight exposure increases risk. Therefore, not only is melanoma incidence not directly correlated with sunlight exposure, but in the case of construction workers and others who work outdoors, chronic sunlight exposure inversely corresponds with melanoma. On the other hand, individuals who spend most of their time indoors and incur sunburn occasionally while vacationing or during recreational activity, suffer more melanoma.[219,220,221,222,223,224,225] Frequency of episodes of painful sunburn during childhood is particularly associated with occurrence of melanoma years later, so protect your children.[226,227,228] Fluorescent lighting has not been ruled-out as a possible cause of melanoma, with at least two studies finding a connection[229,230] (if confirmed, this would help explain why melanoma is much more prevalent among white-collar workers than among blue-collar workers[231,232]). Finally, the following two constitutional factors are associated with heightened risk o melanoma: 1) size, number, and irregularly shaped moles, and 2) low "tannability" (propensity to burn rather than tan).[233,234,235]

The only reason why a "healthy tan" has become an oxymoron is because of moroni pronouncements by health authorities portraying our eons-old ally as a dastardly foe There is no evidence to support the proposition that a suntan is unhealthy - quite th contrary. For example, a study published in the *American Journal of Epidemiolog* found that among tan women, those who wore a bikini more frequently experienced lower incidence of melanoma.[236] The most likely reason why chronic sunlight exposur protects against melanoma is because it enhances sun hormone levels,[237,238] and su hormone has been shown to inhibit cancer[239,240,241] including melanoma.[242,243] * (Chemica analogues of sun hormone are being developed to treat breast cancer[244,245] an leukemia.[246,247]) Sporadic overexposure to sunlight offers no such benefits; rather i reduces immunity,[248,249,250,251] which increases risk of all types of disease including cancer.

Consistent with the anti-carcinogenic properties of sun hormone, sunlight exposure is correlated with lower overall cancer death rates.[252,253,254,255] For example, the geographic epidemiology of prostate cancer parallels the historical distribution of rickets (a vitamin D deficiency disease). The highest death rates from prostate cancer occur in areas that had high prevalence of rickets - regions with winter ultraviolet radiation deficiency due to a combination of high latitude and persistently thick winter cloud cover.[256,257,258] Incidence of pancreatic cancer, one of the most lethal tumors, also rises with distance from the equator.[259,260]

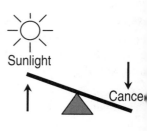

Not only are prostate and pancreatic cancer directly correlated with darkness, but both are also directly correlated with dark skin.[261,262,263,264] Many researchers theorize tha African-Americans are genetically predisposed to these forms of cancer. I subscribe to a different theory, which takes account of the fact that blacks in Africa have much lowe rates of pancreatic and prostate cancer than North American blacks.[265] In my view African-Americans are genetically predisposed to dark skin (there's an astute observation), and dark skin is more resistant to ultraviolet radiation. Therefore, black require more sunlight than whites to produce a given amount of sun hormone.[266,267,268] Fo this reason, the instruction to avoid the sun (which fails to discriminate appropriately based on skin color) has a disproportionate adverse impact on members of races with heavily pigmented skin.

---

* If you think the mythical "balanced diet" will do the trick – it won't. Few foods contain vitamin D, and the ones that do contain small amounts. Supplementation can't substitute for sunlight, either. Dietary supplementation of vitamin D, while advisable for institutionalized, elderly, and other commonly deficien groups, is relatively ineffective at enhancing sun hormone levels.[268a, 268b] Moreover, vitamin D has a much lowe toxicity threshold than most vitamins.[268c] Humans evolved outdoors and we are genetically programmed to ge our vitamin D from the sun - there's no way around this fact.

206

Rickets: An Osteoblast from the Past

Rickets is a vitamin D deficiency disease. It was once a worldwide medical problem, but it has been largely eliminated – largely but not entirely. There are some who will question why I am spending time discussing a relatively rare disease. My answer is that its victims are children.

No child in the 21st century should suffer skeletal deformity from a nutritional deficiency disease that is completely, easily, preventable. Yet it happens every day. Deficiency must be severe and prolonged to cause overt rickets, but milder deficiency can cause subtle skeletal abnormalities. White babies residing at low latitudes are at low risk of vitamin D deficiency, but black babies born during wintertime at high latitudes are at high risk.[269,270,271,272,273] Muslims who don't consume dairy products and who adhere to the custom of covering-up their body are at high risk – which is why rickets is prevalent in Kuwait despite year-round sunshine.[274]

Breast-fed infants nursing from a woman with low sunlight exposure are at higher risk of vitamin D deficiency than formula-fed infants.[275] Therefore, in addition to taking her baby outdoors, nursing mothers should take themselves outdoors. Poor maternal vitamin D status during lactation results in low breast-milk vitamin D.[276,277] Even before the baby is born, poor maternal vitamin D status during pregnancy can adversely affect fetal bone development.[278] If your baby is in a high-risk group, you should consider supplemental vitamin D. But because of the potential toxicity of vitamin D supplements, you should consult your doctor for dosage instructions. If your doctor tells you that rickets no longer exists, find a new doctor.

Natural selection produced a skin color gradient running north and south from the equator, which was subsequently undone by the intercontinental migrations and slave trading of the latter half of the last millennium. Before European expansion rearranged global demographics, darker-skinned people were concentrated closer to the equator and lighter-skinned people were concentrated closer to the poles. When dark-skinned people migrate northward and fair-skinned people southward, from their respective evolutionary homelands, both groups are departing the area of the world for which they are genetically best-suited to thrive. This does not mean that people should not live wherever they please. It simply means that dark-skinned people should make a special effort to expose themselves regularly to sunlight; and fair-skinned people should take special precautions to avoid sunlight overexposure.

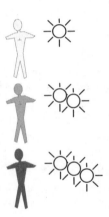

Mention of avoiding sunlight overexposure invokes sunscreen, the widespread availability and use of which began in the 1970's. Since then, steadily rising sales of sunscreen products has coincided with a steadily rising incidence of all types of skin cancer. Now that skin cancer has become the most prevalent tumor in the United States,[279,280] the American public is left wondering what – besides a full-blown skin cancer epidemic – it received in exchange for millions of dollars spent on sunscreen products.

Most sunscreens block "short-wave" UVB radiation, but are virtually transparent to "long-wave" UVA[281] (others advertise UVA protection, but block only a small percentage of UVA solar radiation). From the beginning, the claim that sunscreen protects against skin cancer was dubious because UVB comprises only about 10% of the solar radiation spectrum. The assertion that UVB radiation was solely responsible for skin cancer was based on hopeful speculation supported by unwarranted inferences drawn from limited data. With the recent emergence of evidence implicating UVA radiation in the development of melanoma,[282,283,284] sunscreen has been exposed – just as its users have been all along.

Not only are they not protected, but sunscreen-users may incur a heightened risk of skin cancer. For one, sunscreen fosters a hazardous false sense of security. The skin's alarm system, literally the red flag, is short-circuited by sunscreen.[285] Without skin reddening as a cue to desist sunlight exposure, the sunscreen-user is like a pilot flying without a visible horizon – unable to gauge where optimal ends and excessive begins, and facing potentially catastrophic consequences of misjudgment.

Studies confirm what reason suggests: sunscreen-users spend more time in the sun and have higher rates of melanoma.[286] The higher incidence of lethal skin cancer among sunscreen-users may not be attributable only to greater duration of sunlight exposure. Rather, new research suggests that certain constituents of the chemical cream (sunscreen) with which health authorities advise us to coat our bodies, may turn carcinogenic when struck by ultraviolet radiation.[287,288,289,290] Moreover, since UVB is the portion of the ultraviolet spectrum that initiates vitamin D production, sunscreen, by blocking UVB, inhibits formation of sun hormone.[291,292,293] Increased risk of melanoma, but no sun hormone enhancement and no suntan, is a fool's bargain if ever I've heard one.

Not only does sunlight affect your physical health, but your mental health as well. The rhythm of blues is seasonal, and the relationship between darkness and despair is more than metaphoric. Moods tend to descend with temperature (to the extent that low temperature keeps people indoors) and daylight duration. Approximately 95% of the population experiences some degree of seasonal variation in behavior and mood.[294,295] At its upper extreme, seasonality manifests itself as clinical winter depression, called seasonal affective disorder (SAD). SAD strikes approximately 10% of the population;[296] and in the Northern Hemisphere, it begins in October/November and remits in February/March. The incidence of SAD is three times higher among women,[297,298,299,300] and it is most prevalent in high-latitude areas meterologically prone to cloudy winter days.[301,302,303] The seasonal blues hit particularly hard in Alaska, Antarctica, and other circumpolar regions where winter days are extremely short.[304,305,306]

Phototherapy is highly effective at treating SAD,[307,308,309,310,311] and has produced positive, but less consistent, results at treating other disorders, such as premenstrual syndrome,[312,313] bulimia,[314,315] and nonseasonal depression.[316,317,318,319] An effective phototherapy regimen involves regular exposure to 1) bright light 2) containing all visible wavelengths. Sunlight contains all visible wavelengths; whereas the incandescent and fluorescent lights that illuminate the indoor environs in which modern-day humans spend most of their time lack significant components of the color spectrum. Moreover, not only is a sunny day many times brighter than the most well-lit room, but sunlight also radiates ultraviolet and infrared waves. Light bulbs do not provide these invisible wavelengths, both of which buoy mood and contribute to our general well-being.[320,321] Incidentally, the sun also radiates cosmic rays, gamma rays, x-rays, radio waves, and electric waves – but all of these are intercepted by the atmospheric layers surrounding the Earth, and thus do not reach its surface.

208

From the standpoint of health, light emitted by the bulbs in our homes and offices is inferior to sunlight. In fact, photobiologists suspect that overexposure to "cool-white" indoor light conspires with sunlight deprivation to subtly upset human biochemistry. Research in this area has important implications in view of the trend toward an increasingly indoor society. For inhabitants of higher latitudes, where colder temperatures and shorter daylight hours prevail, the artificial light issue carries added significance.

Besides making you feel better, combating osteoporosis and cancer, and firing sex drive, sunlight can advance fat loss by curbing appetite (and in men by bolstering testosterone, see above). The influence of sunlight on appetite is attributable to the same mechanism that makes sunlight a mood elevator: the neurotransmitter serotonin. Sunlight exposure spurs serotonin production (this is why excessive sunlight exposure makes you sleepy); and sunlight deficiency can lower serotonin levels sufficiently to instigate depressive symptoms and/or carbohydrate craving in susceptible individuals.[322,323,324] This explains why carbohydrate craving is a hallmark symptom of SAD and other serotonin-related forms of depression;[325,326] and it explains why carbohydrate craving responds to phototherapy.[327]

As discussed in Chapter 11, carbohydrate-rich meals boost serotonin levels. But unlike sunlight exposure, medicating the blues with carbs has downside implications for body and mind. So before you reach for a sweet snack or pay for expensive drugs that unnaturally alter brain chemistry, try taking a vigorous walk on a sunny day. You'll be healthier, wealthier, and maybe even wiser given the ability of natural wonders to inspire a transcendent perception of our place and purpose in the universe.

To enhance physical and mental health, regularly expose yourself to moderate doses of sunlight and *don't burn*.

In summary, our biology is wedded to the sun and our physical and mental health depends on it. Since the dawn of human history, we have existed under the sun, relying on it for vision, warmth – even worshipping it. And our world, both figuratively and literally, revolves around the sun. In view of these facts, why have health authorities denounced the sun in recent years, portraying it as a menace to health? Yes, overexposure to sunlight, especially in susceptible individuals, can increase the risk of skin cancer. But moderate, regular sunlight exposure helps protect against many of the deadlier forms of cancer, including melanoma, and provides many other health benefits both physical and mental. According to an article published in a 1993 issue of *Preventive Medicine*, if health authorities would hush their anti-sun advisories and instead encourage regular, moderate sunning, approximately 30,000 U.S. cancer deaths per year could be averted.[328] This is yet another example of the "experts" misrepresenting information to the detriment of public health. What's their excuse this time for their inability to see the larger picture? I suppose the sun got in their eyes.

Alcohol

24 hours in a day, 24 beers in a case. Coincidence?
Stephen Wright

What contemptible scoundrel has stolen the cork to my lunch?
W.C. Fields

To live a long life, stay busy, get plenty of exercise, and don't drink too much
- then again, don't drink too little.
Herman "Jackrabbit" Smith-Johannsen, at 103

Not all chemicals are bad. Without chemicals such as hydrogen and oxygen,
for example, there would be no way to make water, a vital ingredient in beer.
Dave Barry

Abstainer: a weak person who yields to the temptation of denying himself a pleasure.
Ambrose Bierce

I am just smart enough to sound bright at a cocktail party, and just dumb enough to be there.
John Francis Yetter, Professor of Law

My grandmother is eighty and she still doesn't need glasses. Drinks right out of the bottle.
Henny Youngman

To preserve stuff they put it in alcohol; doesn't that mean I'm thoroughly preserved right now?
Drunken friend of the author's, anonymous by request

Alcohol is a lifestyle factor associated with some health benefits and many health hazards. The various and contradictory effects of alcohol on health counsel caution in proposing recommendations regarding whether or not to drink. Until questions pertaining to quantity and type of alcoholic beverage, interaction with pre-existing health conditions, drinking pattern, and co-timing of drinking with meals, cigarette smoking, or drug use are resolved, public health advice on alcohol will be limited in scope and potentially flawed in its impact. With these caveats at the fore, let's canvass the effects of alcohol on health with particular emphasis on hormones.

Moderate alcohol consumption has repeatedly been shown to reduce the risk of cardiovascular disease.[329,330,331,332,333,334,335,336,337,338] By contrast, chronic overindulgence in alcohol can damage the heart[339,340,341] and increase the risk of stroke and sudden cardiac death.[342,343,344] In addition to overall quantity, alcohol ingestion pattern is significant, with binge drinking associated with fewer health benefits and more health risks than steady drinking.[345,346,347]

While the cardioprotective influence of moderate alcohol intake is established, the mechanisms by which it exerts this effect are incompletely understood. One means by which alcohol defends moderate drinkers against diseases of the cardiovascular system is by raising HDL cholesterol.[348,349,350,351,352,353,354,355,356,357] Alcohol also reduces coronary risk by inhibiting platelet aggregation and reducing fibrinogen in the blood.[358,359,360,361] Beyond these factors, it appears that substances found in alcoholic beverages, besides the alcohol itself, contribute to the reported salutary effects of moderate alcohol consumption.

Antioxidants in certain alcoholic beverages, particularly *polyphenols* in red wine, have been proposed as an underlying cardioprotective agent. As explained in Chapter 8, oxidation of LDL cholesterol promotes atherosclerosis. The postulated role of polyphenols is supported by studies correlating drinking habits with heart disease, which consistently find that red wine outperforms beer and liquor.[362,363,364,365,366,367] However, these studies must be viewed skeptically in light of evidence showing that wine drinking is associated with an overall healthier diet than either beer drinking or liquor drinking.[368]

The epidemiological evidence is reinforced by *in vitro* (test tube) evidence clearly demonstrating that polyphenols - such as *resveratrol, quercetin, procyanidin,* and *catechin* - inhibit LDL oxidation.[369,370,371,372] But the impressive evidence generated *in vitro* contrasts with inconsistent results generated *in vivo* (in a living organism). Why haven't the *in vitro* studies, ascribing anti-oxidative properties to alcoholic beverages, been reliably reproduced *in vivo*? Because alcohol acts as a prooxidant *in vivo*.[373,374,375,376]

The pro-oxidative actions of alcohol account for studies showing increased oxidation after consumption of beer or white wine.[377,378] By contrast, studies show decreased oxidation after consumption of red wine.[379,380] Based on studies of the oxidative effects of red wine (high antioxidant content), beer (low antioxidant content, but higher for dark beer), white wine and liquor (low antioxidant content), we can advance the following generalization. For red wine, the anti-oxidative effect outweighs the pro-oxidative effect, but for white wine, liquor, and most types of beer, the pro-oxidative effect outweighs the anti-oxidative effect. In conclusion, all alcoholic beverages, consumed in moderation, protect against cardiovascular disease via multiple physiological mechanisms intrinsic to alcohol, but red wine appears to be more potent in this regard than white wine, beer, or liquor due to its higher content of anti-oxidative polyphenols.

The benefits of alcohol in terms of reducing coronary risk must be considered in light of its metabolic and hormonal effects (see below), and weighed against its potential to promote cancer and liver damage. Remarkably, autopsy studies show that alcoholics have less atherosclerosis than nondrinkers, and in some cases, less than moderate drinkers.[381] As impressive as this finding may be, it does not change the fact that clean arteries are of no benefit to someone with a diseased liver, a terminal malignancy, or who dies an unnatural, alcohol-related death. Many sloppily reported studies of the health effects of alcohol focus on heart disease mortality rate without discussing *overall* mortality. Dead is dead, so consider all the implications of alcohol consumption, in terms of its overall impact on health as well as its social, emotional, and behavioral consequences. And remember: heavy drinking is definitely bad for you.

Mirroring the mixed effects of alcohol on health are its mixed effects on hormones. With respect to insulin, studies show that moderate consumption of alcohol improves insulin sensitivity.[382,383,384,385,386] These studies are contradicted by other studies showing that alcohol impairs insulin sensitivity.[387,388,389,390,391,392] Resolution of this matter awaits further research, but I suspect the conflicting studies can be reconciled by distinguishing the acute from the chronic effects of alcohol. Specifically, it appears

211

that the immediate, transitory (acute) effect of alcohol ingestion on insulin sensitivity is unfavorable; but this may be outweighed by a delayed, lingering (chronic) favorable effect of alcohol on insulin sensitivity. Quantity of alcohol, type of alcohol, and co-timing of alcohol ingestion with meals may also be significant variables underlying the ostensibly discordant studies relating alcohol consumption with insulin function.

Alcohol also bears upon cortisol secretion, depending on dose. Cortisol levels increase during intoxication,[393,394,395,396] but in small quantities alcohol does not stimulate cortisol.[397] It is unclear precisely where is the threshold for alcohol-induced cortisol release, and it probably varies with habituation ("tolerance") and other individualized factors.[398] Moreover, a cortisol-reducing effect of low-level alcohol ingestion cannot be ruled out given the "de-stressing" influence a cocktail-or-two exerts on some people.

The catabolic effect of excessive alcohol intake is demonstrated by the fact that more than half of alcoholics suffer from skeletal myopathy, characterized by selective atrophy of Type II muscle fibers resulting in a loss of up to 20% of total skeletal musculature.[399,400,401] Although cortisol elevation and other hormonal changes engendered by heavy alcohol consumption likely contribute to skeletal myopathy, it is chiefly caused by a direct toxic impact of alcohol on Type II muscle fibers.[402,403,404] Alcohol acutely reduces protein synthesis (anabolism);[405,406,407] but at low intake levels this appears to be offset by an anti-catabolic effect.[408] The bottom line is that at intoxicating doses, alcohol raises cortisol levels and directly thwarts anabolism – bodybuilders, especially, beware.

The news regarding the effect of alcohol on hormones doesn't get much better when we turn our attention to growth hormone and sex hormones. Alcohol suppresses the nocturnal growth hormone surge when ingested at night.[409,410,411] However, alcohol has a less deleterious effect on growth hormone secretion at other times (largely because less growth hormone is secreted at other times), and moderate alcohol consumption does not reduce baseline growth hormone levels.[412,413] These facts lead to the following recommendation: **if you are going to drink, allow ample time between hitting the bottle and hitting the sack**. There is no definite answer to how much time is sufficient, but the more time you put between these two events - finishing your last drink and going to sleep - the better. When attempting to maximize the interval between drinking and sleeping, it is preferable to drink earlier rather than to stay up later and abbreviate your sleep. But, of course, drinking earlier in the day is not always a feasible option.

In addition to inhibiting growth hormone release, alcohol hits men below the belt. With few exceptions, as blood-alcohol levels rise testosterone levels in men fall.[414,415,416,417,418,419,420] In women, the acute effect of alcohol on sex hormones is opposite to its effect in men, and the magnitude of the increase in estrogen and testosterone levels varies with menstrual cycle.[421,422,423,424,425] Whereas chronic moderate alcohol consumption has not been linked to lower baseline testosterone levels in men, it has been linked to higher baseline estrogen levels in women[426,427,428,429,430] - and this fact may have important health implications.

212

Is Alcohol an Aphrodisiac?

The alcohol-induced female sex hormone increase means that for women, but not for men, alcohol is a hormonal aphrodisiac. In both sexes alcohol disinhibits psychological sexual arousal,[431,432] but in men this effect accompanied at higher doses by a reduction in physiological sexual responsiveness owing to reduced testosterone levels.[433] At low doses, the former effect predominates (making alcohol a sexual stimulant); but t higher doses, the latter effect predominates (making alcohol a sexual dampener).

In women, alcohol tends to increase sexual desire across the dose-spectrum due to the positive concordance of hormonal and psychological factors.[434] Furthermore, to the extent that societal mores impose greater constraints on female sexual behavior, the disinhibitory effect of alcohol may have a greater relative effect on women.

While the temporary suppression of testosterone in men caused by a night of drinking is certainly not advantageous, neither does it have a lasting effect. Chronic excessive alcohol consumption, however, is a serious threat to a man's testosterone status, and ultimately, to his masculinity. In women, as well, alcohol abuse gravely threatens hormonal health.

Male alcoholics commonly exhibit symptoms of feminization including impotence, testicular atrophy, sterility, gynecomastia, and changes in bodily hair pattern.[435,436] Feminization in male alcoholics is caused not only by a reduction in baseline testosterone levels due to a toxic effect of alcohol on the testes,[437,438] but also by elevations in estrogen and prolactin.[439,440,441,442,443] Although the liver is not a sex organ per se, it plays an important role in sex hormone metabolism by regulating binding proteins and conversion of androgens to estrogens.

When alcoholism advances to the point of liver damage, hormonal health goes to hell in a handbasket. Specifically, in men, sex-hormone-binding globulin rises (which reduces the bioavailability of testosterone - see Chapter 22) and so do estrogen levels.[444,445,446,447,448] This exacerbates the hormonal alterations associated with long-term alcohol-inflicted testicular damage. The connection between the liver and hormonal health is demonstrated by studies of liver transplantation. After a patient acquires a new liver in place of his diseased one, testosterone and estrogen levels return to near-normal levels, symptoms of feminization subside, and sexual function improves.[449,450,451]

The long-term effects of alcohol abuse in women has received comparatively little attention. We know that chronic excessive alcohol consumption can damage the female reproductive system, causing menstrual disturbances, miscarriages, and infertility.[452,453,454] As with men, alcoholic liver disease in women is associated with profound hormonal derangements beyond those observed in alcoholic women without liver disease.[455,456,457]

While it is clear that chronic excessive alcohol consumption can destroy a woman's health like it can a man's, it is unclear what are the consequences of chronic moderate alcohol consumption in women, given alcohol's estrogen-enhancing effect. An increased risk of hormone-related cancers, such as breast, can be plausibly speculated to accrue to female moderate drinkers; and this hypothesis finds support in the scientific literature.[458,459,460,461,462,463] Overlaid upon this issue is the question of the interaction of alcohol with hormone replacement therapy in postmenopausal women. Insofar as alcohol raises estrogen levels in estrogen users, it may alter the risk/benefit ratio of estrogen replacement in an undesirable direction. The relative paucity of research examining the long-term ramifications of alcohol consumption in connection with hormone levels and hormone-related diseases in women is an unacceptable shortfall in need of rectification.

Another problem with alcohol is that it hampers fat burning. In addition to its potential to suppress lipolytic hormones, incoming alcohol causes a temporary suspension of fat burning.[464,465,466,467,468,469,470] In effect, you become an alcohol-burner, instead of a fat-burner, until the alcohol in your system is either burned for energy or stored as fat. Moreover, you probably have heard alcohol referred to as "empty calories," meaning that it possesses no redeeming nutritional value to offset the calories it contains. This is generally true, but, as discussed above, it is not true with respect to red wine. Red wine does not contain significant amounts of traditional nutrients like vitamins and minerals; but the definition of "nutrient" is rapidly expanding as we discover more about bioflavinoids and phytochemicals. Nonetheless, the net effect of alcohol on fat burning is unfavorable, though in small doses its impact may be negligible.

As you can see, there is no easy answer to the question of whether one should incorporate moderate amount of alcohol into one's diet, notwithstanding conflicting categorical pronouncements by health commentators. One-dimensional reasoning and sound-byte analysis cannot capture the multifarious biological implications of this enigmatic and widely popular drug. Health commentators who recommend regular alcohol consumption to population (the U.S.) in which obesity has reached epidemic proportions and breast cancer is major medical problem are on shaky ground. Granted, moderate alcohol consumption has been shown to protect against cardiovascular disease, but there are many other ways to reduce coronary risk without raising the risk of other infirmities.

Having said that, the history of alcoholic beverage consumption stretches back to biblical times. Even today, beer in Germany, vodka in Russia, and wine in France is for many people a symbol of national heritage. The cultural significance of alcoholic beverages should not be overlooked amid the technical minutiae of scientific investigation – nor should we discount the social import of alcohol or the fact that when used responsibly it makes people feel good.

Nonetheless, the sobering aspects of alcohol must be squarely confronted, because important decisions must not be based upon a selective consideration of facts. In particular "natural hormonal enhancers" have reason to regard alcohol with apprehension given the unhelpful, and potentially harmful, effect of alcohol on testosterone and growth hormone status. Because of its dubious hormonal effects and its direct inhibitory influence on lipolysis and protein synthesis, alcohol is not an ally, but rather a potential nemesis, to individuals seeking to improve their physique.

Fortunately, the antagonistic effects of alcohol on hormones and protein synthesis are dose related and threshold-dependent. And it appears that the threshold for cardiovascular protection (one drink a day) is lower than the threshold for triggering most of alcohol's adverse effects. While more research is needed to delineate precisely the dosage break-point for the various benefits and detriments of alcohol consumption, a fairly strong argument can be made in favor of drinking one glass of dry red wine per day. A much more compelling argument can be made in favor of becoming a drunken fool as infrequently as possible.

214

Cigarette Smoking

Gimme a packa-what-I-am.
Person overheard buying Kool cigarettes at a convenience store

I have every sympathy with the American who was so horrified
by what he had read about smoking that he gave up reading.
Henry G. Strauss

I smoke on ideological grounds.
John Francis Yetter, Professor of Law, who claims that his smoking
is motivated by the recent spate of laws limiting the rights of smokers

It's not cigarettes that are unhealthy, it's the toxic gas emitted by lighters and the
chemicals in the filters; so I smoke Camel non-filters, use matches, and I'm fine.
Bill Ryan, Ph.D.

Adding to the catalogue of misdeeds imputed to cigarette smoking, smoking has recently been charged with causing insulin resistance[471,472,473] and lowering serum testosterone in men. The latter charge is mainly based on data indicating that impotence is higher among smokers than non-smokers.[474,475,476]

First, I am not convinced that cigarette smoking directly causes impotence. Smokers have worse health practices in general than nonsmokers, and this may be the underlying factor accounting for their higher rates of impotence. This may also account for studies showing an association between insulin resistance and smoking, and such an argument against a causal effect of smoking on insulin resistance was advanced recently in *Metabolism*.[477] Because of the systemic damage caused by smoking, it is difficult to differentiate primary effects from secondary ones.

Secondly, even if smoking causes impotence, that does not prove that cigarette smoking lowers testosterone levels. Evidence of a direct effect of cigarette smoking on testosterone levels in humans is lacking, and associational evidence linking smoking with reduced testosterone levels is suspect for the same reason as is the association between smoking and impotence - smokers tend to exercise less and have generally poorer health habits than do nonsmokers. An unhealthy lifestyle can lower a man's testosterone levels, regardless of whether he smokes.

Thirdly, it is not valid to assume that impotence, which afflicts smokers disproportionately, is caused by low testosterone levels. Although low testosterone is likely to produce some impotency symptoms,[478] impotence is not necessarily indicative of low testosterone. This is especially so in the case of cigarette smoking, given that nicotine causes blood vessel constriction while it is in your system.[479] This vasoconstriction effect can impede erections, as demonstrated by a study published in *Addictive Behavior* in which men who smoked two high-nicotine cigarettes prior to watching an erotic film registered a significantly decreased rate of penile diameter change relative to men who had not smoked.[480] Furthermore, cigarette smoking promotes plaque accumulation on arterial walls. In addition to subverting cardiovascular health, clogged arteries represent a grave menace to sexual function.[481,482]

In any event, the testosterone, impotency, and insulin issues are inconsequential with respect to whether or not to smoke. The myriad other health problems connected with smoking, including its carcinogenic influence and its risk to cardiac health, is enough to strongly recommend abstention from smoking. Preaching is not my stock-in-trade, but if you are serious about being healthy, there's a mountain of uncontradicted evidence indicating that you should not smoke.

Sex and Relationships

Lord, give me chastity - but not yet.
St. Augustine

If it weren't for pickpockets I'd have no sex life at all.
Rodney Dangerfield

Eve: *Before we make love, there's something I need to know: do you love me?*
Adam: *You're the only woman for me, sweetheart.*

What do you mean I'm an uncaring father; I was present at the conception wasn't I?
Unknown

Lady Astor to Winston Churchill: *Sir, if you were my husband, I would poison your drink.*
Churchill's reply: *Madam, if you were my wife, I'd drink it.*

We all worry about the population explosion, but we don't worry about it at the right time.
Arthur Hoppe

Any scientist who has ever been in love knows that he may understand everything about sex hormones, but the actual experience is something quite different.
Dame Kathleen Lonsdale

Everyone knows that hormones influence sexual activity, but does sexual activity influence hormones? It can. Animal studies (in cheetahs and stallions) show that sexual stimulation can raise cortisol levels.[483,484] The applicability of these studies to humans must, however, be assessed with reference to the uniqueness of the human sexual experience. Sex between humans often involves emotional factors not present in the case of a mating stud horse or, in the other study cited, a cheetah undergoing electroejaculation.

One virtue of sex from a hormonal standpoint is the potential of sex to act as an anti-stress factor. Sex can be an outlet for tension and a source of satisfaction, fulfillment, and relaxation - all of which counter cortisol. Of course, depending on the person, the relationship between the partners, and attendant circumstances, sex can also be a cause of stress, and this would tend to elevate cortisol levels. For instance, where sex evokes feelings of guilt, apprehension, or anxiety, it will operate to raise cortisol levels for the reasons discussed above in "Stress and Mental Outlook." By the same token, sexual arousal resulting from fantasy or recollection

216

can alter cortisol levels absent a physical act, depending on one's disposition toward sexuality and toward the specific underlying thoughts and images.

As to the inherent physiological effect of sex on hormones, the question is whether sexual activity, or orgasm in particular, affects sex hormone levels. Although it is a basic question, the research addressing it is sparse. In some animal species, females experience a massive post-coital increase in sex hormone output, but males do not.[485,486,487,488] In human males, a recent study found no change in serum testosterone at either 1 or 24 hours after ejaculation.[489] Accordingly, it appears that whereas a higher sex hormone level can increase sexual activity, a higher level of sexual activity does not reliably increase sex hormone levels.

Sexual activity does not directly alter growth hormone levels, either. But it may exert an indirect psychic influence on growth hormone status. Consider that children raised in emotionally deprived environments frequently have lower growth hormone levels; and severely abusive treatment can cause psychosocial dwarfism, a condition marked by growth hormone deficiency and stunted growth.[490,491] Hence, emotional connection is a significant hormonal factor. And to the extent that physical intimacy between adults occurs in the context of a loving relationship and expresses mutual affection, it will tend to enhance growth hormone levels in both partners.

In summary, love, intimacy, companionship, and feelings of security can favorably affect hormone levels. This is the other side of the coin to the negative emotions discussed above in "Stress and Mental Outlook." Accordingly, any personal relationship that fosters these positive feelings and emotions promotes improved hormonal status by lowering cortisol levels (thereby facilitating testosterone production) and raising growth hormone levels. By contrast, relationships characterized by antagonism or mistrust, or which breed feelings of guilt or resentment, can adversely affect your hormonal profile.

References

1. Marin P, et al. Cortisol Secretion in Relation to Body Fat Distribution in Obese Premenopausal Women. *Metabolism* 1992;41:882.

2. Fraser R, et al. Cortisol Effects on Body Mass, Blood Pressure, and Cholesterol in the General Population. *Hypertension* 1999;33:1364.

3. Stewart PM, et al. Cortisol Metabolism in Human Obesity: Impaired Cortisone-->Cortisol Conversion in Subjects with Central Adiposity. *J Clin Endocrinol Metab* 1999;84:1022.

4. Lottenberg SA, et al. Effect of Fat Distribution on the Pharmacokinetics of Cortisol in Obesity. *Int J Clin Pharmacol Ther* 1998;36:501.

5. Plotsky PM, Vale W. Hemorrhage-Induced Secretion of Corticotropin-Releasing Factor-Like Immunoreactivity into the Rat Hypophysial-Portal Circulation and its Inhibition by Glucocorticoids. *Endocrinology* 1984;114:164.

6. Chappell PB, et al. Alterations in Corticotropin-Releasing Factor-Like Immunoreactivity in Discrete Brain Regions after Acute and Chronic Stress. *J Neurosci* 1986;6:2908.

7. Orth DN, Jackson RV, DeCherney GS. Effect of Synthetic Ovine Corticotropin-Releasing Factor: Dose Response of Plasma Adrenocorticotropin and Cortisol. *J Clin Invest* 1983;71:587.

8. Linton EA, et al. Stress-Induced Secretion of Adrenocorticotropin in Rats is Inhibited by Administration of Antisera to Ovine Corticotropin-Releasing Factor and Vasopressin. *Endocrinol* 1985;116:966.

9. Renold AE, et al. The Use of Intravenous ACTH: A Study in Quantitative Adrenocortical Stimulation. *J Clin Endocrinol Metab* 1952;12:763.

10. Amsterdan JD, et al. Cosyntropin (ACTH α1-24) Stimulation Test in Depressed Patients and Healthy Subjects. *Am J Psychiatry* 1983;140:907.

11. Smyth J, et al. Stressors and Mood Measured on Momentary Basis are Associated with Salivary Cortisol Secretion. *Psychoneuroendocrinology* 1998;23:353.

12. Mazzoccoli G, et al. Age-Related Changes of Neuro-Endocrine-Immune Interactions in Healthy Humans. *J Biol Regul Homeost Agents* 1997;11:143.

13. Tomaszewska D, et al. The Immune-Neuro-Endocrine Interactions. *J Physiol Pharmacol* 1997;48:139.

14. Jorgensen C, et al. Modulation of the Immune Response by the Neuro-Endocrine Axis in Rheumatoid Arthritis. *Clin Exp Rheumatol* 1994;12:435.

15. Takao T, et al. Modulation of Interleukin-1 Receptors in the Neuro-Endocrine-Immune Axis. *Int J Dev Neurosci* 1995;13:167.

16. Naliboff BD, et al. Immunological Changes in Young and Old Adults during Brief Laboratory Stress. *Psychosom Med* 1991;53:121.

17. Naliboff BD, et al. Rapid Changes in Cellular Immunity Following a Confrontational Role-Play Stressor. *Brain Behav Immun* 1995;9:207.

18. Ackerman KD, et al. Immunologic Response to Acute Psychological Stress in MS Patients and Controls. *J Neuroimmunol* 1996;68:85.

19. Herbert TB, et al. Cardiovascular Reactivity and the Course of Immune Response to an Acute Psychological Stressor. *Psychosom Med* 1994;56:337.

20. Basso AM, et al. Chronic Restraint Attenuates the Immunosuppressive Response Induced by Novel Aversive Stimuli. *Physiol Behav* 1994;55:1151.

21. Rozlog LA, et al. Stress and Immunity: Implications for Viral Disease and Wound Healing. *J Periodontol* 1999;70:786.

22. Keller SE, et al. Suppression of Immunity by Stress: Effect of a Graded Series of Stressors on Lymphocyte Stimulation in the Rat. *Science* 1981;213:1397.

23. Pezzone MA, et al. Effects of Footshock Stress upon Spleen and Peripheral Blood Lymphocyte Mitogenic Responses in Rats with Lesions of the Paraventricular Nuclei. *J Neuroimmunol* 1994;53:39.

24. Pike JL, et al. Chronic Life Stress Alters Sympathetic, Neuroendocrine, and Immune Responsivity to an Acute Psychological Stressor in Humans. *Psychosom Med* 1997;59:447.

25. Capitanio JP, et al. Social Stress Results in Altered Glucocorticoid Regulation and Shorter Survival in Simian Acquired Immune Deficiency Syndrome. *Proc Natl Acad Sci U S A* 1998;95:4714.

26. Capitanio JP, Lerche NW. Psychosocial Factors and Disease Progression in Simian AIDS: A Preliminary Report. *AIDS* 1991;5:1103.

27. Capitanio JP, Lerche NW. Social Separation, Housing Relocation, and Survival in Simian AIDS: A Retrospective Analysis. *Psychosom Med* 1998;60:235.

28. Leserman J, et al. Progression to AIDS: the Effects of Stress, Depressive Symptoms, and Social Support. *Psychosom Med* 1999;61:397.

29. Evans DL, et al. Severe Life Stress as a Predictor of Early Disease Progression in HIV Infection. *Am J Psychiatry* 1997;154:630.

30. Irwin M, et al. Reduction of Immune Function in Life Stress and Depression. *Biol Psychiatry* 1990;27:22.

31. Irwin M. Immune Correlates of Depression. *Adv Exp Med Biol* 1999;461:1.

32. Irwin M, et al. Depression and Reduced Natural Killer Cytotoxicity: A Longitudinal Study of Depressed Patients and Control Subjects. *Psychol Med* 1992;22:1045.

33. Caldwell CL, Irwin M, Lohr J. Reduced Natural Killer Cell Cytotoxicity in Depression but Not in Schizophrenia. *Biol Psychiatry* 1991;30:1131.

34. Schleifer SJ, et al. Lymphocyte Function in Major Depressive Disorder. *Arch Gen Psychiatry* 1984;41:484.

35. Darko DF, et al. Plasma Beta-Endorphin and Natural Killer Cell Activity in Major Depression: A Preliminary Study. *Psychiatry Res* 1992;43:111.

36. Miller GE, Cohen S, Herbert TB. Pathways Linking Major Depression and Immunity in Ambulatory Female Patients. *Psychosom Med* 1999;61:850.

37. Birmaher B, et al. Cellular Immunity in Depressed, Conduct Disorder, and Normal Adolescents: Role of Adverse Life Events. *J Am Acad Child Adolesc Psychiatry* 1994;33:671.

38. Irwin M, et al. Life Events, Depressive Symptoms, and Immune Function. *Am J Psychiatry* 1987;144:437.

39. Antoni MH. Temporal Relationship between Life Events and Two Illness Measures: A Cross-Lagged Panel Analysis. *J Human Stress* 1985;11:21.

40. Sheehan DV, et al. The Relationship between Response Qualities of Life Change Events and Future Illness Rates. *Int J Psychiatry Med* 1979;9:217.

1. Cleghorn JM, Streiner BJ. Prediction of Symptoms and Illness Behaviour from Measures of Life Change and Verbalized Depressive Themes. *J Human Stress* 1979;5:16.

2. Calvert P, Northeast J, Cunningham E. Death in a Country Area and its Effect on the Health of Relatives. *Med J Aust* 1977;2:635.

3. Van Eijk J, et al. Effect of Bereavement on the Health of the Remaining Family Members. *Fam Pract* 1988;5:278.

4. Jacobs S, Ostfeld A. An Epidemiological Review of the Mortality of Bereavement. *Psychosom Med* 1977;39:344.

5. Lichtenstein P, Gatz M, Berg S. A Twin Study of Mortality after Spousal Bereavement. *Psychol Med* 1998;28:635.

6. Schaefer C, Quesenberry CP Jr, Wi S. Mortality following Conjugal Bereavement and the Effects of a Shared Environment. *Am J Epidemiol* 1995;141:1142.

7. Kaprio J, Koskenvuo M, Rita H. Mortality after Bereavement: A Prospective Study of 95,647 Widowed Persons. *Am J Public Health* 1987;77:283.

8. Martikainen P, Valkonen T. Mortality after Death of Spouse in Relation to Duration of Bereavement in Finland. *J Epidemiol Community Health* 1996;50:264.

9. Helsing KJ, Szklo M. Mortality after Bereavement. *Am J Epidemiol* 1981;114:41.

10. Martikainen P, Valkonen T. Mortality after the Death of a Spouse: Rates and Causes of Death in a Large Finnish Cohort. *Am J Public Health* 1996;86:1087.

11. Lawrence MS, Sapolsky RM. Glucocorticoids Accelerate ATP Loss Following Metabolic Insults in Cultured Hippocampal Neurons. *Brain Res* 1994;646:303.

12. Sapolsky RM. Glucocorticoid Toxicity in the Hippocampus: Temporal Aspects of Neuronal Vulnerability. *Brain Res* 1985;359:300.

13. Sapolsky RM, Krey LC, McEwen BS. Prolonged Glucocorticoid Exposure Reduces Hippocampal Neuron Number: Implications for Aging. *J Neurosci* 1985;5:1222.

14. Stein-Behrens B, et al. Stress Exacerbates Neuron Loss and Cytoskeletal Pathology in the Hippocampus. *J Neurosci* 1994;14:5373.

15. Sapolsky RM. Stress, Glucocorticoids, and Damage to the Nervous System: The Current State of Confusion. *Stress* 1996;1:1.

16. Martignoni E, et al. Dementia of the Alzheimer Type and Hypothalamus-Pituitary-Adrenocortical Axis: Changes in Cerebrospinal Fluid Corticotropin Releasing Factor and Plasma Cortisol Levels. *Acta Neurol Scand* 1990;81:452.

17. Dodt C, et al. Different Regulation of Adrenocorticotropin and Cortisol Secretion in Young, Mentally Healthy Elderly and Patients with Senile Dementia of Alzheimer's Type. *J Clin Endocrinol Metab* 1991;72:272.

18. Masugi F, et al. High Plasma Levels of Cortisol in Patients with Senile Dementia of the Alzheimer's Type. *Methods Find Exp Clin Pharmacol* 1989;11:707.

19. Weiner MF, et al. Cortisol Secretion and Alzheimer's Disease Progression. *Biol Psychiatry* 1997;42:1030.

20. Carroll BJ, Curtis GC, Mendels J. Cerebrospinal Fluid and Plasma Free Cortisol Concentrations in Depression. *Psychol Med* 1976;6:235.

21. Diebold K, Kick H, Schmidt G. Urinary Free Cortisol Excretion in Endogenously Depressed and Schizophrenic Patients. *Psychiatr Clin (Basal)* 1981;14:43.

22. Scott LV, Dinan TG. Urinary Free Cortisol Excretion in Chronic Fatigue Syndrome, Major Depression and in Healthy Volunteers. *J Affect Disord* 1998;47:49.

23. Carroll BJ, et al. Urinary Free Cortisol Excretion in Depression. *Psychol Med* 1976;6:43.

24. Gold PW. Responses to Corticotropin-Releasing Hormone in the Hypercortisolism of Depression and Cushing's Disease. *N Engl J Med* 1986;314:1329.

25. Deuschle M, et al. Effects of Major Depression, Aging and Gender upon Calculated Diurnal Free Plasma Cortisol Concentrations: A Re-Evaluation Study. *Stress* 1998;2:281.

26. Dinan TG, et al. Lowering Cortisol Enhances Growth Hormone Response to Growth Hormone Releasing Hormone in Healthy Subjects. *Acta Physiol Scand* 1994;151:413.

27. Sartin JL, et al. Cortisol Inhibition of Growth Hormone-Releasing Hormone-Stimulated Growth Hormone Release from Cultured Sheep Pituitary Cells. *J Endocrinol* 1994;141:517.

28. Thompson K, et al. Effects of Short-Term Cortisol Infusion on Growth Hormone-Releasing Hormone Stimulation of Growth Hormone Release in Sheep. *Am J Vet Res* 1995;56:1228.

29. See Chapter 22, notes 90-92.

30a. Johansson GG, et al. Examination Stress Decreases Plasma Level of Luteinizing Hormone in Male Students. *Psychosom Med* 1988;50:286.

30b. Sapolsky RM, Krey LC. Stress-Induced Suppression of Luteinizing Hormone Concentrations in Wild Baboons: Role of Opiates. *J Clin Endocrinol Metab* 1988;66:722.

30c. Norman RL, Smith CJ. Restraint Inhibits Luteinizing Hormone and Testosterone Secretion in Intact Male Rhesus Macaques: Effects of Concurrent Naloxone Administration. *Neuroendocrinology* 1992;55:405.

69d. Johnson BH, Welsh TH, Juniewicz PE. Suppression of Luteinizing Hormone and Testosterone Secretion in Bulls Following Adrenocorticotropin Hormone Treatment. *Biol Reprod* 1982;26:305.

69e. Hangaard J, et al. Pulsatile Luteinizing Hormone Secretion in Patients with Addison's Disease. Impact of Glucocorticoid Substitution. *J Clin Endocrinol Metab* 1998;83:736.

69f. Bambino TH, Hsueh AJW. Direct Inhibitory Effect of Glucocorticoids upon Testicular Luteinizing Hormone Receptor and Steroidogenisis In Vivo and In Vitro. *Endocrinol* 1981;108:2142.

69g. Sapolsky RM. Stress-Induced Suppression of Testicular Function in the Wild Baboon: Role of Glucocorticoids. *Endocrinology* 1985;116:2273.

69h. Orr TE, Mann DR. Role of Glucocorticoids on the Stress-Induced Suppression of Testicular Steroidogenesis in Adu Male Rats. *Horm Behav* 1992;26:350.

69i. Charpenet G, et al. Stress-Induced Testicular Hyposensitivity to Gonadotropin in Rats. Role of the Pituitary Gland. *Biol Reprod* 1982;27:616.

69j. Fenske M. Role of Cortisol in the ACTH-Induced Suppression of Testicular Steroidogenesis in Guinea Pigs. *J Endocrinol* 1997;154:407.

69k. Cumming DC, Quigley ME, Yen SSC. Acute Suppression of Circulating Testosterone Levels by Cortisol Levels in Men. *J Endocrinol Metab* 1983;57:671.

70. Weber C. Cortisol's Purpose. *Med Hypotheses* 1998;51:289.

71. Gal R, et al. The Role of Activity in Anticipating and Confronting Stressful Situations. *J Human Stress* 1975;1:4.

72. Olff M. Stress, Depression and Immunity: The Role of Defense and Coping Styles. *Psychiatry Res* 1999;85:7.

73. Aspinwall LG, et al. A Stitch in Time: Self-Regulation and Proactive Coping. *Psychol Bull* 1997;121:417.

74. Billings AG, et al. The Role of Coping Responses and Social Resources in Attenuating the Stress of Life Events. *J Behav Med* 1981;4:139.

75. Segerstrom SC, et al. Optimism is Associated with Mood, Coping, and Immune Change in Response to Stress. *J Per Soc Psychol* 1998;74:1646.

76. Cohen F, et al. Differential Immune System Changes with Acute and Persistent Stress for Optimists vs. Pessimists. *Brain Behav Immun* 1999;13:155.

77. van Eck MM, et al. Individual Differences in Cortisol Responses to a Laboratory Speech Task and their Relationship to Responses to Stressful Daily Events. *Biol Psychol* 1996;43:69.

78. van Eck M, et al. The Effects of Perceived Stress, Traits, Mood States, and Stressful Daily Events on Salivary Cortisol. *Psychosom Med* 1996;58:447.

79. Pansera F. Sleep as Vegetation: A Tautological Theory of Sleep. *Med Hypotheses* 1996;46:312.

80. Morgan L, et al. Effects of the Endogenous Clock and Sleep Time on Melatonin, Insulin, Glucose and Lipid Metabolism. *J Endocrinol* 1998;157:443.

81. Goichot B, et al. Effect of the Shift of the Sleep-Wake Cycle on Three Robust Endocrine Markers of the Circadian Clock. *Am J Physiol* 1998;275:E243.

82. Pietrowsky R, et al. Effects of Diurnal Sleep on Secretion of Cortisol, Luteinizing Hormone, and Growth Hormone i Man. *J Clin Endocrinol Metab* 1994;78:683.

83. Opstad K. Circadian Rhythm of Hormones is Extinguished during Prolonged Physical Stress, Sleep and Energy Deficiency in Young Men. *Eur J Endocrinol* 1994;131:56.

84. Everson CA. Functional Consequences of Sustained Sleep Deprivation in the Rat. *Behav Brain Res* 1995;69:43.

85. Everson CA. Sustained Sleep Deprivation Impairs Host Defense. *Am J Physiol* 1993;265:R1148.

86. Rechtschaffen A, et al. Physiological Correlates of Prolonged Sleep Deprivation in Rats. *Science* 1983;221:182.

87. Weibel L, et al. Growth Hormone Secretion in Night Workers. *Chronobiol Int* 1997;14:49.

88. Weibel L, Brandenberger G. Disturbances in Hormonal Profiles of Night Workers during their Usual Sleep and Wor Times. *J Biol Rhythms* 1998;13:202.

89. Ribeiro DC, et al. Altered Postprandial Hormone and Metabolic Responses in a Simulated Shift Work Environment. *Endocrinol* 1998;158:305.

90. Motohashi Y. Alteration of Circadian Rhythm in Shift-Working Ambulance Personnel. Monitoring of Salivary Cortisol Rhythm. *Ergonomics* 1992;35:1331.

91. Weibel L, Follenius M, Brandenberger G. [Biologic Rhythms: Their Changes in Night-Shift Workers]. *Presse Med* 1999;28:252. French.

92. Weitzman ED, et al. Cortisol Secretion is Inhibited during Sleep in Normal Man. *J Clin Endocrinol Metab* 1983;56:352.

93. Spiegel K, Leproult R, Van Cauter E. Impact of Sleep Debt on Metabolic and Endocrine Function. *Lancet* 1999;354:1435.

220

94. von Treuer K, et al. Overnight Human Plasma Melatonin, Cortisol, Prolactin, TSH, under Conditions of Normal Sleep, Sleep Deprivation, and Sleep Recovery. *J Pineal Res* 1996;20:7.

95. Vgontzas AN, et al. Sleep Deprivation Effects on the Activity of the Hypothalamic-Pituitary-Adrenal and Growth Axes: Potential Clinical Implications. *Clin Endocrinol (Oxf)* 1999;51:205.

96. Leproult R, et al. Sleep Loss Results in an Elevation of Cortisol Levels the Next Evening. *Sleep* 1997;20:865.

97. Weibel L, et al. Comparative Effect of Night and Daytime Sleep on the 24-Hour Cortisol Secretory Profile. *Sleep* 1995;18:549.

98. Radomski MW, et al. Aerobic Fitness and Hormonal Responses to Prolonged Sleep Deprivation and Sustained Mental Work. *Aviat Space Environ Med* 1992;63:101.

99. See, supra, note 93.

100. Scheen AJ, et al. Relationships between Sleep Quality and Glucose Regulation in Normal Humans. *Am J Physiol* 1996;271:E261.

101. VanHelder T, et al. Effects of Sleep Deprivation and Exercise on Glucose Tolerance. *Aviat Space Environ Med* 1993;64:487.

102. Kasper S, et al. Nocturnal TSH and Prolactin Secretion during Sleep Deprivation and Prediction of Antidepressant Response in Patients with Major Depression. *Biol Psychiatry* 1988;24:631.

103. Sadamatsu M, et al. The 24-Hour Rhythms in Plasma Growth Hormone, Prolactin and Thyroid Stimulating Hormone: Effect of Sleep Deprivation. *J Neuroendocrinol* 1995;7:597.

104. Palmblad J, et al. Thyroid and Adrenomedullary Reactions during Sleep Deprivation. *Acta Endocrinol (Copenh)* 1979;90:233.

105. See, supra, note 98.

106. Baumgartner A, et al. Neuroendocrinological Investigations during Sleep Deprivation in Depression. I. Early Morning Levels of Thyrotropin, TH, Cortisol, Prolactin, LH, FSH, Estradiol, and Testosterone. *Biol Psychiatry* 1990;28:556.

107. Mathur PP, Chattopadhyay S. Effect of Sleep Deprivation on the Physiological Status of Rat Testis. *Andrologia* 1991;23:49.

108. Opstad PK, Aakvaag A. The Effect of Sleep Deprivation on the Plasma Levels of Hormones during Prolonged Physical Strain and Calorie Deficiency. *Eur J Appl Physiol* 1983;51:97.

109. Remes K, Kuoppasalmi K, Adlercreutz H. Effect of Physical Exercise and Sleep Deprivation on Plasma Androgen Levels: Modifying Effect of Physical Fitness. *Int J Sports Med* 1985;6:131.

110. Monk TH. Sleep Disorders in the Elderly. Circadian Rhythm. *Clin Geriatr Med* 1989;5:331.

111. van Coevorden A, et al. Neuroendocrine Rhythms and Sleep in Aging Men. *Am J Physiol* 1991;260:E651.

112. Van Cauter E, et al. Alterations of Circadian Rhythmicity and Sleep in Aging: Endocrine Consequences. *Horm Res* 1998;49:147.

113. Dijk DJ, Duffy JF. Circadian Regulation of Human Sleep and Age-Related Changes in its Timing, Consolidation and EEG Characteristics. *Ann Med* 1999;31:130.

114. Van Cauter E, Plat L. Physiology of Growth Hormone Secretion during Sleep. *J Pediatr* 1996;128:S32.

115. Holl RW, et al. Thirty-Second Sampling of Plasma Growth Hormone in Man: Correlation with Sleep Stages. *J Clin Endocrinol Metab* 1991;72:854.

116. Prinz PN, et al. Plasma Growth Hormone during Sleep in Young and Aged Men. *J Gerontol* 1983;38:519.

117. Van Cauter E, et al. A Quantitative Estimation of Growth Hormone Secretion in Normal Man: Reproducibility and Relation to Sleep and Time of Day. *J Clin Endocrinol Metab* 1992;74:1441.

118. Spath-Schwalbe E, et al. Nocturnal Wakefulness Inhibits Growth Hormone (GH)-Releasing Hormone-Induced GH Secretion. *J Clin Endocrinol Metab* 1995;80:214.

119. Van Cauter E, et al. Sleep, Awakenings, and Insulin-Like Growth Factor-I Modulate the Growth Hormone (GH) Secretory Response to GH-Releasing Hormone. *J Clin Endocrinol Metab* 1992;74:1451.

120. Van Cauter E, Plat L, Copinschi G. Interrelations between Sleep and the Somatotropic Axis. *Sleep* 1998;21:553.

121. Born J, Fehm HL. Hypothalamus-Pituitary-Adrenal Activity during Human Sleep: A Coordinating Role for the Limbic Hippocampal System. *Exp Clin Endocrinol Diabetes* 1998;106:153.

122. Fehm HL, et al. Relationships between Sleep Stages and Plasma Cortisol: A Single Case Study. *Acta Endocrinol (Copenh)* 1986;111:264.

123. Spath-Schwalbe E, et al. Corticotropin-Releasing Hormone-Induced Adrenocorticotropin and Cortisol Secretion Depends on Sleep and Wakefulness. *J Clin Endocrinol Metab* 1993;77:1170.

124. Born J, Muth S, Fehm HL. The Significance of Sleep Onset and Slow Wave Sleep for Nocturnal Release of Growth Hormone (GH) and Cortisol. *Psychoneuroendocrinology* 1988;13:233.

125. Steiger A, Herth T, Holsboer F. Sleep-Electroencephalography and the Secretion of Cortisol and Growth Hormone in Normal Controls. *Acta Endocrinol (Copenh)* 1987;116:36.

221

126. Kern W, et al. Changes in Cortisol and Growth Hormone Secretion during Nocturnal Sleep in the Course of Aging. *J Gerontol A Biol Sci Med Sci* 1996;51:M3.

127. Deuschle M, et al. Effects of Major Depression, Aging and Gender upon Calculated Diurnal Free Plasma Cortisol Concentrations: A Re-Evaluation Study. *Stress* 1998;2:281.

128. Copinschi G, Van Cauter E. Effects of Ageing on Modulation of Hormonal Secretions by Sleep and Circadian Rhythmicity. *Horm Res* 1995;43:20.

129. Parker DC, Rossman LG. Human Growth Hormone in Sleep: Nonsuppression by Acute Hyperglycemia. *J Clin Endocrinol* 1971;32:65.

130. Serrano Rios M, et al. Nocturnal Growth Hormone Surges in Type 1 Diabetes Mellitus are Both Sleep- and Glycemia-Dependent: Assessment under Continuous Sleep Monitoring. *Diabetes Res Clin Pract* 1990;10:1.

131. Parker DC, Rossman LG, VanderLaan EF. Persistence of Rhythmic Human Growth Hormone Release during Sheep in Fasted and Nonisocalorically Fed Normal Subjects. *Metabolism* 1972;21:241.

132. Reynolds CF 3d, et al. Sleep Deprivation in Healthy Elderly Men and Women: Effects on Mood and on Sleep during Recovery. *Sleep* 1986;9:492.

133. Aeschbach D, et al. Homeostatic Sleep Regulation in Habitual Short Sleepers and Long Sleepers. *Am J Physiol* 1996;270:R41.

134. Lucidi F, et al. Effects of Different Sleep duration on Delta Sleep in Recovery Nights. *Psychophysiology* 1997;34:227.

135. Endo T, et al. Selective REM Sleep Deprivation in Humans: Effects on Sleep and Sleep EEG. *Am J Physiol* 1998;274:R1186.

136. Dijk DJ, Beersma DG. Effects of SWS Deprivation on Subsequent EEG Power Density and Spontaneous Sleep Duration. *Electroencephalogr Clin Neurophysiol* 1989;72:312.

137. Bonnet MH, Arand DL. We are Chronically Sleep Deprived. *Sleep* 1995;18:908.

138. Kripke DF, et al. Short and Long Sleep and Sleeping Pills. Is Increased Mortality Associated? *Arch Gen Psychiatry* 1979;36:103.

139. Wingard DL, Berkman LF. Mortality Risk Associated with Sleeping Patterns among Adults. *Sleep* 1983;6:102.

140. Fehm HL, et al. Entrainment of Nocturnal Pituitary-Adrenocortical Activity to Sleep Processes in Man--A Hypothesis. *Exp Clin Endocrinol* 1993;101:267.

141. See, supra, note 82.

142. Karacan I, et al. Growth Hormone Levels during Morning and Afternoon Naps. *Behav Neuropsychiatry* 19741975;6:67.

143. See, supra, note 140.

144. See, supra, note 82.

145. Dijk DJ, Duffy JF. Circadian Regulation of Human Sleep and Age-Related Changes in its Timing, Consolidation and EEG Characteristics. *Ann Med* 1999;31:130.

146. Van Cauter E, et al. Alterations of Circadian Rhythmicity and Sleep in Aging: Endocrine Consequences. *Horm Res* 1998;49:147.

147. Bremner WJ, Vitiello MV, Prinz PN. Loss of Circadian Rhythmicity in Blood Testosterone Levels with Aging in Normal Men. *J Clin Endocrinol Metab* 1983;56:1278.

148. van Coevorden A, et al. Neuroendocrine Rhythms and Sleep in Aging Men. *Am J Physiol* 1991;260:E651.

149. Waterhouse JM, Minors DS. Circadian Rhythms in the Neonate and in Old Age: What Do They Tell Us about the Development and Decay of the Body Clock in Humans? *Braz J Med Biol Res* 1996;29:87.

150. Turek FW. Circadian Rhythms. *Recent Prog Horm Res* 1994;49:43.

151. Krieger DT. "Circadian and Pituitary Adrenal Rhythms" In: Hedlund LW, Franz JM, Kenny AD, eds. *Biological Rhythms and Endocrine Function*. Advances in Experimental Medicine and Biology Vol. 54, NY: Plenum Press 1974.

152. Weitzman ED, et al. "The Relationship of Sleep and Sleep Stages to Neuroendocrine Secretion and Biological Rhythms in Man" In: *Recent Progress in Hormone Research, Proceedings of the 1974 Laurentian Hormone Conference* 1975;31.

153. Webb WB, Bonnet MH. The Sleep of 'Morning' and 'Evening' Types. *Biol Psychol* 1978;7:29.

154. Taub JM. Behavioral and Psychophysiological Correlates of Irregularity in Chronic Sleep Routines. *Biol Psychol* 1978;7:37.

155. Taub JM, Berger RJ. The Effects of Changing the Phase and Duration of Sleep. *J Exp Psychol [Hum Percept]* 1976;2:30.

156. Manber R, et al. The Effects of Regularizing Sleep-Wake Schedules on Daytime Sleepiness. *Sleep* 1996;19:432.

157. Hoch CC, et al. The Superior Sleep of Healthy Elderly Nuns. *Int J Aging Hum Dev* 1987;25:1.

158. Duffy JF, Kronauer RE, Czeisler CA. Phase-Shifting Human Circadian Rhythms: Influence of Sleep Timing, Social Contact and Light Exposure. *J Physiol (Lond)* 1996;495:289.

159. Czeisler CA. The Effect of Light on the Human Circadian Pacemaker. *Ciba Found Symp* 1995;183:254.

160. Ralph MR, Hurd MW. Pacemaker Interactions in the Mammalian Circadian System. *Braz J Med Biol Res* 1996;29:77.

161. Gillette MU, Tischkau SA. Suprachiasmatic Nucleus: The Brain's Circadian Clock. *Recent Prog Horm Res* 1999;54:33.

162. Golombek DA, Ralph MR. Let There Be Light: Signal Transduction in a Mammalian Circadian System. *Braz J Med Biol Res* 1996;29:131.

163. Olcese J. The Mammalian Pineal Gland and Reproduction. Controversies and Strategies for Future Research. *Adv Exp Med Biol* 1995;377:1.

164. Weaver DR, et al. Melatonin Receptors in Human Hypothalamus and Pituitary: Implications for Circadian and Reproductive Responses to Melatonin. *J Clin Endocrinol Metab* 1993;76:295.

165. Korf HW, Schomerus C, Stehle JH. The Pineal Organ, its Hormone Melatonin, and the Photoneuroendocrine System. *Adv Anat Embryol Cell Biol* 1998;146:1.

166. Cassone VM, et al. Melatonin, the Pineal Gland, and Circadian Rhythms. *J Biol Rhythms* 1993;(8 Suppl):S73.

167. Stetson MH, Watson-Whitmyre M. Effects of Exogenous and Endogenous Melatonin on Gonadal Function in Hamsters. *J Neural Transm Suppl* 1986;21:55.

168. Miernicki M, Karp JD, Powers JB. Pinealectomy Prevents Short Photoperiod Inhibition of Male Hamster Sexual Behavior. *Physiol Behav* 1990;47:293.

169. Turek FW, Losee-Olson SH, Ellis GB. Pinealectomy and Lesions of the Suprachiasmatic Nucleus Affect the Castration Response in Hamsters Exposed to Short Photoperiods. *Neuroendocrinology* 1983;36:335.

170. Wallen EP, et al. Photoperiodic Response in the Male Laboratory Rat. *Biol Reprod* 1987;37:22.

171. Swaab DF, et al. Biological Rhythms in the Human Life Cycle and their Relationship to Functional Changes in the Suprachiasmatic Nucleus. *Prog Brain Res* 1996;111:349.

172. Swaab DF, Gooren LJ, Hofman MA. Brain Research, Gender and Sexual Orientation. *J Homosex* 1995;28:283.

173. Swaab DF, Gooren LJ, Hofman MA. Gender and Sexual Orientation in Relation to Hypothalamic Structures. *Horm Res* 1992;38(Suppl):51S.

174. Swaab DF, Hofman MA. An Enlarged Suprachiasmatic Nucleus in Homosexual Men. *Brain Res* 1990 Dec 24;537:141.

175. Bartke A, Klemcke H, Amador A. Effects of Testosterone, Pregnenolone, Progesterone and Cortisol on Pituitary and Testicular Function in Male Golden Hamsters with Gonadal Atrophy Induced by Short Photoperiods. *J Endocrinol* 1981;90:97.

176. Blank JL, Desjardins C. Photic Cues Induce Multiple Neuroendocrine Adjustments in Testicular Function. *Am J Physiol* 1986;250:R199.

177. Steger RW, Bartke A, Goldman BD. Alterations in Neuroendocrine Function during Photoperiod Induced Testicular Atrophy and Recrudescence in the Golden Hamster. *Biol Reprod* 1982;26:437.

178. Chandrashekar V, Bartke A. The Influence of Short Photoperiod on Testicular and Circulating Levels of Testosterone Precursors in the Adult Golden Hamster. *Biol Reprod* 1989;40:300.

179. Stanisiewski EP, et al. Effect of Photoperiod and Castration on Prolactin, Testosterone and Luteinizing Hormone Concentrations in Male Calves. *J Anim Sci* 1987;65:1306.

180. Saboureau M, Dutourne B. The Reproductive Cycle in the Male Hedgehog (Erinaceus Europaeus L.): A Study of Endocrine and Exocrine Testicular Functions. *Reprod Nutr Dev* 1981;21:109.

181. Johnson L, Thompson DL Jr. Age-Related and Seasonal Variation in the Sertoli Cell Population, Daily Sperm Production and Serum Concentrations of Follicle-Stimulating Hormone, Luteinizing Hormone and Testosterone in Stallions. *Biol Reprod* 1983;29:777.

182. Malecki IA, et al. Endocrine and Testicular Changes in a Short-Day Seasonally Breeding Bird, the Emu (Dromaius Novaehollandiae), in Southwestern Australia. *Anim Reprod Sci* 1998;53:143.

183. Gemmell RT, Johnston G, Barnes A. Seasonal Variations in Plasma Testosterone Concentrations in the Male Marsupial Bandicoot Isoodon Macrourus in Captivity. *Gen Comp Endocrinol* 1985;59:184.

184. Beck W, Wuttke W. Annual Rhythms of Luteinizing Hormone, Follicle-Stimulating Hormone, Prolactin and Testosterone in the Serum of Male Rhesus Monkeys. *J Endocrinol* 1979;83:131.

185. Delgadillo JA, Leboeuf B, Chemineau P. Maintenance of Sperm Production in Bucks during a Third Year of Short Photoperiodic Cycles. *Reprod Nutr Dev* 1993;33:609.

186. Saboureau M, Dutourne B. The Reproductive Cycle in the Male Hedgehog (Erinaceus Europaeus L.): A Study of Endocrine and Exocrine Testicular Functions. *Reprod Nutr Dev* 1981;21:109.

187. Burns PJ, et al. Effect of Increased Photoperiod on Hormone Concentrations in Thoroughbred Stallions. *J Reprod Fertil Suppl* 1982;32:103.

188. Clay CM, et al. Influences of Season and Artificial Photoperiod on Stallions: Testicular Size, Seminal Characteristics and Sexual Behavior. *J Anim Sci* 1987;64:517.

223

189. Byers SW, Dowsett KF, Glover TD. Seasonal and Circadian Changes of Testosterone Levels in the Peripheral Blood Plasma of Stallions and their Relation to Semen Quality. *J Endocrinol* 1983;99:141.

190. Malpaux B, et al. Regulation of the Onset of the Breeding Season of the Ewe: Importance of Long Days and of an Endogenous Reproductive Rhythm. *J Endocrinol* 1989;122:269.

191. Cox JE, Redhead PH, Jawad NM. The Effect of Artificial Photoperiod at the End of the Breeding Season on Plasma Testosterone Concentrations in Stallions. *Aust Vet J* 1988;65:239.

192. Kostoglou-Athanassiou I, et al. Bright Light Exposure and Pituitary Hormone Secretion. *Clin Endocrinol (Oxf)* 1998;48:73.

193. Czeisler CA, et al. Bright Light Resets the Human Circadian Pacemaker Independent of the Timing of the Sleep-Wake Cycle. *Science* 1986;233:667.

194. Smals AG, Kloppenborg PW, Benraad TJ. Circannual Cycle in Plasma Testosterone Levels in Man. *J Clin Endocrinol Metab* 1976;42:979.

195. Bellastella A, et al. [Annual Variations in Plasma Testosterone Levels in Prepuberal Subjects]. *Boll Soc Ital Biol Sper* 1980;56:2001. Italian.

196. Bellastella A, et al. Circannual Rhythms of Plasma Luteinizing Hormone, Follicle-Stimulating Hormone, Testosterone, Prolactin and Cortisol in Prepuberty. *Clin Endocrinol (Oxf)* 1983;19:453.

197. Kauppila A, et al. Inverse Seasonal Relationship between Melatonin and Ovarian Activity in Humans in a Region with a Strong Seasonal Contrast in Luminosity. *J Clin Endocrinol Metab* 1987;65:823.

198. Kauppila A, et al. The Effect of Season on the Circulating Concentrations of Anterior Pituitary, Ovarian and Adrenal Cortex Hormones and Hormone Binding Proteins in the Subarctic Area; Evidence of Increased Activity of the Pituitary-Ovarian Axis in Spring. *Gynecol Endocrinol* 1987;1:137.

199. Holick MF. Environmental Factors that Influence the Cutaneous Production of Vitamin D. *Am J Clin Nutr* 1995;61(3 Suppl):638S.

200. Chevalier G, et al. Was the Formation of 1,25-Dihydroxyvitamin D3 Initially a Catabolic Pathway? *Med Hypotheses* 1997;48:325.

201. DeLuca HF. New Concepts of Vitamin D Functions. *Ann N Y Acad Sci* 1992;669:59.

202. DeLuca HF, Krisinger J, Darwish H. The Vitamin D System: 1990. *Kidney Int Suppl* 1990;29:S2.

203. Dusso AS, Brown AJ. Mechanism of Vitamin D Action and its Regulation. *Am J Kidney Dis* 1998;32(Suppl):S13.

204. DeLuca HF, Zierold C. Mechanisms and Functions of Vitamin D. *Nutr Rev* 1998;56:S4.

205. Norman AW. The Vitamin D Endocrine System: Manipulation of Structure-Function Relationships to Provide Opportunities for Development of New Cancer Chemopreventive and Immunosuppressive Agents. *J Cell Biochem Suppl* 1995;22:218.

206. Henry HL, Norman AW. Vitamin D: Metabolism and Biological Actions. *Annu Rev Nutr* 1984;4:493.

207. Green A. Changing Patterns in Incidence of Non-Melanoma Skin Cancer. *Epithelial Cell Biol* 1992;1:47.

208. Lee JA. Declining Effect of Latitude on Melanoma Mortality Rates in the United States. A Preliminary Study. *Am J Epidemiol* 1997;146:413.

209. Balzi D, Carli P, Geddes M. Malignant Melanoma in Europe: Changes in Mortality Rates (1970-90) in European Community Countries. *Cancer Causes Control* 1997;8:85.

210. Podda M, et al. UV-Irradiation Depletes Antioxidants and Causes Oxidative Damage in a Model of Human Skin. *Free Radic Biol Med* 1998;24:55.

211. Shindo Y, et al. Dose-Response Effects of Acute Ultraviolet Irradiation on Antioxidants and Molecular Markers of Oxidation in Murine Epidermis and Dermis. *J Invest Dermatol* 1994;102:470.

212. Shindo Y, Witt E, Packer L. Antioxidant Defense Mechanisms in Murine Epidermis and Dermis and their Responses to Ultraviolet Light. *J Invest Dermatol* 1993;100:260.

213. Leccia MT, et al. Protective Effect of Selenium and Zinc on UV-A Damage in Human Skin Fibroblasts. *Photochem Photobiol* 1993;58:548.

214. Emonet-Piccardi N, et al. Protective Effects of Antioxidants against UVA-Induced DNA Damage in Human Skin Fibroblasts in Culture. *Free Radic Res* 1998;29:307.

215. Darr D, et al. Effectiveness of Antioxidants (Vitamin C And E) with and without Sunscreens as Topical Photoprotectants. *Acta Derm Venereol* 1996;76:264.

216. English DR, et al. Sunlight and Cancer. *Cancer Causes Control* 1997;8:271.

217. Pathak MA. Ultraviolet Radiation and the Development of Non-Melanoma and Melanoma Skin Cancer: Clinical and Experimental Evidence. *Skin Pharmacol* 1991;(4 Suppl 1):85.

218. Christophers AJ. Melanoma is Not Caused by Sunlight. *Mutat Res* 1998;422:113.

219. Garland FC, et al. Occupational Sunlight Exposure and Melanoma in the U.S. Navy. *Arch Environ Health* 1990;45:261.

224

220. Elwood JM. Melanoma and Sun Exposure: Contrasts between Intermittent and Chronic Exposure. *World J Surg* 1992;16:157.

221. Gallagher RP, et al. Socioeconomic Status, Sunlight Exposure, and Risk of Malignant Melanoma: The Western Canada Melanoma Study. *J Natl Cancer Inst* 1987;79:647.

222. Elwood JM, et al. Cutaneous Melanoma in Relation to Intermittent and Constant Sun Exposure--The Western Canada Melanoma Study. *Int J Cancer* 1985;35:427.

223. Osterlind A. Epidemiology on Malignant Melanoma in Europe. *Acta Oncol* 1992;31:903.

224. Nelemans PJ, et al. Effect of Intermittent Exposure to Sunlight on Melanoma Risk among Indoor Workers and Sun-Sensitive Individuals. *Environ Health Perspect* 1993;101:252.

225. Osterlind A, et al. The Danish Case-Control Study of Cutaneous Malignant Melanoma. II. Importance of UV-Light Exposure. *Int J Cancer* 1988;42:319.

226. Elwood JM, Jopson J. Melanoma and Sun Exposure: An Overview of Published Studies. *Int J Cancer* 1997;73:198.

227. Lee JA. The Relationship between Malignant Melanoma of Skin and Exposure to Sunlight. *Photochem Photobiol* 1989;50:493.

228. Marks R. Photoprotection and Prevention of Melanoma. *Eur J Dermatol* 1999;9:406.

229. Beral V, et al. Malignant Melanoma and Exposure to Fluorescent Lighting at Work. *Lancet* 1982;2:290.

230. Walter SD, et al. The Association of Cutaneous Malignant Melanoma and Fluorescent Light Exposure. *Am J Epidemiol* 1992;135:749.

231. Cooke KR, Skegg DC, Fraser J. Socio-Economic Status, Indoor and Outdoor Work, and Malignant Melanoma. *Int J Cancer* 1984;34:57.

232. Pion IA, et al. Occupation and the Risk of Malignant Melanoma. *Cancer* 1995;75(2 Suppl):637.

233. Elwood JM, Williamson C, Stapleton PJ. Malignant Melanoma in Relation to Moles, Pigmentation, and Exposure to Fluorescent and other Lighting Sources. *Br J Cancer* 1986;53:65.

234. Dubin N, et al. Sun Exposure and Malignant Melanoma among Susceptible Individuals. *Environ Health Perspect* 1989;81:139.

235. Chamlin SL, Williams ML. Moles and Melanoma. *Curr Opin Pediatr* 1998;10:398.

236. Weinstock MA, et al. Melanoma and the Sun: The Effect of Swimsuits and a "Healthy" Tan on the Risk of Nonfamilial Malignant Melanoma in Women. *Am J Epidemiol* 1991;134:462.

237. Matsuoka LY, Wortsman J, Hollis BW. Suntanning and Cutaneous Synthesis of Vitamin D3. *J Lab Clin Med* 1990;116:87.

238. Wilske J. Plasma Concentrations of 25-Hydroxyvitamin-D3 (Calcifediol) as an Indicator of Ultraviolet Radiation. *Arctic Med Res* 1993;52:166.

239. DeLuca HF, Ostrem V. The Relationship between the Vitamin D System and Cancer. *Adv Exp Med Biol* 1986;206:413.

240. Manolagas SC. Vitamin D and its Relevance to Cancer. *Anticancer Res* 1987;7:625.

241. Eisman JA, Barkla DH, Tutton PJ. Suppression of In Vivo Growth of Human Cancer Solid Tumor Xenografts by 1,25-Dihydroxyvitamin D3. *Cancer Res* 1987;47:21.

242. Yudoh K, Matsuno H, Kimura T. 1alpha,25-Dihydroxyvitamin D3 Inhibits In Vitro Invasiveness through the Extracellular Matrix and In Vivo Pulmonary Metastasis of B16 Mouse Melanoma. *J Lab Clin Med* 1999;133:120.

243. Danielsson C, et al. Differential Apoptotic Response of Human Melanoma Cells to 1 Alpha,25-Dihydroxyvitamin D3 and Its Analogues. *Cell Death Differ* 1998;5:946.

244. James SY, et al. EB1089, a Synthetic Analogue of Vitamin D, Induces Apoptosis in Breast Cancer Cells In Vivo and In Vitro. *Br J Pharmacol* 1998;125:953.

245. Brenner RV, et al. The Antiproliferative Effect of Vitamin D Analogs on MCF-7 Human Breast Cancer Cells. *Cancer Lett* 1995;92:77.

246. Jung SJ, et al. 1,25(OH)2-16ene-vitamin D3 is a Potent Antileukemic Agent with Low Potential to Cause Hypercalcemia. *Leuk Res* 1994;18:453.

247. Pakkala S, et al. Vitamin D3 Analogs: Effect on Leukemic Clonal Growth and Differentiation, and on Serum Calcium Levels. *Leuk Res* 1995;19:65.

248. Falkenbach A, Sedlmeyer A. Travel to Sunny Countries is Associated with Changes in Immunological Parameters. *Photodermatol Photoimmunol Photomed* 1997;13:139.

249. Kripke ML, et al. In Vivo Immune Responses of Mice during Carcinogenesis by Ultraviolet Irradiation. *J Natl Cancer Inst* 1977;59:1227.

250. Norbury KC, Kripke ML, Budmen MB. In Vitro Reactivity of Macrophages and Lymphocytes from Ultraviolet-Irradiated Mice. *J Natl Cancer Inst* 1977;59:1231.

251. Goettsch W, et al. Risk Assessment for the Harmful Effects of UVB Radiation on the Immunological Resistance to Infectious Diseases. *Environ Health Perspect* 1998;106:71.

252. Lefkowitz ES, Garland CF. Sunlight, Vitamin D, and Ovarian Cancer Mortality Rates in US Women. *Int J Epidemiol* 1994;23:1133.

253. Garland FC, et al. Geographic Variation in Breast Cancer Mortality in the United States: A Hypothesis Involving Exposure to Solar Radiation. *Prev Med* 1990;19:614.

254. Gorham ED, Garland FC, Garland CF. Sunlight and Breast Cancer Incidence in the USSR. *Int J Epidemiol* 1990;19:820.

255. Garland CF, Garland FC. Do Sunlight and Vitamin D Reduce the Likelihood of Colon Cancer? *Int J Epidemiol* 1980;9:227.

256. Schwartz GG. Multiple Sclerosis and Prostate Cancer: What do their Similar Geographies Suggest? *Neuroepidemiology* 1992;11:244.

257. Kafadar K. Geographic Trends in Prostate Cancer Mortality: An Application of Spatial Smoothers and the Need for Adjustment. *Ann Epidemiol* 1997;7:35.

258. Hanchette CL, Schwartz GG. Geographic Patterns of Prostate Cancer Mortality. Evidence for a Protective Effect of Ultraviolet Radiation. *Cancer* 1992;70:2861.

259. Tominaga S, Kuroishi T. Epidemiology of Pancreatic Cancer. *Semin Surg Oncol* 1998;15:3.

260. Kato I, et al. Latitude and Pancreatic Cancer. *Jpn J Clin Oncol* 1985;15:403.

261. Merrill RM, Brawley OW. Prostate Cancer Incidence and Mortality Rates among White and Black Men. *Epidemiology* 1997;8:126.

262. Morton RA Jr. Racial Differences in Adenocarcinoma of the Prostate in North American Men. *Urology* 1994;44:637.

263. Gold EB, Goldin SB. Epidemiology of and Risk Factors for Pancreatic Cancer. *Surg Oncol Clin N Am* 1998;7:67.

264. Levin DL, Connelly RR, Devesa SS. Demographic Characteristics of Cancer of the Pancreas: Mortality, Incidence, and Survival. *Cancer* 1981;47(Suppl):1456.

265. Walker AR, Walker BF, Segal I. Cancer Patterns in Three African Populations Compared with the United States Black Population. *Eur J Cancer Prev* 1993;2:313.

266. Lo CW, Paris PW, Holick MF. Indian and Pakistani Immigrants have the Same Capacity as Caucasians to Produce Vitamin D in Response to Ultraviolet Irradiation. *Am J Clin Nutr* 1986;44:683.

267. Clemens TL, et al. Increased Skin Pigment Reduces the Capacity of Skin to Synthesise Vitamin D3. *Lancet* 1982;1:74.

268. Matsuoka LY, et al. Racial Pigmentation and the Cutaneous Synthesis of Vitamin D. *Arch Dermatol* 1991;127:536.

268a. Kessenich CR, Rosen CJ. Vitamin D and Bone Status in Elderly Women. *Orthop Nurs* 1996;15:67.

268b. Gloth FM III, et al. Vitamin D Deficiency in Homebound Elderly Persons. *JAMA* 1995;274:1683.

268c. Holmes RP, Kummerow FA. The Relationship of Adequate and Excessive Intake of Vitamin D to Health and Disease. *J Am Coll Nutr* 1983;2:173.

269. Pettifor JM, et al. The Effect of Season and Latitude on In Vitro Vitamin D Formation by Sunlight in South Africa. *S Afr Med J* 1996;86:1270.

270. Gessner BD, et al. Nutritional Rickets among Breast-Fed Black and Alaska Native Children. *Alaska Med* 1997;39:72.

271. Specker BL, Tsang RC, Hollis BW. Effect of Race and Diet on Human-Milk Vitamin D and 25-Hydroxyvitamin D. *Am J Dis Child* 1985;139:1134.

272. Atiq M, et al. Maternal Vitamin-D Deficiency in Pakistan. *Acta Obstet Gynecol Scand* 1998;77:970.

273. Garabedian M, Ben-Mekhbi H. [Deficiency Rickets: The Current Situation in France and Algeria]. *Pediatrie* 1989;44:259. French.

274. Lubani MM, et al. Vitamin-D-Deficiency Rickets in Kuwait: The Prevalence of a Preventable Disease. *Ann Trop Paediatr* 1989;9:134.

275. Zeghoud F, et al. [Effects of Sunlight Exposure on Vitamin D Status in Pregnant Women in France]. *J Gynecol Obstet Biol Reprod (Paris)* 1991;20:685. French.

276. Specker BL. Do North American Women Need Supplemental Vitamin D during Pregnancy or Lactation? *Am J Clin Nutr* 1994;59(Suppl):484S.

277. Daaboul J, et al. Vitamin D Deficiency in Pregnant and Breast-Feeding Women and their Infants. *J Perinatol* 1997;17:10.

278. Brunvand L, et al. Vitamin D Deficiency and Fetal Growth. *Early Hum Dev* 1996 Jul 5;45:27.

279. Epstein JH. Experimental Models for Primary Melanoma. *Photodermatol Photoimmunol Photomed* 1992;9:91.

280. Garland CF, Garland FC, Gorham ED. Rising Trends in Melanoma. An Hypothesis Concerning Sunscreen Effectiveness. *Ann Epidemiol* 1993;3:103.

281. Gasparro FP, Mitchnick M, Nash JF. A Review of Sunscreen Safety and Efficacy. *Photochem Photobiol* 1998;68:243.

282. Moan J, Dahlback A, Setlow RB. Epidemiological Support for an Hypothesis for Melanoma Induction Indicating a Role for UVA Radiation. *Photochem Photobiol* 1999;70:243.

283. Schmitz S, et al. [Long-Wave Ultraviolet Radiation (UVA) and Skin Cancer]. *Hautarzt* 1994;45:517. German.

284. Setlow RB. Spectral Regions Contributing to Melanoma: A Personal View. *J Investig Dermatol Symp Proc* 1999;4:46.

285. Wolf P, Donawho CK, Kripke ML. Effect of Sunscreens on UV Radiation-Induced Enhancement of Melanoma Growth in Mice. *J Natl Cancer Inst* 1994;86:99.

286. Autier P, et al. Sunscreen Use and Duration of Sun Exposure: A Double-Blind, Randomized Trial. *J Natl Cancer Inst* 1999;91:1304.

287. Knowland J, et al. Sunlight-Induced Mutagenicity of a Common Sunscreen Ingredient. *FEBS Lett* 1993;324:309.

288. Dunford R, et al. Chemical Oxidation and DNA Damage Catalysed by Inorganic Sunscreen Ingredients. *FEBS Lett* 1997;418:87.

289. Wamer WG, Yin JJ, Wei RR. Oxidative Damage to Nucleic Acids Photosensitized by Titanium Dioxide. *Free Radic Biol Med* 1997;23:851.

290. McHugh PJ, Knowland J. Characterization of DNA Damage Inflicted by Free Radicals from a Mutagenic Sunscreen Ingredient and its Location Using an In Vitro Genetic Reversion Assay. *Photochem Photobiol* 1997;66:276.

291. Matsuoka LY, Wortsman J, Hollis BW. Use of Topical Sunscreen for the Evaluation of Regional Synthesis of Vitamin D3. *J Am Acad Dermatol* 1990;22:772.

292. Matsuoka LY, et al. Chronic Sunscreen Use Decreases Circulating Concentrations of 25-Hydroxyvitamin D. A Preliminary Study. *Arch Dermatol* 1988;124:1802.

293. Matsuoka LY, et al. Sunscreens Suppress Cutaneous Vitamin D3 Synthesis. *J Clin Endocrinol Metab* 1987;64:1165.

294. Spoont MR, Depue RA, Krauss SS. Dimensional Measurement of Seasonal Variation in Mood and Behavior. *Psychiatry Res* 1991;39:269.

295. Kasper S, et al. Epidemiological Findings of Seasonal Changes in Mood and Behavior. A Telephone Survey of Montgomery County, Maryland. *Arch Gen Psychiatry* 1989;46:823.

296. Gysin F, Gysin F, Gross F. [Winter Depression and Phototherapy. The State of the Art]. *Acta Med Port* 1997;10:887. Portugese.

297. Lee TM, Chan CC. Vulnerability by Sex to Seasonal Affective Disorder. *Percept Mot Skills* 1998;87:1120.

298. Hansen V, Lund E, Smith-Sivertsen T. Self-Reported Mental Distress under the Shifting Daylight in the High North. *Psychol Med* 1998;28:447.

299. Hegde AL, Woodson H. Prevalence of Seasonal Changes in Mood and Behavior during the Winter Months in Central Texas. *Psychiatry Res* 1996;62:265.

300. Low KG, Feissner JM. Seasonal Affective Disorder in College Students: Prevalence and Latitude. *J Am Coll Health* 1998;47:135.

301. Dilsaver SC, Jaeckle RS. The Naturally Occurring Rhythm of Blues: Winter Depression. *Ohio Med* 1990;86:58.

302. Okawa M, et al. Seasonal Variation of Mood and Behaviour in a Healthy Middle-Aged Population in Japan. *Acta Psychiatr Scand* 1996;94:211.

303. Suhail K, Cochrane R. Seasonal Changes in Affective State in Samples of Asian and White Women. *Soc Psychiatry Psychiatr Epidemiol* 1997;32:149.

304. Booker JM, Hellekson CJ. Prevalence of Seasonal Affective Disorder in Alaska. *Am J Psychiatry* 1992;149:1176.

305. Palinkas LA, Houseal M, Rosenthal NE. Subsyndromal Seasonal Affective Disorder in Antarctica. *J Nerv Ment Dis* 1996;184:530.

306. Haggag A, et al. Seasonal Mood Variation: An Epidemiological Study in Northern Norway. *Acta Psychiatr Scand* 1990;81:141.

307. Meesters Y, et al. Early Light Treatment Can Prevent an Emerging Winter Depression from Developing into a Full-Blown Depression. *J Affect Disord* 1993;29:41.

308. Lingjaerde O, et al. Treatment of Winter Depression in Norway. I. Short- and Long-Term Effects of 1500-Lux White Light for 6 Days. *Acta Psychiatr Scand* 1993 Oct;:292.

309. McIntyre IM, et al. Treatment of Seasonal Affective Disorder with Light: Preliminary Australian Experience. *Aust N Z J Psychiatry* 1989;23:369.

310. Grota LJ, et al. Phototherapy for Seasonal Major Depressive Disorder: Effectiveness of Bright Light of High or Low Intensity. *Psychiatry Res* 1989;29:29.

311. Hellekson CJ, Kline JA, Rosenthal NE. Phototherapy for Seasonal Affective Disorder in Alaska. *Am J Psychiatry* 1986;143:1035.

312. Lam RW, et al. A Controlled Study of Light Therapy in Women with Late Luteal Phase Dysphoric Disorder. *Psychiatry Res* 1999;86:185.

313. Parry BL, et al. Light Therapy of Late Luteal Phase Dysphoric Disorder: An Extended Study. *Am J Psychiatry* 1993;150:1417.

314. Lam RW, et al. A Controlled Study of Light Therapy for Bulimia Nervosa. *Am J Psychiatry* 1994;151:744.

Natural Hormonal Enhancement

315. Braun DL, et al. Bright Light Therapy Decreases Winter Binge Frequency in Women with Bulimia Nervosa: A Double-Blind, Placebo-Controlled Study. *Compr Psychiatry* 1999;40:442.

316. Yamada N, et al. Clinical and Chronobiological Effects of Light Therapy on Nonseasonal Affective Disorders. *Biol Psychiatry* 1995;37:866.

317. Rao ML, et al. Blood Serotonin, Serum Melatonin and Light Therapy in Healthy Subjects and in Patients with Nonseasonal Depression. *Acta Psychiatr Scand* 1992;86:127.

318. Kripke DF, et al. Controlled Trial of Bright Light for Nonseasonal Major Depressive Disorders. *Biol Psychiatry* 1992;31:119.

319. Mackert A, et al. Effect of Bright White Light on Non-Seasonal Depressive Disorder. *Pharmacopsychiatry* 1990;23:151.

320. Lam RW, et al. Ultraviolet Versus Non-Ultraviolet Light Therapy for Seasonal Affective Disorder. *J Clin Psychiatry* 1991;52:213.

321. Meesters Y, et al. Prophylactic Treatment of Seasonal Affective Disorder (SAD) by Using Light Visors: Bright White or Infrared Light? *Biol Psychiatry* 1999;46:239.

322. See, supra, note 317.

323. Rao ML, et al. The Influence of Phototherapy on Serotonin and Melatonin in Non-Seasonal Depression. *Pharmacopsychiatry* 1990;23:155.

324. Danilenko KV, et al. Diurnal and Seasonal Variations of Melatonin and Serotonin in Women with Seasonal Affective Disorder. *Arctic Med Res* 1994;53:137.

325. Ghadirian AM, et al. Seasonal Mood Patterns in Eating Disorders. *Gen Hosp Psychiatry* 1999;21:354.

326. Saeed SA, Bruce TJ. Seasonal Affective Disorders. *Am Fam Physician* 1998;57:1340.

327. Bylesjo EI, Boman K, Wetterberg L. Obesity Treated with Phototherapy: Four Case Studies. *Int J Eat Disord* 1996;20:443.

328. Ainsleigh HG. Beneficial Effects of Sun Exposure on Cancer Mortality. *Prev Med* 1993;22:132.

329. Gaziano JM, et al. Moderate Alcohol Intake, Increased Levels of High-Density Lipoprotein and its Subfractions, and Decreased Risk of Myocardial Infarction. *N Engl J Med* 1993;329:1829.

330. Suh I, et al. Alcohol Use and Mortality from Coronary Heart Disease: The Role of High-Density Lipoprotein Cholesterol. The Multiple Risk Factor Intervention Trial Research Group. *Ann Intern Med* 1992;116:881.

331. Hammar N, Romelsjo A, Alfredsson L. Alcohol Consumption, Drinking Pattern and Acute Myocardial Infarction. A Case Referent Study Based on the Swedish Twin Register. *J Intern Med* 1997;241:125.

332. McElduff P, Dobson AJ. How Much Alcohol and How Often? Population Based Case-Control Study of Alcohol Consumption and Risk of a Major Coronary Event. *BMJ* 1997;314:1159.

333. Rimm EB, et al. Prospective Study of Alcohol Consumption and Risk of Coronary Disease in Men. *Lancet* 1991;338:464.

334. Kitamura A, et al. Alcohol Intake and Premature Coronary Heart Disease in Urban Japanese Men. *Am J Epidemiol* 1998;147:59.

335. Jackson R, Scragg R, Beaglehole R. Alcohol Consumption and Risk of Coronary Heart Disease. *BMJ* 1991;303:211.

336. Stampfer MJ, et al. A Prospective Study of Moderate Alcohol Consumption and the Risk of Coronary Disease and Stroke in Women. *N Engl J Med* 1988;319:267.

337. Miller GJ, et al. Alcohol Consumption: Protection against Coronary Heart Disease and Risks to Health. *Int J Epidemiol* 1990;19:923.

338. Klatsky AL, Armstrong MA, Friedman GD. Red Wine, White Wine, Liquor, Beer, and Risk for Coronary Artery Disease Hospitalization. *Am J Cardiol* 1997;80:416.

339. Richardson PJ, Patel VB, Preedy VR. Alcohol and the Myocardium. *Novartis Found Symp* 1998;216:35.

340. Patel VB, et al. Protein Profiling in Cardiac Tissue in Response to the Chronic Effects of Alcohol. *Electrophoresis* 1997;18:2788.

341. Preedy VR, Richardson PJ. Alcoholic Cardiomyopathy: Clinical and Experimental Pathological Changes. *Herz* 1996;21:241.

342. Iso H, et al. Alcohol Intake and the Risk of Cardiovascular Disease in Middle-Aged Japanese Men. *Stroke* 1995;26:767.

343. Wannamethee G, Shaper AG. Alcohol and Sudden Cardiac Death. *Br Heart J* 1992;68:443.

344. Wilhelmsen L, Elmfeldt D, Wedel H. Cause of Death in Relation to Social and Alcoholic Problems among Swedish Men Aged 35-44 Years. *Acta Med Scand* 1983;213:263.

345. McKee M, Britton A. The Positive Relationship between Alcohol and Heart Disease in Eastern Europe: Potential Physiological Mechanisms. *J R Soc Med* 1998;91:402.

346. Puddey IB, et al. Influence of Pattern of Drinking on Cardiovascular Disease and Cardiovascular Risk Factors--A Review. *Addiction* 1999;94:649.

347. Kauhanen J, et al. Pattern of Alcohol Drinking and Progression of Atherosclerosis. *Arterioscler Thromb Vasc Biol* 1999;19:3001.

348. Angelico F, et al. Further Considerations on Alcohol Intake and Coronary Risk Factors in a Rome Working Population Group: HDL-Cholesterol. *Ann Nutr Metab* 1982;26:73.

349. LaPorte R, et al. The Relationship between Alcohol Consumption, Liver Enzymes and High-Density Lipoprotein Cholesterol. *Circulation* 1981;64:67.

350. Razay G, et al. Alcohol Consumption and its Relation to Cardiovascular Risk Factors in British Women. *BMJ* 1992;304:80.

351. Dai WS, et al. Alcohol Consumption and High Density Lipoprotein Cholesterol Concentration among Alcoholics. *Am J Epidemiol* 1985;122:620.

352. Linn S, et al. High-density Lipoprotein Cholesterol and Alcohol Consumption in US White and Black Adults: Data from NHANES II. *Am J Public Health* 1993;83:811.

353. Ernst N, et al. The Association of Plasma High-Density Lipoprotein Cholesterol with Dietary Intake and Alcohol Consumption. The Lipid Research Clinics Prevalence Study. *Circulation* 1980;62:41.

354. Luoma PV, et al. High-Density Lipoproteins and Hepatic Microsomal Enzyme Induction in Alcohol Consumers. *Res Commun Chem Pathol Pharmacol* 1982;37:91.

355. Barboriak JJ, Anderson AJ, Hoffmann RG. Interrelationship between Coronary Artery Occlusion, High-Density Lipoprotein Cholesterol, and Alcohol Intake. *J Lab Clin Med* 1979;94:348.

356. See, supra, note 329.

357. See, supra, note 330.

358. Renaud S, de Lorgeril M. Wine, Alcohol, Platelets, and the French Paradox for Coronary Heart Disease. *Lancet* 1992;339:1523.

359. Mennen LI, et al. Fibrinogen: A Possible Link between Alcohol Consumption and Cardiovascular Disease? DESIR Study Group. *Arterioscler Thromb Vasc Biol* 1999;19:887.

360. Hendriks HF, van der Gaag MS. Alcohol, Coagulation and Fibrinolysis. *Novartis Found Symp* 1998;216:111.

361. Pellegrini N, et al. Effects of Moderate Consumption of Red Wine on Platelet Aggregation and Haemostatic Variables in Healthy Volunteers. *Eur J Clin Nutr* 1996;50:209.

362. Nanji AA. Alcohol and Ischemic Heart Disease: Wine, Beer or Both? *Int J Cardiol* 1985;8:487.

363. Renaud SC, et al. Wine, Beer, and Mortality in Middle-Aged Men from Eastern France. *Arch Intern Med* 1999;159:1865.

364. Gronbaek M, et al. Mortality Associated with Moderate Intakes of Wine, Beer, or Spirits. *BMJ* 1995;310:1165.

365. Messner T, Petersson B. Alcohol Consumption and Ischemic Heart Disease Mortality in Sweden. *Scand J Soc Med* 1996;24:107.

366. Truelsen T, et al. Intake of Beer, Wine, and Spirits and Risk of Stroke: The Copenhagen City Heart Study. *Stroke* 1998;29:2467.

367. Gronbaek MN, et al. [Mortality Differences Associated with Moderate Consumption of Beer, Wine and Spirits]. *Ugeskr Laeger* 1996;158:2258. Danish.

368. Tjonneland A, et al. Wine Intake and Diet in a Random Sample of 48763 Danish Men and Women. *Am J Clin Nutr* 1999;69:49.

369. Frankel EN, et al. Inhibition of Oxidation of Human Low-Density Lipoprotein by Phenolic Substances in Red Wine. *Lancet* 1993;341:454.

370. Kerry NL, Abbey M. Red Wine and Fractionated Phenolic Compounds Prepared from Red Wine Inhibit Low Density Lipoprotein Oxidation In Vitro. *Atherosclerosis* 1997;135:93.

371. Abu-Amsha R, et al. Phenolic Content of Various Beverages Determines the Extent of Inhibition of Human Serum and Low-Density Lipoprotein Oxidation In Vitro: Identification and Mechanism of Action of Some Cinnamic Acid Derivatives from Red Wine. *Clin Sci (Colch)* 1996;91:449.

372. Rifici VA, et al. Red Wine Inhibits the Cell-Mediated Oxidation of LDL and HDL. *J Am Coll Nutr* 1999;18:137.

373. Renis M, et al. Nuclear DNA Strand Breaks during Ethanol-Induced Oxidative Stress in Rat Brain. *FEBS Lett* 1996;390:153.

374. Nordmann R. Oxidative Stress from Alcohol in the Brain. *Alcohol Alcohol* 1987;(Suppl)1:75.

375. Lecomte E, et al. Effect of Alcohol Consumption on Blood Antioxidant Nutrients and Oxidative Stress Indicators. *Am J Clin Nutr* 1994;60:255.

376. Bondy SC. Ethanol Toxicity and Oxidative Stress. *Toxicol Lett* 1992;63:231.

377. Croft KD, et al. Oxidative Susceptibility of Low-Density Lipoproteins--Influence of Regular Alcohol Use. *Alcohol Clin Exp Res* 1996;20:980.

378. Aviram M, Lavy A, Fuhrman B. [Plasma Lipid Peroxidation: Inhibited by Drinking Red Wine but Stimulated by White Wine]. *Harefuah* 1994;127:517. Hebrew.

379. Id.

380. Nigdikar SV, et al. Consumption of Red Wine Polyphenols Reduces the Susceptibility of Low-Density Lipoproteins to Oxidation In Vivo. *Am J Clin Nutr* 1998;68:258.

381. Thomsen JL. Atherosclerosis in Alcoholics. *Forensic Sci Int* 1995;75:121.

382. Kiechl S, et al. Insulin Sensitivity and Regular Alcohol Consumption: Large, Prospective, Cross Sectional Population Study. *BMJ* 1996;313:1040.

383. Facchini F, Chen YD, Reaven GM. Light-to-Moderate Alcohol Intake is Associated with Enhanced Insulin Sensitivity. *Diabetes Care* 1994;17:115.

384. Mayer EJ, et al. Alcohol Consumption and Insulin Concentrations. Role of Insulin in Associations of Alcohol Intake with High-Density Lipoprotein Cholesterol and Triglycerides. *Circulation* 1993;88:2190.

385. Lazarus R, Sparrow D, Weiss ST. Alcohol Intake and Insulin Levels. The Normative Aging Study. *Am J Epidemiol* 1997;145:909.

386. See, supra, note 350.

387. Boden G, et al. Effects of Ethanol on Carbohydrate Metabolism in the Elderly. *Diabetes* 1993;42:28.

388. Yki-Jarvinen H, Nikkila EA. Ethanol Decreases Glucose Utilization in Healthy Man. *J Clin Endocrinol Metab* 1985;61:941.

389. Singh SP, Patel DG. Effects of Ethanol on Carbohydrate Metabolism: I. Influence on Oral Glucose Tolerance Test. *Metabolism* 1976;25:239.

390. Shah JH. Alcohol Decreases Insulin Sensitivity in Healthy Subjects. *Alcohol Alcohol* 1988;23:103.

391. Avogaro A, et al. Alcohol Impairs Insulin Sensitivity in Normal Subjects. *Diabetes Res* 1987;5:23.

392. Shelmet JJ, et al. Ethanol Causes Acute Inhibition of Carbohydrate, Fat, and Protein Oxidation and Insulin Resistance. *J Clin Invest* 1988;81:1137.

393. Ylikahri RH, et al. Acute Effects of Alcohol on Anterior Pituitary Secretion of the Tropic Hormones. *J Clin Endocrinol Metab* 1978;46:715.

394. Valimaki MJ, et al. Sex Hormones and Adrenocortical Steroids in Men Acutely Intoxicated with Ethanol. *Alcohol* 1984;1:89.

395. Ylikahri RH, Huttunen MO, Harkonen M. Hormonal Changes during Alcohol Intoxication and Withdrawal. *Pharmacol Biochem Behav* 1980;13 (Suppl):131.

396. Valimaki M, et al. The Pulsatile Secretion of Gonadotropins and Growth Hormone, and the Biological Activity of Luteinizing Hormone in Men Acutely Intoxicated with Ethanol. *Alcohol Clin Exp Res* 1990;14:928.

397. Prinz PN, et al. Effect of Alcohol on Sleep and Nighttime Plasma Growth Hormone and Cortisol Concentrations. *J Clin Endocrinol Metab* 1980;51:759.

398. Wall TL, et al. Cortisol Responses Following Placebo and Alcohol in Asians with Different ALDH2 Genotypes. *J Stud Alcohol* 1994;55:207.

399. Preedy VR, et al. Oxidants, Antioxidants and Alcohol: Implications for Skeletal and Cardiac Muscle. *Front Biosci* 1999;4:58.

400. Martin F, et al. Alcoholic Skeletal Myopathy, a Clinical and Pathological Study. *Q J Med* 1985;55:233.

401. Preedy VR, Salisbury JR, Peters TJ. Alcoholic Muscle Disease: Features and Mechanisms. *J Pathol* 1994;173:309.

402. Preedy VR, Peters TJ. Alcohol and Skeletal Muscle Disease. *Alcohol Alcohol* 1990;25:177.

403. Martin F, Peters TJ. Alcoholic Muscle Disease. *Alcohol Alcohol* 1985;20:125.

404. Duane P, Peters TJ. Glucocorticosteroid Status in Chronic Alcoholics With and Without Skeletal Muscle Myopathy. *Clin Sci* 1987;73:601.

405. Reilly ME, et al. Studies on the Time-Course of Ethanol's Acute Effects on Skeletal Muscle Protein Synthesis: Comparison with Acute Changes in Proteolytic Activity. *Alcohol Clin Exp Res* 1997;21:792.

406. Tiernan JM, Ward LC. Acute Effects of Ethanol on Protein Synthesis in the Rat. *Alcohol Alcohol* 1986;21:171.

407. Preedy VR, Peters TJ. The Effect of Chronic Ethanol Ingestion on Protein Metabolism in Type-I- and Type-II-Fibre-Rich Skeletal Muscles of the Rat. *Biochem J* 1988;254:631.

408. Berneis K, Ninnis R, Keller U. Ethanol Exerts Acute Protein-Sparing Effects during Postabsorptive but Not during Anabolic Conditions in Man. *Metabolism* 1997;46:750.

409. See, supra, note 396.

410. See, supra, note 397.

411. Ekman AC, et al. Ethanol Decreases Nocturnal Plasma Levels of Thyrotropin and Growth Hormone but Not those of Thyroid Hormones or Prolactin in Man. *J Clin Endocrinol Metab* 1996;81:2627.

412. See, supra, note 393.

230

413. Leppaluoto J, et al. Secretion of Anterior Pituitary Hormones in Man: Effects of Ethyl Alcohol. *Acta Physiol Scand* 1975;95:400.

414. See, supra, note 394.

415. Gordon GG, Southren AL, Lieber CS. The Effects of Alcoholic Liver Disease and Alcohol Ingestion on Sex Hormone Levels. *Alcohol Clin Exp Res* 1978;2:259.

416. Mendelson JH, Mello NK, Ellingboe J. Effects of Acute Alcohol Intake on Pituitary-Gonadal Hormones in Normal Human Males. *J Pharmacol Exp Ther* 1977;202:676.

417. Mello NK, et al. Alcohol Effects on Luteinizing Hormone and Testosterone in Male Macaque Monkeys. *J Pharmacol Exp Ther* 1985;233:588.

418. Badr FM, et al. Suppression of Testosterone Production by Ethyl Alcohol. Possible Mode of Action. *Steroids* 1977;30:647.

419. Cicero TJ, Bernstein D, Badger TM. Effects of Acute Alcohol Administration on Reproductive Endocrinology in the Male Rat. *Alcohol Clin Exp Res* 1978;2:249.

420. Gordon GG, et al. Effect of Alcohol (Ethanol) Administration on Sex-Hormone Metabolism in Normal Men. *N Engl J Med* 1976;295:793.

421. Ginsburg ES, et al. The Effect of Acute Ethanol Ingestion on Estrogen Levels in Postmenopausal Women Using Transdermal Estradiol. *J Soc Gynecol Investig* 1995;2:26.

422. Mendelson JH, et al. Acute Alcohol Effects on Plasma Estradiol Levels in Women. *Psychopharmacology (Berl)* 1988;94:464.

423. Sarkola T, et al. Acute Effect of Alcohol on Androgens in Premenopausal Women. *Alcohol Alcohol* 2000;35:84.

424. Ginsburg ES, et al. Effects of Alcohol Ingestion on Estrogens in Postmenopausal Women. *JAMA* 1996;276:1747.

425. Ellingboe J. Acute Effects of Ethanol on Sex Hormones in Non-Alcoholic Men and Women. *Alcohol Alcohol* 1987;(Suppl)1:109.

426. Muti P, et al. Alcohol Consumption and Total Estradiol in Premenopausal Women. *Cancer Epidemiol Biomarkers Prev* 1998;7:189.

427. Reichman ME, et al. Effects of Alcohol Consumption on Plasma and Urinary Hormone Concentrations in Premenopausal Women. *J Natl Cancer Inst* 1993;85:722.

428. Gavaler JS, Van Thiel DH. The Association between Moderate Alcoholic Beverage Consumption and Serum Estradiol and Testosterone Levels in Normal Postmenopausal Women: Relationship to the Literature. *Alcohol Clin Exp Res* 1992;16:87.

429. Martin CA, et al. Alcohol Use in Adolescent Females: Correlates with Estradiol and Testosterone. *Am J Addict* 1999;8:9.

430. Gavaler JS, et al. An International Study of the Relationship Between Alcohol Consumption and Postmenopausal Estradiol Levels. *Alcohol Alcohol Suppl* 1991;1:327.

431. Crowe LC, George WH. Alcohol and Human Sexuality: Review and Integration. *Psychol Bull* 1989;105:374.

432. Wilson GT, Niaura R. Alcohol and the Disinhibition of Sexual Responsiveness. *J Stud Alcohol* 1984;45:219.

433. Rubin HB, Henson DE. Effects of Alcohol on Male Sexual Responding. *Psychopharmacologia* 1976;47:123.

434. Lindman RE, Koskelainen BM, Eriksson CJ. Drinking, Menstrual Cycle, and Female Sexuality: A Diary Study. *Alcohol Clin Exp Res* 1999;23:169.

435. Lester R, Van Thiel DH. Gonadal Function in Chronic Alcoholic Men. *Adv Exp Med Biol* 1977;85A:399.

436. Van Thiel DH, Lester R. Alcoholism: Its Effect on Hypothalamic Pituitary Gonadal Function. *Gastroenterology* 1976;71:318.

437. Cobb CF, et al. Is Ethanol a Testicular Toxin? *Clin Toxicol* 1981;18:149.

438. Van Thiel DH, et al. Alcohol-Induced Testicular Atrophy. An Experimental Model for Hypogonadism Occurring in Chronic Alcoholic Men. *Gastroenterology* 1975;69:326.

439. Andersson SH, Cronholm T, Sjovall J. Effects of Ethanol on the Levels of Unconjugated and Conjugated Androgens and Estrogens in Plasma of Men. *J Steroid Biochem* 1986;24:1193.

440. Andersson SH, Cronholm T, Sjovall J. Effects of Ethanol on Conjugated Gonadal Hormones in Plasma of Men. *Alcohol Alcohol* 1987;(Suppl)1:529.

441. Lindholm J, et al. Pituitary-Testicular Function in Patients with Chronic Alcoholism. *Eur J Clin Invest* 1978;8:269.

442. Valimaki M, et al. Liver Damage and Sex Hormones in Chronic Male Alcoholics. *Clin Endocrinol (Oxf)* 1982;17:469.

443. Van Thiel DH, et al. Plasma Estrone, Prolactin, Neurophysin, and Sex Steroid-Binding Globulin in Chronic Alcoholic Men. *Metabolism* 1975;24:1015.

444. Bahnsen M, et al. Pituitary-Testicular Function in Patients with Alcoholic Cirrhosis of the Liver. *Eur J Clin Invest* 1981;11:473.

445. Kolster J, et al. [Pituitary-Gonadal Hormonal Evaluation in Male Patients with Alcoholic Liver Cirrhosis]. *GEN* 1990;44:203. Spanish.

446. Gluud C. Testosterone and Alcoholic Cirrhosis. Epidemiologic, Pathophysiologic and Therapeutic Studies in Men. *Dan Med Bull* 1988;35:564.

447. Madersbacher S, et al. The Impact of Liver Transplantation on Endocrine Status in Men. *Clin Endocrinol (Oxf)* 1996;44:461.

448. Gordon GG, et al. Conversion of Androgens to Estrogens in Cirrhosis of the Liver. *J Clin Endocrinol Metab* 1975;40:1018.

449. See, supra, note 447.

450. Van Thiel DH, et al. Effect of Liver Transplantation on the Hypothalamic-Pituitary-Gonadal Axis of Chronic Alcoholic Men with Advanced Liver Disease. *Alcohol Clin Exp Res* 1990;14:478.

451. Guechot J, et al. Effect of Liver Transplantation on Sex-Hormone Disorders in Male Patients with Alcohol-Induced or Post-Viral Hepatitis Advanced Liver Disease. *J Hepatol* 1994;20:426.

452. Mello NK, et al. Alcohol Self-Administration Disrupts Reproductive Function in Female Macaque Monkeys. *Science* 1983;221:677.

453. Mello NK, Mendelson JH, Teoh SK. Neuroendocrine Consequences of Alcohol Abuse in Women. *Ann N Y Acad Sci* 1989;562:211.

454. Mendelson JH, Mello NK. Chronic Alcohol Effects on Anterior Pituitary and Ovarian Hormones in Healthy Women. *J Pharmacol Exp Ther* 1988;245:407.

455. Gavaler JS, et al. Alcohol and Estrogen Levels in Postmenopausal Women: The Spectrum of Effect. *Alcohol Clin Exp Res* 1993;17:786.

456. Becker U. The Influence of Ethanol and Liver Disease on Sex Hormones and Hepatic Oestrogen Receptors in Women. *Dan Med Bull* 1993;40:447.

457. Gavaler JS, Van Thiel DH. Hormonal Status of Postmenopausal Women with Alcohol-Induced Cirrhosis: Further Findings and a Review of the Literature. *Hepatology* 1992;16:312.

458. Ferraroni M, et al. Alcohol Consumption and Risk of Breast Cancer: A Multicentre Italian Case-Control Study. *Eur J Cancer* 1998;34:1403.

459. Ferraroni M, et al. Alcohol Consumption and Risk of Breast Cancer: A Multicentre Italian Case-Control Study. *Eur J Cancer* 1998;34:1403.

460. Longnecker MP, et al. Risk of Breast Cancer in Relation to Lifetime Alcohol Consumption. *J Natl Cancer Inst* 1995;87:923.

461. Hiatt RA, Klatsky A, Armstrong MA. Alcohol and Breast Cancer. *Prev Med* 1988;17:683.

462. Smith-Warner SA, et al. Alcohol and Breast Cancer in Women: A Pooled Analysis of Cohort Studies. *JAMA* 1998;279:535.

463. Toniolo P, et al. Breast Cancer and Alcohol Consumption: A Case-Control Study in Northern Italy. *Cancer Res* 1989;49:5203.

464. See, supra, note 392.

465. Suter PM, Schutz Y, Jequier E. The Effect of Ethanol on Fat Storage in Healthy Subjects. *N Engl J Med* 1992;326:983.

466. Sonko BJ, et al. Effect of Alcohol on Postmeal Fat Storage. *Am J Clin Nutr* 1994;59:619.

467. Murgatroyd PR, et al. Alcohol and the Regulation of Energy Balance: Overnight Effects on Diet-Induced Thermogenesis and Fuel Storage. *Br J Nutr* 1996;75:33.

468. Siler SQ, Neese RA, Hellerstein MK. De Novo Lipogenesis, Lipid Kinetics, and Whole-Body Lipid Balances in Humans after Acute Alcohol Consumption. *Am J Clin Nutr* 1999;70:928.

469. Heikkonen E, et al. Effect of Alcohol on Exercise-Induced Changes in Serum Glucose and Serum Free Fatty Acids. *Alcohol Clin Exp Res* 1998;22:437.

470. Contaldo F, et al. Short-Term Effects of Moderate Alcohol Consumption on Lipid Metabolism and Energy Balance in Normal Men. *Metabolism* 1989;38:166.

471. Ronnemaa T, et al. Smoking is Independently Associated with High Plasma Insulin Levels in Nondiabetic Men. *Diabetes Care* 1996;19:1229.

472. Eliasson B, et al. Smoking Cessation Improves Insulin Sensitivity in Healthy Middle-Aged Men. *Eur J Clin Invest* 1997;27:450.

473. Attvall S, et al. Smoking Induces Insulin Resistance--A Potential Link with the Insulin Resistance Syndrome. *J Intern Med* 1993;233:327.

474. Jeremy JY, et al. Cigarette Smoking and Erectile Dysfunction. *J R Soc Health* 1998;118:151.

475. Mannino DM, et al. Cigarette Smoking: an Independent Risk Factor for Impotence? *Am J Epidemiol* 1994;140:1003.

476. Condra M, et al. Prevalence and Significance of Tobacco Smoking in Impotence. *Urology* 1986;27:495.

232

477. Wareham NJ, et al. Cigarette Smoking is Not Associated with Hyperinsulinemia: Evidence Against a Causal Relationship between Smoking and Insulin Resistance. *Metabolism* 1996;45:1551.

478. Magoha GA. Effect of Ageing on Androgen Levels in Elderly Males. *East Afr Med J* 1997;74:642.

479. Mayhan WG. Acute Infusion of Nicotine Potentiates Norepinephrine-Induced Vasoconstriction in the Hamster Cheek Pouch. *J Lab Clin Med* 1999;133:48.

480. Gilbert DG, et al. The Effects of Cigarette Smoking on Human Sexual Potency. *Addict Behav* 1986;11:431.

481. Adams MR, et al. Erectile Failure in Cynomolgus Monkeys with Atherosclerosis of the Arteries Supplying the Penis. *J Urol* 1984;131:571.

482. Rosen RC, et al. Cardiovascular Disease and Sleep-Related Erections. *J Psychosom Res* 1997;42:517.

483. Rabb MH, et al. Effects of Sexual Stimulation, With and Without Ejaculation, on Serum Concentrations of LH, FSH, Testosterone, Cortisol and Prolactin in Stallions. *J Anim Sci* 1989;67:2724.

484. Wildt DE, et al. Adrenal-Testicular-Pituitary Relationships in the Cheetah Subjected to Anesthesia/Electroejaculation. *Biol Reprod* 1984;30:665.

485. Younglai EV, Moor BC, Dimond P. Effects of Sexual Activity on Luteinizing Hormone and Testosterone Levels in the Adult Male Rabbit. *J Endocrinol* 1976;69:183.

486. Phoenix CH, Dixson AF, Resko JA. Effects of Ejaculation on Levels of Testosterone, Cortisol, and Luteinizing Hormone in Peripheral Plasma of Rhesus Monkeys. *J Comp Physiol Psychol* 1977;91:120.

487. Hilliard J, et al. Effect of Coitus on Serum Levels of Testosterone and LH in Male and Female Rabbits. *Proc Soc Exp Biol Med* 1975;149:1010.

488. Berger M, et al. Sexual Stimulation Does Not Affect Plasma LH Nor Testosterone Levels in New-Zealand Male Rabbits. *Arch Int Physiol Biochim* 1983;91:59.

489. Heidenreich A, et al. The Influence of Ejaculation on Serum Levels of Prostate Specific Antigen. *J Urol* 1997;157;209.

490. Doeker B, et al. [Psychosocially Stunted Growth Masked as Growth Hormone Deficiency]. *Klin Padiatr* 1999;211:394. German.

491. Stanhope R, Wilks Z, Hamill G. Failure to Grow: Lack of Food or Lack of Love? *Prof Care Mother Child* 1994;4:234.

Chapter 21

Hormonally Intelligent Exercise

The best time to begin exercising is sometime between yesterday and tomorrow.
Rob Faigin

Why is it that those people who never have time for exercise always have time to eat?
Unknown

It's better to make time for exercise in your schedule now than to be forced out of your schedule by illness later.
Rob Faigin

Too many people confine their exercise to jumping to conclusions, running up bills, stretching the truth, bending over backwards, sidestepping responsibility, pushing their luck, and ducking questions.
Unknown

The problem with the average self-appointed workout expert is not that he's ignorant, but that he knows so much that isn't true.
Rob Faigin

A vigorous five-mile walk will do more good for an unhappy but otherwise healthy adult than all the medicine and psychology in the world.
Paul Dudley White, M.D.

Popular Exercise Myths

Myth: More is better.
Truth: Better is better.

Myth: The ideal workout lasts more than one hour.
Truth: The ideal workout lasts less than one hour.

Myth: Aerobic exercise is the best form of exercise for burning fat.
Truth: Hormonally correct resistance exercise is the best form of exercise for burning fat.

Myth: It is okay to lift weights every day as long as you allow ample time between training individual bodyparts.
Truth: It is not okay to lift weights every day, regardless of which bodyparts you train.

Myth: The best way to improve muscle definition and burn fat when weight training is to do very high repetitions with very light weight.
Truth: The worst way to improve muscle definition and burn fat when weight training is to do very high repetitions with very light weight.

Myth: To maximize fat loss, aerobic exercise should performed slower and longer.
Truth: To maximize fat loss, aerobic exercise should be performed faster and shorter.

Myth: The key to success from exercise is hard work - the harder you work-out, the better the results.
Truth: No brain, no gain - overtrain, no gain.

Myth: Stretching is a great way to warm-up, and it reduces the likelihood of injury.
Truth: Stretching is a terrible way to warm-up, and it increases the likelihood of injury (never stretch a cold muscle).

Myth: Lifting weights will generally make women bigger.
Truth: Lifting weights will generally make women smaller.

How do you know if you are too old to start exercising?

Perform this test, devised by George Burns.

One, put your hands up over your head. Two, put your hands in front of your chest and push outward as if you were doing a pushup. Are your hands touching anything? No? Then you're not in your coffin, and you're still able to work-out.

Why all the fuss about exercise. . . ?

Hans - How many calories do I burn as a result of jogging three miles?

Frans - It varies with your body weight and intensity level, but probably not more than 300.

Hans - WHAT?! Three miles of hell for a lousy 300 calories. That's about as many calories as I get from a bagel with cream cheese. Why all the fuss about exercise if that's all it's good for? Why can't I just skip the bagel and cream cheese? There's got to be more to this story.

You're right there is. . .

A New Dimension in Exercise

The calories burned while exercising are relatively few in quantity and small in significance. The major benefits of exercise are metabolic and hormonal, and they accrue after the exercise session has ended. For this reason, it is remarkable that so much emphasis is placed on "burning calories." If you surf the TV channels at night you no doubt see good-looking, charismatic actors and actresses promoting the latest newfangled home-workout gismo claiming that it burns more calories than its competitor gismo. They just don't get it (or perhaps they *do* get it but they are hoping *you* don't get it so they can get your money). This quantitative conception of exercise, focusing exclusively on the amount of calories burned while exercising, fails to acknowledge a supremely important fact: **exercise alters your metabolism and profoundly influences your internal hormonal environment**.

Exercise has the ability to unleash powerful hormonal forces, either powerfully beneficial or powerfully detrimental. Exercise can increase insulin sensitivity; or it can decrease insulin sensitivity (by raising cortisol levels). Exercise is potentially the most powerful natural growth hormone stimulator known to science, and, therefore, an unmatched anti-aging force, fat burner, and immune booster; or it can suppress growth hormone levels. Exercise can raise testosterone levels in men, opening the door to all the physiological and psychological qualities of youth; or it can suppress testosterone so low that mating and building muscle are near-impossibilities. Exercise can suppress cortisol; or it can cause a catabolic jailbreak, loosing this hostile hormone to assault your immune system, eat-away at precious muscle tissue, and create generalized havoc within your body.

235

The reason why most people achieve sub-optimal results from exercise is that their workouts are hormonally incorrect. In terms of results, exercising in a hormonally advantageous manner, as opposed to "flying blind" which is what people are doing who do not understand the impact of exercise on hormones and metabolism, can produce three times the results in half the time. What are the factors that influence fat burning and muscle building hormones? Intensity, volume, duration, frequency, load, and exercise selection. *Coordinating these six variables for optimal hormonal response is the key to achieving great results from exercise.*

First, I will explain how energy is generated during exercise. This brief discussion of "bioenergetic pathways" is helpful to understanding how your body works (and you will see later how bioenergetic pathways relate to hormones). But it is also a bit technical, so if you wish to skip it that's okay.

Bioenergetic Pathways

There are two basic families of exercise: aerobic and anaerobic. Each of these two types of exercise entails the use of different bioenergetic pathways to produce energy. To simplify, aerobic exercise primarily taxes the cardiovascular system and utilizes the "with oxygen" pathway. Most of your daily energy needs, including your energy needs right now while reading this book, are fulfilled through the aerobic pathway. The aerobic pathway is the slowest, and thus it is not suited to explosive, high-intensity exercise. This pathway can, however, produce energy indefinitely because 1) it taps into the richest energy source available to the human body, fat, and 2) it does not generate waste byproducts, such as lactic acid, which at high concentrations cause momentary muscle failure.

The other family of exercise, anaerobic, primarily taxes the musculoskeletal system and utilizes the "without oxygen" bioenergetic pathways: ATP/CP and glycolysis. At first blush, it may seem peculiar that muscular work can proceed in the absence of oxygen. But recall from Chapter 18 that ATP is the fundamental energy unit for all living things. The human body has a limited supply of ATP (conveniently located along with glycogen and creatine phosphate in the muscles) on hand for immediate energy needs.[1] You have only enough immediately available stored ATP for one momentary, maximal burst of muscular output.[2] After that, a compound called creatine phosphate (CP) swings into action "donating" phosphate molecules to convert spent adenosine diphosphate (ADP) back into adenosine triphosphate (ATP), thereby regenerating your ATP supply. From the moment readily available ATP becomes depleted, available energy per second declines and so does maximal muscle contraction force, as other fuel sources must be converted to ATP.[3]

In practical terms, if you are straining at maximal effort to lift a weight, and it has not gone up within 4 seconds, it's not going up. During the brief period of time in which high-energy phosphates (ATP/CP) are utilized exclusively, neither protein, nor fat, nor carbohydrate, nor even oxygen is required. Within seconds, the window of wholly anaerobic activity closes, at which point, if maximal effort persists, a different bioenergetic pathway is engaged.

236

After about 10 seconds of maximal muscular effort, both ATP and CP become depleted, and glycogen becomes the dominant fuel source; this is the *glycolytic* bioenergetic pathway. At this point, with glycogen being used to "phosphorylate" ADP into ATP, muscular power output drops-off further because of the slower rate of energy transfer via glycolysis. When glycolysis is the chief pathway utilized, maximal *effort* produces 45%-70% maximal *output*.[4] This is why in track and field, the 100-meter sprint lasts 10-12 seconds - after that, it is no longer a sprint. Technically, since maximal muscle contraction cannot be maintained beyond 4 or 5 seconds, even the 100-meter sprint is not a maximal output competition (in contrast to powerlifting, the javelin, the shot-put, and the 40-yard dash). Accordingly, the victor in a 100-meter sprint, who typically prevails by a fraction-of-a-second, is often the person who slows down the least from the midway point to the finish line.

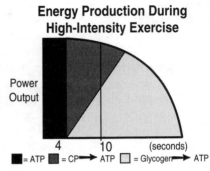

Energy Production During High-Intensity Exercise

Power Output

4   10   (seconds)

■ = ATP   ■ = CP ➡ ATP   □ = Glycogen ➡ ATP

One byproduct of glycolysis is lactic acid, which is responsible for the familiar "burn" that accompanies high-intensity exercise and which is a cause of the momentary muscle failure that occurs with this type of exercise.[5,6,7] The accumulation of lactic acid indicates that you are incurring an "oxygen debt."[8] Oxygen debt results from the fact that glycolysis allows for energy formation even though oxygen supply is inadequate relative to the demands of the activity. Heavy breathing following a short burst of intense activity signifies paying off the "oxygen debt" accrued during the anaerobic period.

If you weight train, you know that you can lift more weight if you rest longer between sets. This is because lactic acid is removed and high-energy phosphates are regenerated during these brief mini-recovery periods, commensurately with oxygen uptake.[9,10] Low-intensity exercise, by contrast, uses the "pay-as-you-go" aerobic pathway, in which no oxygen debt is incurred.* Thus, with low-intensity exercise, lactic acid does not accumulate, respiratory rate remains stable, and abrupt muscle failure does not occur.**

---

* Technically, some degree of oxygen debt is always incurred as a result of exercise, even low-intensity exercise, because during the initial minutes oxygen uptake increases sharply but lags behind energy expenditure. After the first few minutes of exercise, the oxygen uptake curve flattens-out, and, assuming you are working within your aerobic capacity, a "steady state" is achieved in which energy requirements and ATP production via aerobic metabolism are equivalent. In steady state metabolic conditions, lactic acid does not accumulate because it is cleared at the same rate it is produced. Accordingly, steady state exercise can continue indefinitely, until fluid loss, electrolyte depletion, or flagging willpower intervenes. One of the training-induced metabolic advantages enjoyed by endurance athletes is that a steady state is attained sooner and with a correspondingly lesser oxygen debt than in untrained individuals.

** In case you are wondering how our earlier discussion of "metabolic pathways" in connection with diet, and "bioenergetic pathways" relate to each other, it's simple. As noted above, fat can be burned only in the presence of oxygen (i.e., the aerobic bioenergetic pathway, utilized for approximately 95% of daily energy needs). Glucose (sugar) also can be burned in the presence oxygen (although, as I explained above, for brief periods sugar can be burned in the absence of oxygen, as well). The proportion of sugar/fat burned to fulfill roughly 95% of your daily energy needs depends on which metabolic pathway is dominant, the sugar-burning pathway or the fat-burning pathway. And, of course, whether you are a sugar-burner or a fat-burner depends on hormones.

Trained athletes incur less oxygen debt at a given intensity level and have a higher "blood lactate threshold" due to enhanced lactate clearance.[11,12] The difference in lactate threshold between highly trained and untrained individuals is vast; and along with improvements in neuromuscular efficiency, lactate threshold accounts for much of what is commonly termed "strength" and "endurance" (see Appendix B). Heightened lactate threshold is one of the many stress-specific adaptations that occur in response to exercise. Weight training is a classic example of an activity that draws heavily on the ATP/CP and glycolytic pathways and which, thereby, promotes greater efficiency of these pathways. There are hormonal implications, as well, to activating each of these pathways, which we will address shortly.

The Pre-Workout Meal: Priming the Hormonal Environment

Few people fully appreciate the importance of the pre-workout meal. Among those who do, even fewer possess an accurate understanding of its optimal composition. The fact of the matter is that **what you eat or drink prior to beginning your workout strongly influences how much fat you burn during your workout**. Based on what you learned in Chapter 10, about the functions of insulin and glucagon, you are probably a bit perplexed by a contradiction between the facts presented in that chapter and the conventional wisdom on this subject. Specifically, recall that insulin is lipogenic, which means fat-storing, and anti-lipolytic, which means it shifts metabolism away from fat burning toward sugar burning.[13,14,15,16] In view of these fundamental and indisputable facts that can be found in any biochemistry textbook, why are all the "experts" urging us to consume carbohydrate, which stimulates insulin, before exercising? The answer to that question in a moment.

The anti-lipolytic effect of insulin is compounded by the growth-hormone-blocking effect of high blood sugar, which we discussed in Chapter 20 and will return to in a moment. Furthermore, in Chapter 18 I explained how sugar derived from ingested carbohydrate influences the enzymes that regulate sugar-/fat-burning. As you can see, a high-carbohydrate pre-workout meal operates through various physiological mechanisms to shift metabolism away from fat burning toward sugar burning. The practical effect is clear and has been repeatedly demonstrated by clinical studies: *consuming carbohydrate before or during a workout reduces the amount of fat burned during the workout.*[17,18,19,20,21]

More specifically, when carbohydrate is consumed before or during exercise, the magnitude of the inhibitory effect on fat burning directly corresponds with the extent to which blood sugar and insulin levels are raised.[22,23,24] And what determines the blood sugar/insulin response to carbohydrate ingestion? Three factors: insulin sensitivity, total amount of carbohydrate consumed, and the glycemic index of the carbs consumed (Glycemic index is a measure of the blood-sugar-raising potential of a particular type of carbohydrate.)

The NHE Eating Plan eliminates this problem. Carbohydrate intake is limited at all meals except for the carb-load, which, as the last meal(s) of the day, should never be a

238

pre-workout meal. By eschewing pre-workout carbohydrate in favor of protein/fat, you enable greater use of fat for fuel during exercise.

The Glycemic Index Should Not be Accidentally Overlooked, Rather it Should be Deliberately Disregarded

I am critical of the widely endorsed and increasingly popular glycemic index, because it is misleading and obscures more significant considerations. To illustrate, carrots have a higher glycemic rating than do cookies; however, because the glycemic index is calculated for a given quantity of carbohydrate, it fails to account for the fact that cookies are far more carbohydrate-dense than carrots. In practical terms, because of the vast difference in carbohydrate-density between these two foods, you would have to eat a far greater quantity of carrots to produce a blood sugar response equivalent to that produced by a far lesser quantity of cookies. From a broader perspective, the glycemic index, as it is promoted by many authors, justifies a high-carbohydrate diet by implying that the type of carbohydrate ingested is more important than the amount; this is false. Moreover, to the extent that a useful basis of distinction among different kinds of carbohydrate exists, sugary carbs vs. starchy carbs, not glycemic rating, is it (see Chapter 15). And because glycemic ratings do not always correspond with the sugary/starchy distinction, following the glycemic index is not merely an unnecessary inconvenience but may actually prove counterproductive to fat loss.

For these reasons, the glycemic index should be diligently ignored by adherents of the NHE Eating Plan, despite the enthusiasm this flawed concept is garnering among an American public ever susceptible to a "one-glove-fits-all" approach to diet. Such one-dimensional dietary strategies sell books, but they provide ineffective assistance to readers of such books striving to reduce bodyfat. Instead of the glycemic index, focus on daily and per-meal carb limits during the downcycle and on the starchy-carb/sugary-carb distinction during the upcycle. These considerations are far more important than the glycemic index.

Another benefit of consuming protein, rather than carbohydrate, pre-workout is that it can help preserve muscle protein during exercise.[25] An underappreciated fact is that amino acids supply a small percentage of the energy used during exercise (especially prolonged exercise).[26,27,28] Although the *percentage* is small, the absolute amount of muscle broken down is significant, especially for individuals who are attempting not merely to maintain muscle but to build muscle. *By consuming a protein-based pre-workout meal, you supply amino acids that might otherwise be extracted from working muscles, thereby offsetting the catabolic effects of exercise.* Protein shakes are advantageous in this regard, because they are more easily digested than food and thus can be consumed immediately prior to training.

Recall the growth-hormone-blocking effect of high blood sugar from Chapter 20, where it was discussed in connection with sleep-related growth hormone release. This growth-hormone-blocking effect has been observed by Dr. Douglas Crist, who reported that ingestion of only three ounces of fruit juice immediately prior to a growth-hormone-inducing exercise session negated growth hormone secretion in a person who, weeks earlier, had registered a significant growth hormone elevation in response to an identical exercise session.[29] Dr. Crist's finding is supported by a large body of scientific literature solidly establishing that elevated blood sugar inhibits growth hormone release and showing, specifically, that a carbohydrate-rich pre-workout meal squelches exercise-

239

induced growth hormone secretion.[30,31,32,33,34] Keep this in mind next time you see someone at the gym sipping one of those "performance drinks" between sets - a mad scientist could not concoct a better potion for stifling growth hormone release. So why are these drinks so popular (to the tune of millions upon millions of dollars in sales)?

Carbohydrate consumed before or during exercise restrains growth hormone release.

The fact is that a highly profitable industry has emerged to sell uninformed people ultra-cheap sugar-water disguised as "performance drinks." The popularity of these products is due in large part to the dominant influence of the major fitness magazines (all of which are owned by, or have close financial ties to, dietary supplement companies) on the public's perception of health and fitness issues. The problem with these magazines is not the clearly identifiable advertisements, but rather the underhanded propaganda masquerading as objective articles. Some publications are worse than others in this regard, but financially inspired bias and back-door salesmanship are pervasive in the fitness industry, and reach a pinnacle in fitness magazines.

WARNING! You Can't Trust What You Read in Fitness Magazines

Most readers take what a fitness magazine writer says at face value, having no idea that the writer is often being either directly or indirectly paid by a supplement manufacturer. This contributes substantially to the "misinformation problem" that I have decried throughout this book. I am not suggesting that all fitness writers are biased - but many are. Nor am I suggesting that all fitness magazines are publishing lies - but some are. What I am saying is that there lurks a hidden commercial agenda, which manifests itself as publication bias. What I mean by publication bias is that if there is one study indicating that "X" helps you burn fat and there are 10 studies indicating that "X" serves no useful purpose whatsoever in the human body; and a particular fitness magazine is owned by the same company that owns ABC supplement company, which sells "X" - *guess which study you are going to read about.*

Collectively, fitness magazines and other media exert a commanding influence over what the public perceives to be truth regarding health and fitness - and this is a major reason why the public guzzles millions of gallons of growth-hormone-suppressing-sugar-water (a.k.a., "energy" or "performance" drinks) per year even though, as you learned in Chapter 18, carbohydrate is neither optimal nor even necessary for energy. Moreover, fluids with a high-sugar concentration empty from the stomach at a slower rate than plain water.[35] With some "performance drinks" containing more than 100 grams of carbohydrate, gastric emptying can be slowed to a snail's pace, forcing the "performance drinker" to compete or train with a distended gut. By hindering fat burning, blocking growth hormone release, and bloating you, these drinks reduce both performance and the beneficial effects of exercise.

Publication bias and "creative interpretation" of scientific studies have contaminated the information pool to such an egregious extent that all magazine articles pertaining to fat loss/bodybuilding supplements must be taken with a grain of salt the size of an ice cube.

Another disadvantage of a pre-workout meal rich in carbohydrate pertains to its effect on brain chemistry, described in Chapters 10 and 11. By elevating serotonin, a neurotransmitter with sedative properties, a carbohydrate-rich meal can adversely affect motivation and energy levels. A protein-based pre-workout meal has the opposite effect on brain chemistry. (See "Better Living Through Better Brain Chemistry: Using Food to Enhance Mental Performance and Emotional Well-Being," in Chapter 19.) In addition to blunting alertness, serotonin, which increases during exercise, may directly precipitate exercise-related fatigue.[36,37,38] In any event, practical experience counsels that consuming a high quantity of carbohydrate prior to a scheduled workout renders it less likely that you will get off the couch and into the gym.

A concern commonly expressed by individuals who read this book after a lifetime of pro-carb indoctrination is that reducing carbohydrate intake will diminish exercise performance. While it is true that glycogen is the primary energy source utilized during high-intensity exercise and low glycogen levels can limit one's ability to perform this type of exercise,[39,40] it does not follow that reducing carbohydrate intake will diminish glycogen levels/performance. To the contrary, studies show that: 1) an overall reduction in carbohydrate intake, combined with 2) a proportional increase in fat intake, and 3) a cyclical carbohydrate consumption pattern, can enhance both anaerobic and aerobic exercise performance.[41,42,43,44,45,46,47,48,49] (That sounds a lot like the NHE Eating Plan, doesn't it?)

The physiological factors responsible for this performance increment are: 1) a glycogen-sparing effect, and 2) greater access to fat for energy (see "Increasing Energy Levels and Improving Athletic Performance," in Chapter 11). Not only can a higher-fat diet improve fat utilization in general by making free fatty acids more available to working muscles, but it can also increase levels of intramuscular triglyceride.[50]* This is advantageous because, whereas free fatty acids can supply energy only for low-/moderate-intensity exercise, intramuscular triglyceride can be tapped to fuel higher-intensity work.[51,52] Greater triglyceride storage in muscles combined with glycogen-loading, produces a condition optimal for maximizing high-intensity muscular output.

The foregoing research has electrifying implications, because it suggests that world-class athletic performances to date have been limited by diet! Studies ostensibly proving a high-carb/low-fat diet superior to a lower-carb/higher-fat diet, *have uniformly failed to allow for a sufficient period of adaptation.* It takes time to make the transition to a fat-burning state. Accordingly, the immediate consequence of cutting carbohydrate intake is a downturn in exercise performance. But once the metabolic shift is made, exercise performance improves, sometimes dramatically. The *Journal of Sports Science* reports that adaptation to a high-fat diet for a period of four weeks can increase by two-fold, resistance to fatigue during prolonged, low-to-moderate intensity exercise.[53] The *Journal* reports even greater performance enhancement resulting from adaptation to a high-fat diet combined with carb-loading[54] (this sounds a lot like the bodybuilders' NHE Eating Plan, doesn't it?).

I call upon athletes to heed these findings and switch to a higher-fat/lower-carbohydrate/cyclical diet. Whether the general NHE Eating Plan or the bodybuilders'

---

* Don't confuse intramuscular triglyceride with serum triglyceride. The latter refers to fat in the blood and is a coronary risk factor discussed in Chapters 8 and 18.

version is best for you depends not only upon your performance goals but also upon whether building muscle or reducing bodyfat is your principal objective. By embracing scientific wisdom over conventional wisdom, we can ascend to glorious new heights of athletic achievement.

Although all of your pre-workout-NHE-Eating-Plan meals will be medium-sized or smaller, you should allow at least 75 minutes between eating and exercising. This is a good general rule, but it is especially applicable to a protein-based meal, which takes longer to digest than a carbohydrate-based meal. If your schedule does not permit you to wait that long between eating and exercising (as is often the case if you are working-out in the morning before going to work), you can counter this circumstance by consuming easier-to-digest protein foods. These include: egg, yogurt, tofu, cottage cheese, and the homemade pre-workout drinks described below.

The Post-Workout Meal: More of the Same, Please

Much of the same reasoning that applies to the pre-workout meal applies to the post-workout meal. If you consumed a hormonally correct pre-workout meal and performed your workout in a hormonally intelligent fashion, you boosted your metabolic rate and stimulated a surge of growth hormone that shifted your metabolism into a heightened fat-burning mode. *It is now time to reap the fat-burning/muscle-enhancing benefits of your time and energy investment in the gym.*

All the misinformed "experts" and the ones with hidden commercial agendas would have you drink a "recovery" drink or shake (which is the post-workout version of the pre-workout "performance" drink). The insulin spike produced by these high-carbo concoctions will, literally within seconds of swallowing your first gulp, kick you out of the heightened fat-burning state that you worked so hard during your workout to attain. You will still enjoy the benefit of the post-exercise metabolic elevation, which is independent of hormonal factors, but the percentage of fat burned to fulfill the increased post-exercise energy requirement will be reduced significantly.

By contrast, a medium-sized protein or protein/fat meal will not thwart post-exercise fat burning. Rather, it perpetuates fat-burning momentum generated by your workout. Moreover, post-workout protein consumption is useful in replenishing amino acids in the wake of exercise-induced amino acid oxidation (see p. 240). In addition, by consuming protein immediately after exercise, you capitalize upon a "window of opportunity" in which amino acid transport into muscles and protein synthesis are accelerated.[55,56] *By taking advantage of this metabolic "window of opportunity," you get post-workout recovery off to a strong start by counteracting the catabolic conditions that prevail in the aftermath of an intense training session.* (See also, regarding the post-workout meal, p. 292-293.)

How to Save Tons of Money by Making Your Own Homemade Performance Drink that Blows Away Anything You'll Find in Health Food Stores!

Most commercial performance/recovery drinks are loaded with carbohydrate, often appearing on the label with the impressive-sounding names "glucose polymers" or "maltodextrin." As explained above, these drinks block growth hormone release and impede fat burning. Protein-only drinks are available, but the gastrointestinal distress caused by these pure protein drinks can make you a prisoner in your own bathroom. Adding insult to stomach cramps, the average growth-hormone-suppressing carbohydrate drink or diarrhea-inducing protein drink costs between three and four dollars, a ludicrously high price considering the low-grade ingredients most of them contain.

I recommend making your own pre-workout performance drink or post-workout recovery drink. First, buy high-quality protein powder. (Be careful - the protein supplement industry, like the dietary supplement industry in general, is bursting at the seams with impure, inferior products slickly marketed as the ultimate breakthrough in human nutrition.) The protein powder can be whichever flavor you favor. If it is sweetened, be wary of the carbohydrate content. If it is unsweetened, you can sweeten it yourself with a zero-carb sweetener. Add a few tablespoons of whipping cream and ice and blend for a low-carb, high-protein, moderate-fat, rich, creamy, frosty, shake. You can substitute a tablespoon of olive oil and/or flaxseed oil for a tablespoon of cream to provide even more health and fat loss benefits (see Chapter 18). Using oil will also allow you to use less saturated fat in the form of cream. However, too little cream relative to oil may ruin the taste, so experiment to find a happy medium.

The saturated and monounsaturated fat in this shake supports testosterone production in men (see Chapter 22). Thus, not only will it promote growth hormone release due to the absence of carbohydrate and the presence of protein, but it will also give men a testosterone boost when they need it most, after an intense workout when testosterone levels are depressed.

The caliber of these ingredients - high-quality protein powder, fresh whipping cream, extra virgin olive oil, and/or flaxseed oil - is far superior to the ingredients that comprise most commercial performance/recovery drinks. And while it is never as convenient to make something yourself as it is to buy it, the money savings is considerable. I estimate that the total cost to you, per homemade shake, is about $1.50. This $1.50 is much greater than the per-unit cost to the manufacturer of the ingredients in a typical performance/recovery drink, but much less than the retail cost of the same product.

What Kind of Exercise Should You Do?

This is one of the more basic questions concerning exercise, and yet most people have it wrong. Of the two categories of exercise discussed earlier - aerobic exercise and resistance exercise - which is more effective for reducing bodyfat? If you believe that aerobic exercise is superior in this regard, then you're among 99% of the population - and dead wrong.

Cardiovascular health is a critical component of fitness. However, aerobic exercise ranks second to progressive resistance training as a tool for shedding excess bodyfat and keeping it off permanently.

The notion that treadmills and stairclimbers are the best means of reducing bodyfat and that weight training is beneficial solely toward the objective of building muscle, is a time-honored and unfortunate misconception. At the core of this false belief is the fact that, as explained above, aerobic exercise engages a bioenergetic pathway that is conducive to fat burning; whereas resistance exercise engages the anaerobic pathway, which entails the burning of fuel sources other than fat. In other words, aerobic exercise burns more fat than resistance exercise, *while you are exercising*. But that is not the end of the story - it's the beginning. The greater portion of fat loss benefits accrue *between* not *during* exercise sessions. The hormonal and metabolic forces set into motion as a result of your motions in the gym can have an effect for many hours after your workout ends.

Both aerobic and resistance exercise raise metabolic rate for a period of time after exercise ceases. But studies show that resistance exercise is substantially more powerful in this regard, with post-exercise metabolic elevation persisting for 15 hours[57,58] and sometimes for as long as 24 or even 48 hours after a resistance training session ends.[59,60] Intensity is the key factor accounting for why weight training outdistances endurance training as a metabolic stimulus. Evidence suggests that duration is linearly,[61] whereas intensity is exponentially,[62] related to post-exercise metabolic elevation. The practical import is that:

1) Higher-intensity/lower-duration exercise will burn more calories *after the workout* than will lower-intensity/higher-duration exercise, even where the amount of calories burned *during the workout* is equivalent.[63,64,65]

2) Two, more intense training sessions of lesser duration will burn more calories overall (during + after) than will one less intense training session of greater duration.[66,67]

NOTE - We are discussing the *metabolic* effects of exercise. Later in this chapter we will discuss the *hormonal* effects of exercise. In this context, metabolic refers to total calories burned; whereas *hormonal* refers to the relative contribution of fat/carbohydrate to fulfilling metabolic demands. As you will see later, the prescription for optimizing the hormonal effects of exercise mirrors the prescription for optimizing the metabolic effects of exercise. This makes it simple, doesn't it? As you might suspect, this happy coincidence is not a product of chance. Rather, it results from the interrelationship between hormones and metabolism.

The extensive post-exercise metabolic elevation that prevails in the wake of an intense resistance training session stems from the fact that if done properly, resistance training initiates a restoration/recovery process in which depleted energy compounds, like glycogen and creatine phosphate, are replenished and muscle tissue is repaired and rebuilt. Anabolic and catabolic hormones orchestrate this energy-intensive recovery process. "Energy-intensive" means requires additional energy (calories) = higher metabolic rate. But resistance training does not stop there.

Not only does resistance training increase your overall metabolic rate, but it can also increase the percentage of fat burned relative to sugar. How can resistance training accomplish this? By prompting the release of growth hormone, which shifts your metabolism into a fat-burning mode. A *well-designed* resistance training program is a potent stimulator of growth hormone (whereas a poorly designed one can suppress growth hormone). In men, resistance training can also increase testosterone levels; and testosterone, like growth hormone, is a lipolytic (fat-mobilizing) hormone. Aerobic exercise, too, can positively influence hormone levels, but not nearly as effectively as resistance training. The post-exercise metabolic increase and the hormonal enhancement effects are the short-term-fat-loss benefits of resistance exercise. The long-term benefits are even more impressive.

In addition to giving your body shape and firmness, and imparting functional ability, muscle is intimately involved in fat burning. At the cellular level, muscle is the locus of fat burning. Specifically, muscle cells contain structures called *mitochondria,* which are tiny organic furnaces that produce energy from fatty acids and glucose. And as you learned in Chapter 4, a direct relationship exists between muscle mass and metabolic rate. Therefore, **the more muscle you have**, **the more calories you burn**, **even at rest**.

Muscle is vital, dynamic tissue churning with busy activity: protein synthesis, glycolysis, ATP regeneration, and fatty acid oxidation are just a few of the activities that regularly go on inside muscle cells. Fat, on the other hand, is basically inert - it just sits there. Per ounce, muscle takes-up less space and uses-up more calories. Muscle enhances the functional ability of the body; fat diminishes the functional ability of the body by saddling it with dead weight. Muscle tissue possesses an extensive capillary network allowing the heart to pump blood through the muscles with relative ease; adipose tissue is much less vascular and thus taxes the heart.

As you can see, muscle is "high-maintenance tissue," requiring a steady supply of energy (calories) and oxygenated blood. By contrast, fat is "low-maintenance tissue," requiring less energy and less blood. Not only does muscle "cost" more energy to maintain than fat, but also muscle contributes less energy to your survival. In other words, whereas fat is an excellent energy source, muscle is a poor energy source. Muscle must be broken down to its constituent amino acids, and the amino acids must be converted to glucose - and after all that work, glucose yields less than half as much energy as does fat. This explains why, when under duress, the body readily jettisons muscle. Faced with the potentially life-threatening specter of calorie restriction (which is how your body perceives it), the body eagerly unloads "energy-costly" muscle.[68,69,70]

As fasting progresses to bona fide starvation and after "unnecessary muscle" (that which helps you excel athletically and look good in a swimsuit) has been unloaded, counterregulatory adaptive mechanisms, including thyroid downregulation and ketosis, come into play to conserve remaining "necessary muscle" (the heart, other organs, and a minimal amount of skeletal muscle requisite for basic movement).[71,72,73,74] At this point, even if adequate caloric intake is restored, a severe metabolic disadvantage has been incurred. And while lost fat is never far from home, a portion of lost muscle often proves irretrievable, especially among females, the aged, and the sedentary.

In light of the foregoing discussion, it is clear that, whether male or female, **building a calorically "high-maintenance" body is the best strategy for achieving maximum** *permanent* **fat loss** - and that means a high muscle/fat ratio. Women are limited in this regard, due to their relative lack of testosterone. Nevertheless, within this narrow window of muscle growth potential, building muscle will greatly assist a woman in her effort to lose fat permanently, while giving her a firm, toned, shapely look to go along with low bodyfat.

Relying solely on aerobic exercise to reduce bodyfat, which many people (especially women) do, can actually have a *negative* long-term effect, by reducing muscle mass. Prolonged, high-volume aerobic exercise is catabolic, raising cortisol levels and causing muscle loss in both men and women.[75,76,77,78,79,80] * And it appears that women, who can less afford to lose muscle than men (see Appendix A), are more susceptible to the catabolic effects of endurance training.[81,82] *Even the loss of one ounce of muscle reduces your metabolic rate and your ability to burn fat.* Hence, those highly motivated men and women who spend hours laboring-away on the treadmill or stairclimber, rather than allocating an appropriate proportional amount of energy to this mode of exercise, are committing a costly error.

Take a look at the body of a world class long-distance runner: do you see a shapely, lean body with impressive muscle tone and fullness? No, in most cases you see a stick-figure physique, emaciated and weak. "Some runners are so weak they can't carry their own luggage," comments Dr. William Evans of the USDA Human Nutrition Center on Aging.[83] Dr. Michael Colgan of the Colgan Institute concurs, observing that "30 push-ups are beyond many of the elite runners that we test."[84]

Even if, like those individuals whose mindset has been distorted by the popular media and the fashion industry's obsession with rail-thinness, you aspire to the skeleton look rather than the lean and sculpted look, a skinny, muscleless** body does not age well. By burning-off muscle tissue, you accelerate the physical degeneration associated with aging and the age-related metabolic slowdown. Conversely, by building muscle you counteract these adverse physiological trends. In this connection, a study published in the *Journal of Applied Physiology* reported an 8% increase in resting metabolic rate in 50- to 65-year-old men after 16 weeks of weight training.[85] Another study, published in the *American Journal of Clinical Nutrition*, found a similar metabolic increase in men and women, aged 56-80, after 12 weeks of resistance training.[86] Moreover, researchers find that in addition to producing strength gains, progressive resistance training consistently improves body composition in both men and women by increasing lean mass and decreasing bodyfat[87,88,89,90,91] - even when subjects trained only twice a week.[92]

The point is not that you should dispense with aerobic exercise - quite the contrary. Cardiovascular fitness is essential to good health, and aerobic exercise promotes cardiovascular fitness. Furthermore, endurance training enhances the body's capacity to use fat for fuel[93,94,95,96,97] by positively altering fat-burning enzymes, called *lipases.*[98,99,100,101,102] Thus, aerobic training and resistance training work together synergistically. **By combining aerobic training with resistance training, you multiply the benefits of each, while avoiding the muscle loss associated with high-volume aerobic-only exercise**. And, by applying the principles of hormonally intelligent exercise, you can achieve optimal results from only 2-4 hours total, per week. Is a couple of hours a week - out of 119 waking hours - too much to ask when the rewards are a stronger, sexier, healthier, more energized, better functioning body? It sounds like the bargain of the century to me.

---

* It is true that *any* type of exercise, including resistance training, can have a net catabolic effect if frequency, intensity, duration, and load are not properly modulated. However, resistance training, if done properly, generates a compensatory anabolic response that outweighs the catabolic response. By contrast, with aerobic exercise, the catabolic effects are unopposed by a countervailing anabolic stimulus.

** I know this word looks strange - it's my humble contribution to the English language.

The lack of appreciation of the remarkable anti-aging, health, and fat loss benefits of resistance training is due, in large part, to the tardiness of health authorities in endorsing resistance training (there are still many benighted health authorities and doctors who have yet to awaken to its many benefits). Among its benefits, resistance training not only builds muscle, but bone too. The importance of weight-bearing exercise for the skeletal system became evident when America sent men into space. Without gravity, astronauts rapidly lost bone mass.[103] Efforts to prevent bone loss by having astronauts pedal exercycles while in orbit met with failure; despite being young and exceptionally healthy, the astronauts' bones disintegrated.[104] This illustrated the need for weight stress in maintaining skeletal health. Unfortunately, aerobic exercise performed on Earth also fails to maintain bone mass.[105,106,107]

Resistance Training as a Means of Warding-Off the Deadly Crippler

In the face of aging and the attendant drop-off in anabolic hormones, gravity alone is not enough to maintain bone mass, as evidenced by the prevalence of osteoporosis - the deadly crippler of older men and women. Millions of older men and women are afflicted with this merciless disease, which breaks approximately 1.5 million bones per year in the U.S.[108] The million-and-a-half fractures of the spine, hip, and forearm attributable to osteoporosis account for an estimated $13 billion in medical costs.[109] Demographic changes in the U.S. toward an older population herald an enormous public health burden in coming decades, with the cost of osteoporosis-related morbidity projected to exceed $60 billion by the year 2020. [110]

Women are disproportionately affected by osteoporosis due to menopausal loss of estrogen, smaller bones than men, greater propensity to engage in restrictive dieting throughout life, and lesser propensity to lift weights. For many elderly people, the trauma of a hip fracture and the consequent stay at that extremely dangerous place called the hospital proves fatal.[111] Even when elderly hip-fracture-victims survive, protracted agony and disability often mar the rest of their days.[112] Once the crippler strikes, it's too late. The only cure is prevention.

While gravity alone is not sufficient to maintain bone mass in the face of aging, neither is the popular medical recommendation of calcium supplementation. True, calcium (and many other nutrients) is vital to bone health. But the ultimate issue is not how much calcium you ingest, but how much calcium is retained and incorporated into your bone structure. This is why calcium supplements, alone, fail to maintain bone.

Weight stress, which can be effectively applied by resistance exercise, influences calcium metabolism by promoting retention and incorporation of minerals into bone.[113] This mineral synthesis process is analogous to protein synthesis, in which amino acids are retained and incorporated into muscle. Both of these processes are mediated by hormones, particularly growth hormone,[114,115,116] which can be stimulated by resistance training. And just as resistance training can reverse muscle loss, it can also reverse bone loss.[117,118,119]

Although osteoporosis is a life-threatening and debilitating disease that affects millions of Americans, the good news is - it is almost completely preventable. Like most chronic conditions that become manifest later in life, the crippler does not go in for the kill until after decades of stalking. Osteoporosis is a creeping degenerative process, which can be arrested or reversed at any point along the way. The current medical approach of calcium supplements and estrogen replacement is woefully inadequate, a fact to which the statistics readily attest.

The widespread prevalence of the human tragedy known as osteoporosis despite the existence of effective means of prevention, represents yet another piteous failing on the part of a medical establishment focused on treating rather than preventing disease. To prevent osteoporosis, employ resistance exercise and appropriate nutritional supplementation.

247

The Times, They are A-Changin'

For the last decade, I have been advocating resistance training for fat loss, health, and as an anti-aging strategy. I became convinced, early on, of the efficacy of resistance training as a hormonal enhancement vehicle. For much of that period, I was a lone voice in the wilderness. In support of my recommendation of resistance training, I could not cite the American College of Sports Medicine, nor the National Academy of Sciences, nor famous exercise authorities like Dr. Kenneth Cooper, the man who coined the term "aerobics." The prevailing view of resistance training ranged from unnecessary to inadvisable.

The times, they are a-changin.' Both the National Academy of Sciences and the American College of Sports Medicine have revised their positions and now recommend resistance training. Dr. Kenneth Cooper, as well, after seeing too many people with great cardiovascular systems and crumpling bones, has recanted his longstanding denunciation of resistance training and has redesigned his facilities at the Cooper Clinic to accommodate this form of exercise. With new discoveries being made almost daily concerning the impact of hormones on body composition, health, aging, and mental well-being, resistance training will only grow in popularity. I recommend you start now, if you have not already.

Having discussed exercise on a general level, it is time to focus on how to structure your workouts for optimal hormonal response. A large percentage of people who exercise, and many trainers, have not the faintest inkling of the hormonal effects of exercise or how to modulate exercise variables to optimize these effects. Most exercise practices are the product of tradition, convention, and imitation - not science. Personal trainers can be of some benefit, especially in the areas of motivation and proper exercise execution. But for your cash per hour, you are unlikely to learn much about using exercise as a means of hormonal enhancement - this technology is the razor-sharp-cutting-edge of exercise science.

A Quick Word about Personal Trainers

The substantive material that must be mastered in order to become a "certified" personal trainer is largely theoretical and makes only passing reference to hormones. Furthermore, there exists an alphabet soup of certifying organizations with widely varying legitimacy (including nil). Certification emerged for insurance purposes to ensure an irreducible minimum of knowledge among personal trainers. From this standpoint, the emphasis on certification has been a positive development: on a random basis, it is less likely that a "certified" personal trainer will commit malpractice than an uncertified trainer because the certified trainer at least knows *something* about which he or she is instructing.

I raise the issue of trainers by way of disclaimer: there is a limit to how much can be taught via the written word, and there is no substitute for a wise mentor/coach.

The Six Exercise Variables

The following factors determine the hormonal response to exercise: frequency, intensity, duration, load, volume, and exercise selection. Hormonally intelligent exercise entails strategically manipulating these variables for optimal hormonal response.

EXERCISE SELECTION

We have already discussed exercise selection in broad terms, comparing aerobic exercise with resistance exercise. To review: whereas resistance exercise is superior for achieving permanent fat loss and is a more effective means of hormonal enhancement, aerobic exercise promotes cardiovascular health. As well, aerobic exercise can significantly increase the rate of fat loss when properly integrated into a resistance-training-based exercise program.

On a more specific level, the issue is exactly which exercises to do. Free weights or machines? Compound exercises or isolation exercises? Jogging or jumping? Dumbells or barbells? Sit-ups or crunches? Pulldown or pullup? This is a vast topic that could easily occupy a book of its own – and does. All exercises are not created equal.

FREQUENCY

This variable refers to how often you exercise and relates to recovery in the following way: the more frequently you work-out, the shorter will be recovery periods between workouts.

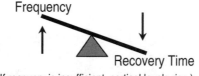

Frequency

Recovery Time

(If recovery is insufficient, cortisol levels rise.)

As you know by now, exercise sets into motion powerful hormonal forces. By stimulating secretion of anabolic (muscle-building) and lipolytic (fat-burning) hormones, vigorous exercise creates a *potential* for favorable body composition changes. If you train too frequently, however, this potential cannot be realized. What is worse, under these circumstances catabolic hormone levels escalate, overwhelming "good" hormones and assaulting your physique and health. Specifically, "king catabolic" - the hormone cortisol - eats-away at muscle, reduces insulin sensitivity, and impairs immune function (see p. 92). Chronic overstimulation of cortisol leads to adrenal insufficiency, a condition in which the endocrine system cannot respond properly to stress.[120,121]

In addition, overtraining dramatically increases the likelihood of injury, especially connective-tissue injuries, the kind that can keep you out of the gym for months.[122] And, as many athletes can attest, inability to train heralds the unraveling of hard-earned progress. In the words of Olympian long-distance runner Jeff Galloway, "the single greatest cause of improvement is remaining injury-free to train."

The obvious question is how frequently is too frequently. Unfortunately, the answer is not as obvious as the question. It depends on the other variables: exercise selection, intensity, duration, and load.

You can perform a given volume of aerobic exercise (like jogging) more frequently than weight lifting because aerobic exercise is less intense. Therefore, the greater the resistance training component of your workout regimen relative to the aerobic training component, the less frequently you should work-out and vice versa.

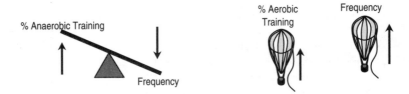

EXAMPLE: It is okay to jog for 30 minutes every day. But it is *not* okay to weight train for 30 minutes every day. Resistance training, when performed properly, is, by its nature, much more intense than jogging. This illustrates the interplay between exercise selection, intensity, and frequency. Every day is not too frequent for lower-intensity exercise (jogging); but it is too frequent for higher-intensity exercise (resistance training).

NOTE - I am employing a convenient distinction between low-/moderate-intensity cardiovascular exercise and resistance exercise. What about high-intensity cardiovascular exercise, like interval training (e.g., wind sprints, discussed later)? Interval training is a hybrid, and should be accounted as such in determining frequency. Like resistance training, interval training entails high effort intensity. But like jogging, interval training does not involve added load and it chiefly engages the cardiovascular system, as opposed to the musculoskeletal system. In terms of bioenergetic pathways, interval training is more-aerobic/less-anaerobic than resistance training and less-aerobic/more-anaerobic than continuous, moderate-intensity cardiovascular exercise.

LOAD

This variable refers to amount of weight or resistance against which force is applied. Weight lifting, by definition, involves added load. Pull-ups, push-ups, and sit-ups, like jogging, entail moving a fixed load (your body) through space against gravity. The primary significance of load is that it provides a means of *quantitative progression.* At a given level of strength, more effort is required to lift 300 pounds than to lift 150 pounds, *per time*.

Why isn't it accurate to simply say "more effort is required to lift 300 pounds than to lift 150 pounds"? Because the relationship between load and effort intensity is modified by time (duration) such that effort intensity is greater when lifting 50 pounds 3 times successively (i.e., 1 set of 3 reps with 50 lbs. = 150 lbs.) than when lifting 50 pounds 2 times successively then resting 2 minutes then lifting 50 pounds 2 times again then resting again then lifting 50 pounds 2 times again (i.e., 3 sets of 2 reps with 50 lbs. = 300 lbs.). And *the hormonal implications of each of these workouts are markedly different.* Similarly, it is not accurate to say more effort is required to roll a 16-pound bowling ball than to roll a 12-pound bowling ball. Why? Because more effort is required to roll a 12-pound bowling ball at 40 mph than to roll a 16-pound bowling ball at 4 mph. (When rolling a 12-pound bowling ball at 40 mph, the duration from when the arm holding the ball begins moving forward to when the ball is released is less than when rolling a 16-pound bowling ball at 4 mph.)

Hence, at a given duration and level of strength, load is directly correlated with effort intensity. (You must exert more effort to carry fifty 2-pound bricks a given distance in 10 minutes than to carry fifty 1-pound bricks the same distance in 10 minutes.)

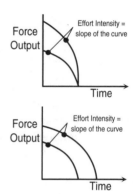

And, at a given level of effort intensity and strength, load is directly correlated with duration. (If you do not increase effort to match the greater load, then it will take you longer to carry fifty 2-pound bricks a given distance than to carry fifty 1-pound bricks the same distance.)

INTENSITY

There are two basic types of intensity - effort intensity and relative intensity - and a third that encompasses both - anabolic intensity. At a given level of fitness, an increase in effort intensity increases relative intensity. But relative intensity can increase absent a change in effort intensity. I will define each of the different types of intensity and explain the hormonal significance of each.

Effort Intensity (e-intensity)

Effort intensity is a measure of the quantum of effort exerted while performing an exercise. More precisely, e-intensity is *the percentage of momentary muscular capability exerted at a given moment.* During the course of taxing physical activity, absolute muscular capability diminishes and thus a correspondingly greater *percentage* of momentary muscular capability (effort) is required in order to perform the activity. Ultimately, 99% momentary muscular capability is required, and a moment later, 100% is insufficient - this terminal moment is called "point of failure."

Increasing e-intensity, like increasing load, constitutes quantitative progression.

251

EXAMPLE: If you can lift 100 pounds twice, and you hit the "point of failure" while attempting the 2nd repetition with that load, you are, at the point of failure, exercising at 100% e-intensity. If you are lifting only 50 pounds, a much lesser load, your e-intensity level will be much lower during the 2nd repetition, as compared with the 2nd repetition with the greater load. With the lesser load, you may hit the point of failure on the 8th repetition; at that moment, you are exercising at 100% e-intensity (a greater load causes you to become fatigued – lose muscular capability - at a more rapid rate).

Repetitions to Failure

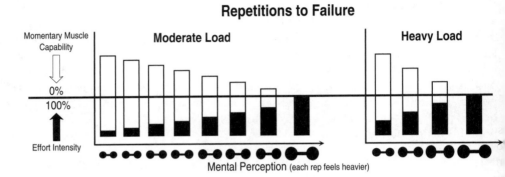

EXAMPLE: As you can see from the previous example, there is an inverse relationship between duration and e-intensity such that at a given volume more of one means less of the other. To illustrate, if you are told that Bullet Bob ran 100 meters in 15 seconds you know that he was "loafing" (running at low e-intensity); but if you are told that Slo Mo ran it in 15 seconds you can conclude that Slo Mo was putting forth mo' effort (higher e-intensity) than Bullet Bob.

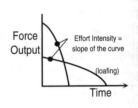

NOTE - You have greater control over e-intensity than over load (load progression is largely constrained by strength gains, whereas e-intensity is chiefly a function of the will). Therefore, your ability to err in modulating e-intensity is greater. When beginning an exercise regimen, or resuming exercise following a layoff, you must *gradually*, over a period of weeks (and sometimes months depending on biological age and fitness level), work up to the point where the last repetition of each set (except for warm-up sets) is performed at 100% e-intensity. Failure to increase e-intensity inevitably results in stagnation (due to a drop in *relative intensity*, discussed below), whereas a too rapid rise in e-intensity is counterproductive and potentially injurious (see below).

Hormonal Significance: Effort intensity determines the *anabolic potential* of exercise. "Anabolic potential" can be defined as the extent to which the anabolic impetus created by a particular exercise outweighs the catabolic impetus created by that exercise. "Potential" denotes the fact that the anabolic period follows the catabolic period and is contingent upon adequate nutrition and recovery time. For example, weight lifting (high e-intensity) has greater anabolic potential than jogging (low e-intensity). Very low e-intensity exercise has zero anabolic potential – meaning it can have either a net catabolic effect, or a net effect that is neither catabolic nor anabolic, but it cannot have a net anabolic effect.

Activity	Anabolic Potential
Weight Lifting (least likely to have net catabolic effect and capable of having substantial net anabolic effect)	high
Vigorous Running	moderate
Slow Jogging (most likely to have net catabolic effect and incapable of having net anabolic effect)	zero

Relative Intensity (r-intensity)

Relative intensity is a measure of physical stress. Relative intensity is "relative" because stress is relative. For example, delivering a speech to an audience of 500 people is likely to be very stressful to someone unaccustomed to public speaking, but it would tend to be much less stressful to someone who delivers speeches to large audiences every day. We can generalize about the "stressfulness" of an activity like giving a speech, skydiving, or sprinting 100 yards. But it is impossible to assess the quantum of stress imposed by a particular activity on a particular person unless we know specific facts about that person (like that person's fitness level in the case of sprinting 100 yards). Once you appreciate that stress is relative, you see why relative intensity tends to fall: because a given stressor (e.g., lifting 100 pounds 10 times successively or running a mile in 9 minutes) becomes less stressful each time one encounters it.

By increasing e-intensity and load, you can maintain a high level of r-intensity. But e-intensity and load (quantitative progression) cannot increase indefinitely. As quantitative progression slows then ceases, r-intensity accelerates downward because the stress of exercise slackens (see diagram, p. 277). Falling r-intensity translates to diminished hormonal response and, consequently, diminished results from exercise. This is why most people who work-out enjoy positive results initially, then stagnate. Can the downward trend in r-intensity/hormonal response/results be countered? Yes.

Hormonal Significance: Relative intensity determines the relative (relative to other occasions) hormonal response (catabolic and anabolic) to exercise. Where hormonal response is equal to or greater than on previous occasions, the body will change (either for the better or worse). Where hormonal response is lesser than on previous occasions, the body will either remain the same or will change in the opposite direction to the direction it changed on previous occasions, depending on the magnitude of the reduction in hormonal response (the "detraining effect" discussed on p. 260 is an example of an "opposite direction" change). Hence, r-intensity determines whether A) physical change will occur B) physical change will not occur C) previous physical change will be undone.

253

Anabolic Intensity (a-intensity)

Anabolic intensity encompasses both e-intensity and r-intensity.

$$AI = RI \times EI^n *$$

Hormonal Significance: Anabolic intensity describes the relative (relative to other occasions) anabolic potential of exercise, and it determines the *actual amount* of anabolic hormones secreted in response to exercise. Therefore, a-intensity determines whether (assuming adequate nutrition and rest) you will A) gain muscle mass, or in the case of women, "muscle tone" B) neither gain nor lose muscle mass/tone C) lose previously gained muscle mass/tone.

DURATION

Generally, this variable refers to time spent exercising; but there are two distinct usages.

1) When used to discuss how long a workout session should last (which I will do later in this chapter), duration refers to the interval from when exercise begins to when it ends.

2) When used in the volume equation, duration refers to actual time spent performing exercise, as opposed to resting. According to this definition, there is a significant difference between 40 minutes engaged in continuous exercise (like jogging), and 40 minutes engaged in intermittent exercise (like weight lifting) in which bouts of muscular output are interspersed with rest periods.

When the total amount of work (volume) is the same, duration and load are inversely related. (When transporting bags of groceries from your car into your house you can either carry two bags at a time and be finished in 2 minutes, or carry one bag at a time and be finished in 4 minutes.)

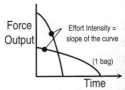

VOLUME

At a given level of fitness, volume is the product of frequency, duration, and load. In essence, volume is a measure of how much exercise you are doing per unit of time.

---

* If you are wondering what "n" is, I am too quite frankly. Someone with mathematical skills superior to mine will crack this mystery someday. How do I know that e-intensity is exponentially related to anabolic hormonal response? Because if one switched from a high e-intensity weight-lifting regimen (to which one were accustomed, thus low relative intensity) to a low e-intensity jogging regimen (to which one were unaccustomed thus high relative intensity) anabolic hormonal response would drop. In other words, a decrease in e-intensity will more effectively blunt anabolic hormonal response than a corresponding increase in r-intensity will enhance it. If you figure-out the quantity of the unknown anabolic exponent, please let me know, I've been pondering this for quite some time.

Volume = Load x Frequency x Duration / Fitness

For example, at a given level of fitness. . .

(Frequency = 3 days per week) x (Duration = 40 min.) (Load = 500 lbs.)

is equal in volume to:

(Frequency = 4 days per week) x (Duration = 30 min.) x (Load = 500 lbs.)

is equal in volume to:

(Frequency = 2 days per week) x (Duration = 40 min.) x (Load = 750 lbs.)

equal volume <u>does not</u> mean equal results.

As a person becomes fitter, the volume of a given workout decreases. . .

less volume = less exercise

less exercise = lower relative intensity (assuming all other variables are constant)

lower relative intensity = less hormonal release

When discussing the volume *of a workout*, as opposed to a period of time encompassing more than one workout, delete frequency.

Volume of a Workout = Load x Duration / Fitness

Excess Volume Impacts Sex Hormones

Where volume is excessive, exercise wreaks havoc on sexual and reproductive function in both sexes.[123] In men, overtraining can depress testosterone levels and reduce sperm count and quality[124,125,126,127,128] with both of these problems more prevalent in endurance athletes than in weight lifters.[129,130,131] In women, overtraining disrupts menstrual cycles, causing irregularity or cessation; and it suppresses production of hormones that regulate ovarian function and fertility.[132,133,134,135,136] Moreover, overtraining-induced alterations in the female reproductive hormones, estrogen, follicle-stimulating hormone, progesterone, and luteinizing hormone,[137,138,139,140,141] and resulting menstrual dysfunction is associated with an increased risk of musculoskeletal injury during exercise[142,143] and accelerated bone loss[144,145,146] (by contrast, properly modulated exercise helps preserve bone, see p. 248). As in men, sex hormone suppression in women is largely caused by excess cortisol.[147]

Excess Volume Reduces Thyroid Output

In Chapter 9, we discussed thyroid hormones in connection with diet, and you learned that thyroid hormone "T3" plays a key role in regulating metabolic rate. Just as calorie restriction and carbohydrate restriction each can lower T3 levels, so can overtraining.[148,149,150] The reduction of T3 in response to excessive exercise is the body's desperate attempt to quell the catabolic uprising instigated by such exercise. Once again, we see the body's innate survival-driven intelligence working at cross-purposes with the body owner's efforts to lose fat. Unfortunately, while T3 reduction slows fat loss, its insufficient to arrest the catabolic action of elevated cortisol. Hence, the restrictive dieter and the excessive exerciser continue to lose muscle even as fat loss slows to a creep. If you are wondering why the body, in its supreme wisdom born of eons of evolutionary experience, would opt to ditch muscle while clinging to fat, see p. 245-246.

The Relationship between Exercise Variables and Hormonal Responses

All Hormones are directly correlated with relative intensity.

Growth Hormone is directly correlated with effort intensity and inversely correlated with excess volume.

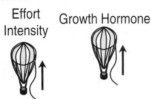
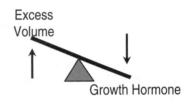

Cortisol is directly correlated with volume.

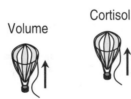

Insulin sensitivity is generally enhanced by exercise (resulting in lower insulin levels). However, insulin sensitivity is reduced (resulting in higher insulin levels) where volume is too high, because excessive volume raises cortisol levels and at high levels cortisol impairs insulin function.

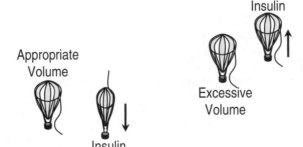

Testosterone is directly correlated with effort intensity and is inversely correlated with excess volume.

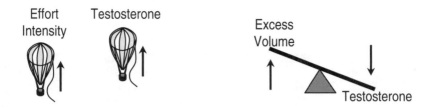

As you can see, the e-intensity/volume ratio influences both growth hormone to cortisol and the ratio of testosterone to cortisol.

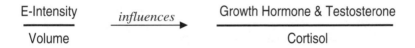

(If you don't like mathematical formulas, here's the English language version: What percentage of the exercise "work" you do is "hard work"?)

A workout that involves a lot of low-intensity/high-duration exercise, like long-distance running, has a low intensity/volume ratio. This type of workout tends to increase cortisol relative to both growth hormone and, in men, testosterone. The superiority of a high-intensity/volume-ratio training regimen is subject to the following qualification: higher intensity corresponds with higher risk of injury.

You can contain the risk of injury (but you can never eliminate it) by *gradually* increasing intensity. In so doing, you allow fitness/recovery ability to increase in lockstep with intensity, which minimizes risk of injury. Conversely, where intensity is increased too rapidly during the first few weeks after beginning an exercise program (or when resuming an exercise program after a layoff), such that intensity outstrips fitness/recovery ability, the risk of injury increases exponentially.

To optimize the hormonal response to exercise, gradually increase e-intensity from low to high and keep the e-intensity/volume ratio high thereafter.

While the intensity/volume ratio is a useful predictive indicator of hormonal response, it applies only *at a given level of volume* – it does not indicate whether volume is excessive or insufficient. To illustrate, a workout consisting of lifting as much

257

weight as possible one time would maximize the intensity/volume ratio; but it would be relatively ineffective because volume is too low (see below). Conversely, overtraining (excess volume) reduces the pituitary output of growth hormone,[161,162,163] in addition to adversely affecting testosterone, insulin, and cortisol levels.

Studies of runners, comparing the effects of increasing mileage while keeping speed constant versus increasing speed while keeping mileage constant, find that the former is more apt to lead to overtraining than the latter.[164,165,166] The former increases volume, whereas the latter keeps volume constant and increases e-intensity. Given that volume is directly correlated with cortisol, whereas e-intensity is directly correlated with growth hormone and, in men, testosterone, the outcome of these experiments was easy to predict.

The following factors determine the volume of exercise that will spark adverse hormonal changes: **nutrition**, **sleep**, **fitness level**, and **emotional stress**. The better your nutrition, the more and sounder your sleep, the fitter you are, and the lower your emotional stress level - the greater volume of exercise you can tolerate without falling prey to overtraining syndrome. Stated differently, the ratio of anabolism to catabolism will be higher over a given period of time when these factors are optimal than when they are sub-optimal.

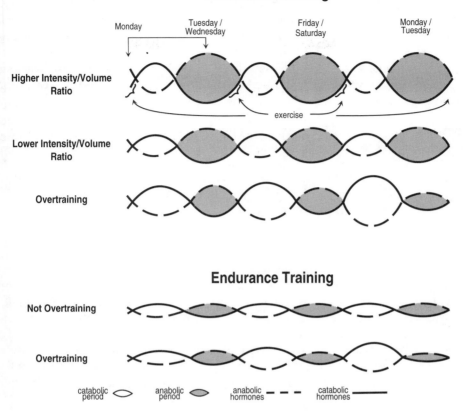

Resistance Training

	Monday	Tuesday / Wednesday	Friday / Saturday	Monday / Tuesday

Higher Intensity/Volume Ratio

exercise

Lower Intensity/Volume Ratio

Overtraining

Endurance Training

Not Overtraining

Overtraining

catabolic period   anabolic period   anabolic hormones - - -   catabolic hormones ———

Modulating Intensity for Maximum Growth Hormone Release

Maximum e-intensity occurs when exerting 100% of momentary muscular capability. As intuition would suggest, there is also a minimum for e-intensity. In fact, it is e-intensity of physical activity that defines exercise. What is the difference between sleeping and running? Why is one considered a form of exercise while the other is not? Because sleeping is non-intense; whereas running has an e-intensity rating greater than zero (it requires an output of force sufficient to prevent it from being performed indefinitely).

The exercise threshold rises commensurately with fitness increments. In other words, whether or not a given activity constitutes exercise for a particular person depends on that person's fitness level. This should also make sense intuitively: whereas brisk walking constitutes exercise for most people, it may not constitute exercise for a world-class runner.

EXAMPLE: Whereas a couch potato who has not exercised in years would experience positive physiological changes (a "training effect") from brisk walking, a world-class endurance athlete, if he or she relied solely on this form of "exercise," would experience negative physiological changes (a "detraining effect"). In this scenario, the world-class athlete would continue to *lose* cardiovascular fitness all the way down to the level at which brisk walking constituted exercise! This illustrates that the exercise threshold moves up or down with fitness level.

Likewise, whether a given activity constitutes "intense exercise" depends on the fitness level of the person doing the activity.

EXAMPLE: In order for "Weak Willy" to bench press 100 pounds, he must exert great effort (high e-intensity); but "Buff Daddy" can manage the lift while exerting minimal effort (low e-intensity).

However, even where e-intensity is high, r-intensity may not be.

EXAMPLE: A highly fit athlete might train at a high level of e-intensity every workout. This person has a high exercise tolerance due to his/her high level of fitness. In other words, his/her body is efficient at managing the stress of high-intensity exercise. For this person, high e-intensity represents moderate r-intensity. For an untrained person, by contrast, exercising at high e-intensity would be traumatic - heightening the risk of injury, causing severe muscle soreness that could last for days, and generating an excessive surge of catabolic hormones. For the untrained person, high e-intensity represents extremely high r-intensity.

Growth hormone release is positively correlated with both effort intensity and relative intensity.

Growth hormone output increases as effort intensity increases.[151,152,153,154,155]
(In other words, the higher the e-intensity level of exercise, the greater the growth hormone response; the lower the e-intensity level of exercise, the lesser the growth hormone response.)

AND

Training diminishes the growth hormone response to exercise.[156,157,158,159,160]
(In other words, the fitter one becomes relative to a given form of physical stress, the lesser the growth hormone response to that form of physical stress.)

Because growth hormone release is positively correlated with both effort intensity (e-intensity) and relative intensity (r-intensity), anabolic intensity (a-intensity, which encompasses both e- and r-intensity, see above) is the most complete and accurate way to depict the basis for physical-activity-related growth hormone output.

Synchronizing the Duration of Your Workouts to Hormonal Responses

Just as there is a minimum for intensity, there is also a minimum for duration. As a practical matter, a workout must be sufficiently lengthy to allow you to complete your exercises, including warm-ups, with the proper form and technique. In addition, there is a lag period from the onset of exercise to the rise in growth hormone (assuming sufficient intensity to stimulate growth hormone in the first place). One brief bout of peak effort exercise can stimulate growth hormone release, but several brief bouts of peak effort exercise performed repetitively generally produces a superior growth hormone response.[167] One reason for this is that certain metabolic byproducts of exercise, like lactic acid[168,169] and/or endorphins,[170,171] catalyze the release of growth hormone. A workout that is too brief limits the build-up of these GH-signaling factors, and does not impart sufficient physical stress to provoke a maximal growth hormone response. Therefore, a training session must go beyond a single exertion of peak effort, and the exerciser must accumulate a significant volume of exercise (which takes some time, but less than commonly believed) in order to achieve an optimal hormonal outcome.

The greater the a-intensity, the lesser the duration of exercise need be for growth hormone to be released.[172,173] Generally, the requisite duration ranges from 10 minutes for more intense exercise to 30 minutes for less intense exercise. [174,175] But this period may be considerably shorter in some instances, as demonstrated by a study published in the *European Journal of Applied Physiology*. The researchers found that after a 30-second sprint, growth hormone levels rose rapidly in both men and women subjects and peaked at approximately 10 minutes post-exercise. [176] This finding, while impressive, is not unprecedented. Similarly robust growth hormone responses to very brief, very intense bouts of exercise have been reported.[177,178,179] While the timing of the growth hormone response to exercise is variable and individualized, the following proposition is firmly supported: where a-intensity is high, it does not take long to stimulate growth hormone release. Therefore, **in terms of growth hormone release, there is no justification for a long workout**.

In most cases, peak growth hormone levels occur 20-50 minutes after the onset of sufficiently intense exercise;[180] after which growth hormone declines, *but cortisol continues to climb*.[181,182,183] **When falling growth hormone intersects with rising cortisol, your workout becomes hormonally incorrect**. And from that point on, your workout becomes progressively more hormonally incorrect with each passing minute that it persists. A-intensity determines when the intersection of growth hormone and cortisol will occur. The less intense the exercise, the slower the rate of increase of both cortisol and growth hormone. Accordingly, where a-intensity is low, an exercise session can run longer before it turns hormonally incorrect; however, less growth hormone is released under these circumstances. And if a-intensity is too low, growth hormone will not be released. Where a-intensity is high, 40-60 minutes after beginning a workout is approximately when growth hormone levels and cortisol levels will begin moving in opposite directions (signifying the impending onset of "hormonal incorrectness").

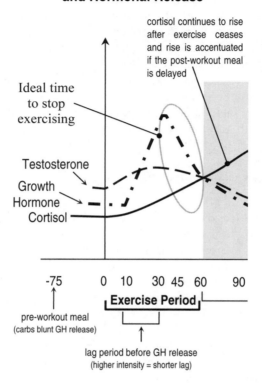

Exercise Duration and Hormonal Release

Even where little or no growth hormone is stimulated (because a-intensity is too low), cortisol will gradually rise and can reach excessive levels if the exercise session is prolonged. This is why I recommend against a workout program that primarily consists of high-duration, low-intensity exercise. This is also why long-distance runners tend to be weak and skinny - their "muscle axis," see Chapter 4, is skewed toward catabolism (promoted by cortisol) as opposed to anabolism (promoted by growth hormone and testosterone); whereas sprinters, *who often have the same bodyfat percentage*, tend to be strong and shapely. (Note the vast difference in the intensity/volume ratio between sprinting and long-distance running. Are you beginning to see how exercise variables affect hormones, which, in turn, affect the shape and composition of the body?)

The bottom line is that to obtain optimal hormonal response, a workout should: 1) be sufficiently intense to prompt growth hormone release, and 2) not last longer than one hour. Remember this: "He who trains then walks away, within one hour, is able to train again another day - sooner, stronger, and more fully recovered." **The goal is to exhaust** *the muscles* **without excessively exhausting** *the body*. As elaborated below, this is one of the training secrets of the Eastern European athletes who dominated world strength competition years ago, before the fall of communism. *A workout that is both intense and long-lasting makes severe inroads into your body's recovery ability by sharply skewing your hormonal profile toward catabolism and depleting energy resources.* Thus, you should train at a high level of a-intensity and limit your training sessions to no longer than one hour.

RULE - Regardless of whether the session is completed in terms of the number of sets or exercises to be performed, THE TRAINING SESSION SHALL TERMINATE WITHIN ONE HOUR AFTER IT BEGINS. But remember: one hour is the durational limit, not necessarily the optimal duration. If you are training at a high level of a-intensity, your workout can turn hormonally incorrect earlier than one hour (see above). Hence, *40 minutes is generally closer to the optimal workout duration than one hour*.

From a psychological standpoint, as well, a shorter workout is advantageous. The specter of a long, grueling workout can be very discouraging, especially where motivation is a problem to begin with (as it is for many people). You are more likely to find a reason to skip a workout if you know that you have a long workout ahead of you. On the other hand, knowing that your workout will be over in 30-45 minutes is a heartening thought - the light at the end of the tunnel is clearly visible from the time you set foot in the gym. Short workouts also negate the ever-popular "I don't have time to work-out" excuse.

For the average person, one exercise session per day is sufficient. Athletes, however, may require additional training time. What is the most effective way to increase volume? Answer: increase frequency and decrease duration of each workout. This facilitates greater per-workout e-intensity, which increases the per-workout intensity/volume ratio. In addition to a higher per-workout intensity/volume ratio (which translates to higher net anabolic potential per workout), chopping-up workouts into smaller pieces provides more occasions for stimulating growth hormone release. Hence, **two shorter more intense workouts**, **separated in time**, **are superior to one longer workout**, both in terms of fat loss (see p. 244) and anabolism/catabolism. When training twice in one day, refrain from directly working the same muscles on both occasions. Doing so leads to *localized overtraining*, discussed later.

Training Secrets from Across the Iron Curtain

The strategy of substituting more frequent, briefer training sessions for less frequent, longer ones was practiced secretly, behind the Iron Curtain, by Eastern Bloc athletes and, particularly, the Bulgarians. If you are not up on international weightlifting history, for years the Bulgarians dominated. Rumors swirled that the Bulgarians had developed an advanced anabolic

263

drug. While there is evidence that Eastern Bloc athletes were subjected to systematic state-sponsored steroid administration, there is also evidence that Eastern training methods were more advanced, from a hormonal standpoint, than Western methods during the period of Eastern domination of Olympic strength competition. (Communism was ideal for keeping secrets because of strict travel restrictions and the absence of a free press.)

In contrast to the prevailing wisdom in the West, the Bulgarians and other Eastern Bloc athletes limited their workouts to 35-45 minutes. A workout of this duration promotes maximum intensity, allows for more frequent training, coincides with growth hormone peaks, and ends on a physical and psychological high rather than with the athlete emotionally drained and physically depleted of critical recovery resources. (Bear in mind that if you are training for a particular sport, like long-distance running for instance, this training methodology may not be appropriate due to the need to conform your training to the demands of the sport.)

The Effect of Recovery Periods on Hormone Levels

When you train at a level of a-intensity sufficient to stimulate growth hormone secretion, the muscle-enhancing and fat-burning effects of such a workout take time to work their magic. (Remember, as explained earlier, the lion's share of benefits accrues *after* the workout ends.) Immediately after such a workout, your internal hormonal environment is catabolic due to exercise-induced cortisol release. This catabolic period, marked by net protein breakdown, gives way to an anabolic period, marked by net protein synthesis.[184,185]

Hormones conduct the transition from catabolism to anabolism. Specifically, cortisol, after being elevated by the workout, falls and ultimately drops below initial levels hours later. Concurrently with cortisol decline, testosterone, in men, after being suppressed by the workout, rebounds, and ultimately rises above initial levels. Growth hormone, meanwhile, trends upward during the recovery period, which is what one would expect given that cortisol is antagonistic (suppressive) to growth hormone and testosterone is complementary (supportive) to growth hormone. Thus, the recovery period begins with catabolism, which yields to anabolism.

It is between workouts, particularly during the anabolic period, that the physical improvements wrought by exercise occur. From a fat-burning standpoint, recall from p. 244-245 that the restoration and rebuilding of the body requires additional energy and thus additional calories are burned for many hours, and sometimes days, after an intense workout. It is crucial that you not short-circuit this physique-renovation process by working the same muscles again too soon <u>or</u> by working different muscles but going overboard with volume such that cortisol remains elevated and energy resources needed for recovery become depleted. Under these circumstances, recovery is derailed. If recovery is chronically impeded, you begin a downward slide leading to

264

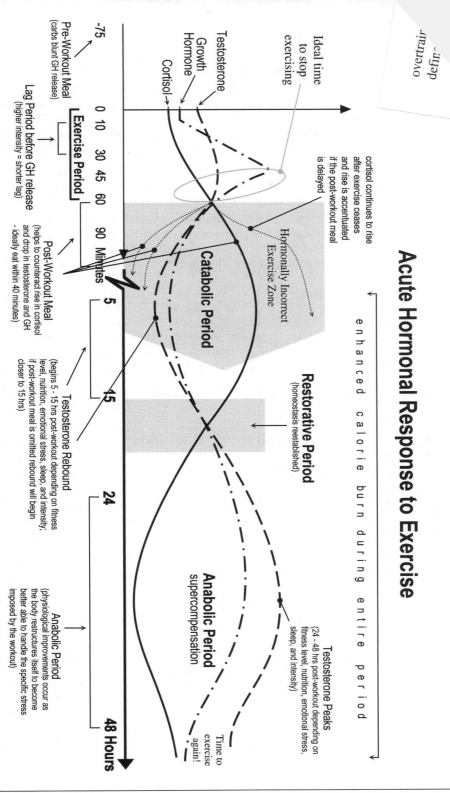

Acute Hormonal Response to Exercise

e n h a n c e d   c a l o r i e   b u r n   d u r i n g   e n t i r e   p e r i o d

Testosterone
Growth
Hormone
Cortisol→

Ideal time
to stop
exercising

-75

0 10 30 45 60 90 Minutes 5 15 24 48 Hours

cortisol continues to rise
after exercise ceases
and rise is accentuated
if the post-workout meal
is delayed

Hormonally
Incorrect
Exercise Zone

Pre-Workout Meal
(carbs blunt GH release)

Lag Period before GH release
(higher intensity = shorter lag)

Exercise Period

Post-Workout Meal
(helps to counteract rise in cortisol
and drop in testosterone and GH
- ideally eat within 40 minutes)

Testosterone Rebound
(begins 5 - 15 hrs post-workout depending on fitness
level, nutrition, emotional stress, sleep, and intensity;
if post-workout meal is omitted rebound will begin
closer to 15 hrs)

Catabolic Period

Restorative Period
(homeostasis reestablished)

Testosterone Peaks
(24 - 48 hrs post-workout depending on
fitness level, nutrition, emotional stress,
sleep, and intensity)

Anabolic Period
supercompensation

Anabolic Period
(physiological improvements occur as
the body restructures itself to become
better able to handle the specific stress
imposed by the workout)

Time to
exercise
again!

overtrain
defin

265

Natural Hormonal Enhancement

ing syndrome, and all the hormonal derangements and health problems that it.*

As you can see, in order for recovery to reach fruition, you must allow sufficient time between workouts. If you do, the anabolic periods will be greater than the catabolic periods and you will advance. Accordingly, more workouts is better than less workouts provided that full recovery occurs after each and every workout. The full-recovery provision is the kicker - without it, you would be left with "more workouts is better than less workouts." This "more is better" mentality is widely prevalent among avid exercisers, and it ensures that they will never achieve the results from exercise they seek. If, conversely, full recovery occurs and you continue not to exercise, you are forgoing the benefits of another workout and eventually you would experience a "detraining effect." This is called undertraining, the opposite of overtraining. Whereas overtraining occurs when volume is too high, undertraining occurs when volume is too low.

The optimal amount of time between workouts is the minimum necessary to allow for maximum recovery.

Earlier, I noted that trained athletes can tolerate higher volume and higher e-intensity. Does this mean that as you become fitter you require less time to recover from your workouts? Yes and no. The fact is that recovery ability increases substantially in response to training, *but the proportional improvement in strength is generally greater than the proportional improvement in recovery ability*. The upshot is that. . .

Contrary to popular belief, the risk of overtraining increases as you become fitter and stronger.

If you were to keep e-intensity and load constant as you became fitter and stronger (which would cause relative intensity to decline), then yes, less recovery time would be needed and you could train more frequently. But the goal is to keep r-intensity high by steadily increasing e-intensity and load. Therefore, since e-intensity and load do not remain constant in a hormonally intelligent exercise program but rather increase; and can increase - along with strength - faster and further than recovery ability, a reduction in frequency, rather than an increase, is often warranted as you become fitter and stronger. Stated differently, your ability to inflict trauma on your body via exercise increases sharply as you become fitter and stronger, and it can outstrip your recovery ability.

In contrast to resistance exercise or intense cardiovascular exercise, low-intensity aerobic exercise can be performed without concern for the recovery process, because

---

* Bear in mind that the definition of volume (see p. 255) includes a time element. There is no such thing as too much exercise in an abstract sense. Running 1000 miles is not necessarily excessive if performed over a period of a year; but running 10 miles can be excessive (depending on fitness level) if performed in one day. But as you will see later, short-term volume excess, which occurs when you weight train intensely two days in a row (because 24 hrs. is not enough time to allow for full recovery) is not necessarily a problem. In fact, short-term volume excess, called *overreaching*, can be beneficial provided that extra recovery time follows. Therefore, "short-term overtraining" is a contradiction in terms. Overtraining describes a condition caused by chronically excessive volume.

266

with such exercise there is no recovery process. Hence, a given duration of weight training is more likely to induce an overtrained state than walking. But just as a given duration of low-intensity exercise is less likely to produce adverse hormonal changes, so it also has much lesser potential to produce positive changes. Furthermore, low-intensity exercise *can* produce adverse hormonal changes if volume is high. In this scenario (low intensity/volume ratio combined with high volume), cortisol levels rise and growth hormone and testosterone levels fall. You can lose some fat when your hormones are arrayed in this unpropitious configuration, but you cannot build the lean, sculpted physique that defines a sexy, fit, strong, healthy body.

We have been talking a lot about resistance training, because it is the centerpiece of a hormonally intelligent training regimen. But as emphasized earlier, cardiovascular exercise is a vital component of any fitness program. Accordingly, let's discuss how the principles of hormonally intelligent exercise can be applied to cardiovascular exercise.

Interval Training for Hormonal and Cardiovascular Enhancement

Although resistance exercise is the ultimate form of exercise for reshaping the contours of your physique, cardiovascular exercise, when done properly, works synergistically with resistance exercise to accelerate fat loss while improving health. As to the issue of "how to," we see that, once again, conventional wisdom is wrong.

The prevailing belief is that to reduce bodyfat you should perform cardiovascular exercise at a low level of intensity in a steady, rhythmic fashion for an extensive duration. However, as discussed above, this lowers the intensity/volume ratio, which, in turn, increases cortisol relative to growth hormone and testosterone - definitely not the hormonal profile you want. Conventional wisdom on this subject reflects the truth in reverse: higher-intensity, lower-duration exercise is superior to lower-intensity, higher-duration exercise for reducing bodyfat[186] (see related discussion on p. 244).

Examining the Conventional Wisdom on How to Exercise for Maximum Fat Loss

The notion that you should trade intensity for duration is based on two premises, both of which are invalid.

1) Higher duration is necessary in order to phase into a fat-burning mode.

2) Lower intensity will keep you in an aerobic rather than anaerobic state, and more fat is burned during aerobic respiration than during anaerobic respiration.

Premise 1 is flawed because it assumes that everyone is in a sugar-burning mode to begin with, and, therefore must exercise continuously for some period of time before fat becomes a significant fuel source. To the extent this is true, it is true only because of misguided dietary practices. Sugar-burners are not born, they are made – self-made. The purpose of the NHE Eating Plan is to put you, and keep you, in a fat-burning mode by activating lipolytic hormones and suppressing lipogenic hormones.

Premise 2 is also faulty. You learned earlier in this chapter that the fat you burn while exercising pales in comparison with the enhanced post-exercise fat-burn that follows a hormonally correct workout and the long-term metabolic advantage of added muscle. Thus, the focus on fat burned during exercise is misplaced.

Furthermore, percentage of fat burned for energy should not be confused with amount of fat burned for energy. A higher-intensity workout uses a lower *percentage* of fat for energy. The real issue, though, is not the proportion of fat burned but rather the amount of fat burned. If you were concerned only with the percentage of fat burned, your best bet would be not to do *any* exercise since the percentage of fat burned is higher when intensity is lower. Does this mean you burn a higher percentage of fat when you are snoozing on the couch than when you are sprinting? Yes. Does it mean you burn more fat? Of course not.

You are probably pleased to learn that, contrary to what you have been told, you need not spend a long time in the gym doing continuous, monotonous exercise in order to burn fat. To the contrary, you should exchange duration for intensity and your cardiovascular training sessions should be composed of short, intermittent bursts of activity interspersed with rest periods. This methodology of brief bouts of high-intensity exercise juxtaposed with pre-established recovery periods is called "interval training"; and it is more effective at stimulating growth hormone release than continuous, lower-intensity exercise.[187,188] In one head-to-head comparison, interval training induced a three-fold greater growth hormone response than an equivalent amount of moderate-intensity continuous exercise.[189] I believe that, while impressive, this study understates the superiority of interval training because in many instances conventional low-/moderate-intensity aerobic exercise produces no growth hormone response at all.

Interval training illustrates the direct relationship between the intensity/volume ratio and growth hormone release. Duration of actual exercise is less for a 30-minute session of interval training (due to the intermittent rest periods) than for a 30-minute session of continuous exercise; therefore, e-intensity is higher. Where volume is equal, higher e-intensity translates to greater growth hormone secretion.

The following dramatizes how interval training increases e-intensity, and demonstrates how interspersing work with rest influences the amount of work that can be performed. Relatively few people can run at a 4-minute per mile pace for longer than 1 minute, much less complete a mile within 4 minutes. However, with correct spacing of running and resting periods, it would not be very difficult to complete a mile in 4 minutes of actual running. In a classic study on this subject, it was found that, when running speed was controlled, a subject who could run for only .8 miles when the run was performed continuously could cover 4 miles when 10 seconds of running was interspersed with 5 seconds of recovery.[190]

In addition to the hormonal advantages of interval training, there are cardiovascular benefits as well. One study that compared improvements in aerobic capacity (as measured by Vo_2max) achieved through interval training to improvements achieved through continuous training, found that interval training resulted in a two-fold greater increment in Vo_2max.[191] Another study comparing these two types of exercise found that

268

while both training modalities improved aerobic capacity to the same degree, interval training increased anaerobic capacity by 28% while continuous exercise failed to improve anaerobic capacity.[192] Furthermore, once aerobic improvements are attained through exercise, interval training is the most effective means of maintaining such improvements. Specifically, studies show that substantial reductions in either frequency (with duration and intensity held constant)[193] or duration (with frequency and intensity held constant)[194] do not result in a loss of aerobic capacity. Remarkably, aerobic improvements were maintained even when frequency alone or duration alone was reduced by two-thirds. But when intensity was reduced by only one-third, and frequency and duration were held constant, Vo_2max declined.[195] Collectively, these studies demonstrate that intensity is the key factor relative to both increasing and maintaining cardiovascular fitness. Interval training accentuates intensity; hence, it affords considerable cardiovascular benefits in addition to hormonal benefits.

"Wind sprints," which involves jogging punctuated by intermittent sprinting, is a popular form of interval training. Because interval training is a high-intensity mode of exercise, I should reemphasize that intensity must be *gradually* increased over time commensurately with fitness increments. A modified version of wind sprints, tailored to the less fit, consists of walking interspersed with jogging. Most cardiovascular training devices, like step machines and stationary bicycles, allow for adjustments in intensity level and therefore are suitable for interval training.

While a full physical examination is an important prelude to any exercise program, it is absolutely imperative where one is beginning a training regimen designed to maximize intensity and thereby maximize demands on the cardiovascular and respiratory systems. The time to discover an undetected cardiac condition or latent defect or irregularity in cardiorespiratory function is in a doctor's office through testing and examination, not in the gym through shooting pain or sudden horror. Having made this clear, I would also make clear that where a doctor's clearance is obtained after a full examination, and where intensity is increased commensurately with fitness increments, no person, no matter how old or unfit, should feel incapable of, or unequal to, interval training, weight training, or any other kind of exercise described in this book.

In support of the foregoing statement, studies show that even elderly people can successfully undertake resistance training.[196,197,198,199,200] In a study published in the *New England Journal of Medicine* an average strength increase of 113% was registered by 100 nursing-home residents (63 women and 37 men, average age = 87 years) after a 10-week program of high-intensity weight training.[201] In another study, published in the *Journal of the American Medical Association*, 8 weeks of resistance training produced a 174% increase in strength in nursing-home residents up to 96 years of age.[202] In yet another study, published in the *Journal of Applied Physiology*, focusing on body composition changes in 76- to 78-year-old women resulting from either weight training or endurance training, the weight-training-women gained muscle and lost fat whereas the endurance-training-women experienced negligible improvement in body composition.[203]

In addition to strengthening their skeletal muscles, elders can strengthen their heart muscle, too, by means of exercise. In fact, older people can increase their aerobic capacity to the same relative degree as younger people.[204] Similarly, cardiac patients, once considered among the permanently disabled, are increasingly using appropriately formulated high-intensity training programs to walk, jog, participate in, and even complete, marathons![205,206,207] The bottom line is that it does not matter whether you are a frail, institutionalized centenarian or someone who has undergone open-heart surgery; you are not foreclosed from the promise of a better, healthier life that hormonally intelligent exercise offers.

Even should you choose not to employ the interval format that I am recommending, you can enjoy a portion of the same benefits by ending your cardiovascular workout with a peak of intensity (your "cool-down" would come after this). For example, if you jog, you can sprint for the last 60 yards. Even a few seconds of high-intensity output added to your aerobic workout can substantially magnify growth hormone release.

The Interval Paradigm Applied to Resistance Training

Resistance exercise is, by its nature, a form of interval training. The vocabulary of resistance exercise is sets, repetitions (reps), and inter-set rest periods. "Reps" refers to how many times in succession you perform a particular lift. After completing your last rep, you rest, then do another set of reps. How many sets and how many reps to do is a time-honored question; it is addressed in broad terms in this book and treated more fully in *Hormonally Intelligent Exercise*. The point here is to show how resistance exercise – bouts of intense muscular work preceded and followed by momentary episodes of recuperative inactivity - is a form of interval training. If your resistance workouts do not conform to this format, you are doing something wrong.

The most common way that people run afoul of the interval framework when weight training is to do ultra-high repetitions with very light weight and very brief rest periods between sets. The belief underlying this wrong-headed practice is that ultra-high repetitions will burn more fat. In fact, *growth hormone* will "burn more fat"; and any load that is so light that you can do 20+ reps with ease is generally too light to generate the intensity requisite to growth hormone release. In addition, excessively light weight results in sub-optimal muscle fiber recruitment, activating only Type I not Type II fibers[208,209] (more about this later). **Don't "make light" of the importance of resistance when doing resistance exercise**.

Adaptation to Stress

In Chapter 9, we discussed the body's adaptive responses to changes in food supply, and I explained the relevance of those responses to your efforts to improve your physique. Now, I will do the same with respect to exercise.

270

Principles of Stress Adaptation

Principle 1 The ability to adapt to stress is the key to survival both from a lifetime and an evolutionary perspective.

Principle 2 The human body responds to stress by restructuring itself to become more capable of handling the particular imposed stress.

Principle 3 The human body is highly efficient at adapting to stress and thus adaptations are narrowly tailored to the specific stress encountered.

Consider a person who, accustomed to working behind a desk, gets a job doing manual construction work. He is likely to develop blisters from the friction on his hands. The damage to his body - signified by inflammation - results from his being unaccustomed to this particular form of stress (i.e., abrasive contact against the skin). His body will repair the damage.

A certain amount of this particular stress, say two weeks at the new job, will induce his body to go beyond merely repairing the damage to taking affirmative measures to "defend" against further stress of this kind. The defense in this instance would be a callus. Hence, the body restructures itself in such a way that further stress of the *same* nature and magnitude will cause *less* harm. By manipulating physical stress factors, we can restructure our bodies in other ways, as well. **This is how you should view exercise - *as the strategic manipulation of physical stress factors designed to induce a beneficial restructuring of the body* - not merely as a means of burning calories**.

The above example illustrates two additional points about how the body adapts to stress, both of which are germane to exercise. For one, stress need not be life-threatening to trigger an adaptive response. Rather, the adaptive response to stress is aimed at offsetting discomfort, promoting efficiency, and averting injury. Exercise is self-imposed, non-life-threatening, physical stress. The other point illustrated by the construction-worker example is that adaptations are stress specific.

Adaptations are Stress Specific

The body responds specifically to each imposed stress. In the example above, the calluses formed only at the contact points; the skin on the entire hand did not thicken. The stress-specificity principle bears important implications for exercise. For example, we discussed earlier how aerobic exercise, while it strengthens the heart and lungs, is ineffective at preserving bone and muscle in the face of aging. This demonstrates that the body does not respond to aerobic exercise by becoming stronger and healthier throughout its entire physiology. Rather, only those systems adapt that are specifically stressed.

The same applies to resistance training. Although resistance training, when done properly, contributes modestly to cardiovascular fitness, aerobic exercise is superior in this regard. The disparity stems from the fact that resistance exercise primarily stresses the skeletal muscles, not the heart and lungs. Accordingly, the adaptive response to resistance training primarily affects the skeletal muscles, not the heart and lungs. This is why, as emphasized earlier, an exercise program should include both of these two different kinds of physical stress - aerobic/cardiovascular and anaerobic/musculoskeletal. In terms of our present discussion, the aim of this two-pronged approach is to trigger two beneficial, but different, adaptations.

The stress-specificity principle transcends the strength/endurance distinction; it applies not only between, but also within, each of these two contexts. For example, recall from earlier in this chapter that both cardiovascular exercise and resistance exercise engage various bioenergetic pathways, depending on intensity and duration. Adaptations are specific to the bioenergetic pathway trained such that an endurance athlete whose training consists of running single miles as fast as possible (thereby engaging the ATP/CP and glycolytic bioenergetic pathways) will enjoy minimal "carry-over benefit" if he/she competes in a 10K run or a marathon (both of which chiefly engage the aerobic bioenergetic pathway), and vice versa. The same limited interchange of benefits occurs in the context of resistance exercise, between higher-rep/lower-load training and lower-rep/higher-load training.

The stress-specificity principle applies to an almost counter-intuitive degree, with limited transfer of benefits occurring among different forms of aerobic exercise. One might reasonably assume the opposite: that there would be complete crossover applicability of fitness increments attained through swimming, running, and bicycling given that all of these modes of exercise impose demands on the cardiovascular system and chiefly engage the aerobic bioenergetic pathway. To the contrary, studies show limited improvement in aerobic capacity when measured during a different mode of aerobic exercise from that which was used to achieve the improvement.[210,211,212,213,214] For example, in the most dramatic finding on this subject, a 10-week swim training program produced significant improvements in Vo_2max among 15 subjects when measured during swimming, but virtually zero improvement was observed when Vo_2max was evaluated during treadmill running![215]

Likewise, when trained male rowers were tested on a cycle ergometer, cardiorespiratory parameters were similar to untrained subjects. But when tested on a rowing ergometer, the same subjects registered readings superior to untrained subjects.[216] Similarly, triathletes (superbly conditioned athletes who compete in an event that includes cycling, running, and swimming) exhibited cardiorespiratory readings inferior to athletes who train and compete only as runners or cyclers, when tested during cycle ergometry and treadmill running.[217] Finally, the stress-specificity principle even applies to the time of day one trains: studies find superior cardiorespiratory performance when the time of day of testing coincides with the time of day of training.[218,219] For the competitive athlete, these findings are of great practical significance; see Appendix B for a discussion of the applicability of stress specificity to sports training. For the average person, the take-home message is: vary your training regimen. (As you will see when we discuss "qualitative progression," there are hormonal advantages, as well, to varying your training regimen.)

272

Exercise Selection and All-in-One Home Fitness Devices

Because it is ideal to vary your mode of cardiovascular training, the concept pushed by the late-night fitness infomercial folks, that there exists one supreme form of cardiovascular exercise (the one they're selling) is inherently false.

Variation is even more important relative to resistance training. The skeletal muscles are many and varied, and they function in intricate patterns of cooperation and opposition. To make matters more complex, there are different muscle fiber types within the muscle which have different firing thresholds such that working a muscle does not necessarily mean working all the fiber types that comprise the muscle. Later, I will discuss how to maximize muscle fiber recruitment. For now, the point to remember is that you should stress each and every muscle to an approximately equal degree. Otherwise, some muscles are forced to adapt while others are not, and this produces a functionally and aesthetically unbalanced body.

The sale of home exercise devices that "work every muscle in the body," while simultaneously providing a cardiovascular workout has become a huge industry, owing to the infomercial revolution and public receptiveness to all-in-one panaceas for getting in shape. Infomercial sales patter notwithstanding, these devices are limited in terms of quality, versatility, and effectiveness. Accordingly, I have a low estimation of the value of most of these contraptions, though I admire the engineering ingenuity they embody.

Unless you are unwilling or unable to exercise away from home, your money would be better spent buying a gym membership. While it may cost more, especially in the long run, there is simply no comparison between one fitness apparatus designed with minimizing production costs a major objective, and a building filled with tens- or hundreds-of-thousands of dollars worth of work-out equipment. Moreover, if you have ever purchased one of these products, upon receiving it you probably acquired a heightened appreciation for the power of lighting, camera angles, music, and an attractive actor/salesperson to make a product look better than it really is. Many people find themselves disappointed in the quality of these products and wind-up using them to hang clothes on - a function for which they often prove more suitable.

Having said all that, applying the principles and techniques of Natural Hormonal Enhancement is much more important than the quality or extent of equipment used. There are millions of people who work-out in exquisitely well-equipped gyms but who, nevertheless, progress at a snail's pace, or not at all, because they are ignorant of the hormonal dynamics of exercise. In the final analysis, tangible tools are of little value if one lacks the intangible tools necessary to apply them properly - specifically, knowledge and commitment.

Strategic Stress

Exercise can be viewed as the strategic application of physical stress as a means of generating desired adaptations. Hormones and their subordinates, enzymes, conduct the remodeling process by which these adaptations are etched into your physique. For example, exercise activates hormones and enzymes that increase fat burning. Not only does this serve to fuel your exercise endeavors, but it also causes a restructuring of your body into a configuration more conducive to physical activity. Earlier, I stated that "the adaptive response to stress is aimed at offsetting discomfort, promoting efficiency, and averting injury" (p. 271). It is discomforting, inefficient, and potentially injurious to carry excess bodyfat with you on a 5-mile run; and the faster you try to run the 5 miles, the more of an encumbrance the excess bodyfat represents.

Just as a construction worker develops calluses on his hands to protect against the stress of abrasive friction, a runner sheds excess bodyfat not only for present fueling purposes but also to protect against the future stress of carrying dead weight (fat) while running.* For the active person, excess fat translates to excess stress. For the sedentary person, this is not the case. Thus, a heightened activity level is a strategically imposed stress designed to make it "impractical" (inefficient) for your body to maintain its current configuration.

The nature and extent of the stress imposed upon the body dictates the nature and extent of changes in body composition and shape. This is why marathon runners tend to be skinny and weak. For their bodies, imposed upon by the extreme stress of running very long distances, not only does bodyfat represent an encumbrance, or stressor, but so does muscle. The point to remember is that exercise-induced adaptations are not necessarily positive, either in terms of health or appearance. Therefore, you must make sure that the nature and extent of the stress you impose upon your body is strategically calculated to produce desired adaptations.

The Principle of Progressivity

You are probably familiar with term "progressive resistance training." Earlier, I defined "training" (demarcated by the "exercise threshold," which varies with fitness level) and I emphasized the importance of resistance (which serves as a vehicle for generating intensity, the key variable in growth hormone release). The "progressive" element is commonly overlooked, but indispensable, to actualizing your physical potential.

Most people who complain about a reduction in their rate of progress or a cessation of progress (known as "plateauing") are training in a manner inconsistent with the principle of progressivity. Simply put, **if you do not exercise progressively, you will not progress**. There are two types of progressivity, *quantitative* and *qualitative*, which we will discuss later.

Progressivity is the practical application of what you learned from "Adaptation to Stress," (above); specifically, that the body responds to each imposed stress, and that adaptations are narrowly tailored. Returning to the previous examples, friction against the skin from construction work causes the skin to toughen at the contact points. Toughness of the skin is an adaptive response, serving as an "antidote" to the stress of abrasive friction. Similarly, long-distance running causes the body to become lighter. Lightweightedness is an "antidote" to the stress of long-distance running. Just as the *kind* of stress dictates the adaptation, so too does the *extent* of stress: the body responds almost exactly to the extent of the stress

---

* There is a subtle and tricky implication of this that holds back many people from achieving continued positive results from cardiovascular training: the adaptations to aerobic exercise, whereby dead weight decreases and metabolic efficiency increases, reduces the stressfulness (i.e., makes easier) a given quantity of aerobic exercise. In other words, running a 10-minute mile might be a good workout for you in January when you begin your exercise program. But in May, when your body has adapted by dropping dead weight in the form of bodyfat, the intensity level (effort intensity and relative intensity) of running the same 10-minute mile will be lower because body weight will be less and metabolic efficiency will be greater. The practical effect is that if you do not increase duration, frequency, or intensity of your cardiovascular workouts, weight loss coupled with heightened metabolic efficiency will spell diminishing returns and eventually no returns. In other words, you will stop progressing or "plateau". Thus, if you are one of those people who, despite making some progress initially, "just can't lose those few extra pounds of fat," your progress and associated adaptations may, ironically, be responsible for the cessation of progress. This illustrates the critical importance of progressivity to achieving positive results from exercise.

274

encountered (i.e., adaptations are "narrowly tailored"). Once the body has effectively responded to a stressor, by becoming stronger, tougher, lighter, etc., it will respond no further to that stressor.

> **EXAMPLE**: The stress of attempting to lift 100 pounds will trigger a "remodeling" of the muscles and an increase in strength, which (assuming adequate nutrition and recovery time) will make the person undergoing this stress ("Stressee") more nearly able to lift 100 pounds. Eventually, if this stress is repeated and nutrition and recovery are adequate, Stressee will be able to lift 100 pounds. However, this particular stressor will not, no matter how many times Stressee is exposed to it, enable Stressee to lift 120 pounds or 150 pounds.

> **ANALOGY**: Think of a restaurant patron who never leaves more than a 15% tip, regardless of the quality of the service. This person pays the necessary amount, the bill, plus the minimum consistent with the mores of society - it's called stingy, and it also describes the way in which the human body adapts to stress. Whereas the stingy restaurant patron strives to conserve money, the body strives to conserve something much more valuable - energy.

Energy is necessary for survival, and all living things conserve energy. Every activity undertaken and everything that goes on inside the body - circulation, digestion, getting out of bed in the morning, brushing your teeth, thinking, breathing, sex, *adaptive responses*, etc. - requires energy. Because the physical restructuring process consumes energy (calories), the body "wants" to do as little restructuring as possible. Not only would a beyond-minimal-adaptation be a waste of energy, but it would also render the body *less*-well-adapted to its environment because the body and the external stressors it encounters would not match as closely as possible. The practical implication of this is that **you must continually <u>increase</u> or <u>vary</u> the stress of exercise in order to continue to progress**. The reluctance of the body to change its shape and composition (a fact all-too-apparent to those who have tried to effect such changes) must be overcome by the insistent prodding of new and/or greater stress.

Qualitative Progression = Introduction of a new stressor

Quantitative Progression = Increase in magnitude of an existing stressor

General Hormonal Response to Exercise

Although adaptations are narrowly tailored to each stressor, exercise also generates overall or systemic improvements. For one, a properly designed exercise program improves endocrine function.

Hormonal output is limited by the functional capacity of the secreting glands. As explained in Chapter 4, absent proper intervention, the entire body, inside and out, deteriorates with advancing age. The deterioration of the glands is part of a self-perpetuating cycle in which weaker glands yield less hormonal output, and less hormonal output results in deterioration of the entire body - including the glands that secrete hormones.

In view of the "use it or lose it" axiom, it is reasonable to posit that exercise, which causes a storm of hormonal activity, would be able to revive a flagging endocrine system. In fact, there is considerable evidence to support this hypothesis. During the 1930's, a series of studies using rats, published in the *American Journal of Anatomy*, found pronounced changes in the weight of glands after a training period lasting 90 days.[220,221,222] Specifically, significant increases in mass were found in the adrenals, pituitary, thyroid, thymus, and gonads as a result of the 90-day exercise program. Exercise was then discontinued, and after 125 days of detraining, the weight of the glands was back to initial levels. Further studies since then have confirmed the revitalizing effect of exercise on the endocrine system.[223,224]

As well, exercise increases blood supply to the glands, and improved blood supply enhances endocrine function.[225] Studies show, moreover, that people who exercise regularly have higher levels of growth hormone;[226] lower levels of insulin (resulting from higher insulin sensitivity);[227] and in men, higher levels of testosterone;[228] than do their sedentary counterparts. Furthermore, it is not uncommon for older, fit individuals to have better hormonal profiles than younger, unfit individuals.[229]

Bringing it all Together: "How Adaptation to Stress" and "Progressivity" Relate to Hormones

As you can see, the "use it or lose it" axiom applies to the endocrine system. However, simply "using it," while sufficient to enhance endocrine function, is not sufficient to elicit continued hormonal response to exercise. Additional hormonal output (i.e., hormonal enhancement) occurs only when an adaptation is *needed*. (Remember: adaptations consume energy and the human body conserves energy; thus, adaptations occur grudgingly not gratuitously.) The only time when an adaptation is needed is when the body encounters stress that it is ill-suited to handle. What kind of stressor is the body ill-suited to handle? New stress.

Progressivity refers to the continuous imposition of new stress on the body. Training progressively means continually increasing and/or continually changing the stress imposed on the body, thereby continually creating new stress. (The astute linguist will note that an "increase" in stress is a "change" in stress; bear with this artificial distinction for now, it will become more meaningful when we discuss quantitative and qualitative progression.)

Absent new stress, the hormonal response to exercise declines.[230,231,232,233] This is because a given stressor becomes decreasingly stressful as the body adapts to it (translating to a fall in relative intensity, which is defined on p. 253 as "a measure of physical stress"). Ultimately, the absence of new stress = no stress = no adaptive stimulus = no hormonal response. Got it?

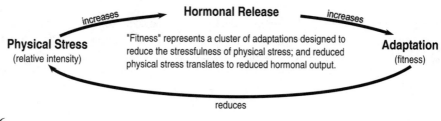

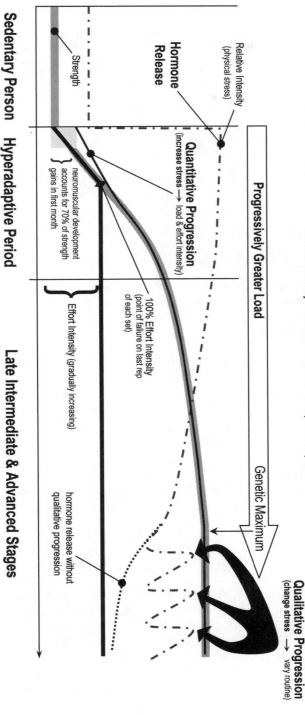

Adaptive Response to Exercise

Relative Intensity = Hormone Release = Adaptive Response

Relative Intensity
(physical stress)

Hormone
Release

Strength

Quantitative Progression
(increase stress → load & effort intensity)

neuromuscular development
accounts for 70% of strength
gains in first month

100% Effort Intensity
(point of failure on last rep
of each set)

Effort Intensity (gradually increasing)

Progressively Greater Load

Genetic Maximum

hormone release without
qualitative progression

Qualitative Progression
(change stress → vary routine)

Sedentary Person

Hyperadaptive Period
6 - 8 months (beginner)

Late Intermediate & Advanced Stages

277

Does Increased Exercise Tolerance Mean You Should Weight Train More Frequently?

As discussed earlier, the answer to this question is no. Although the cortisol response to a given stressor diminishes with repeated exposure and recovery ability increases, it is also true, as discussed above, that as a general rule strength gains exceed improvements in recovery ability. And as strength increases, so does the ability to impose stress on one's own body through exercise. For this reason, if you are increasing e-intensity and load appropriately, frequency of exercise generally does not increase. Remember, too, that the imperative to increase e-intensity must be tempered by prudence. If you increase intensity too rapidly, the increased stress will outpace the increase in recovery ability. Consequently, cortisol levels escalate, and you experience negative results including muscle loss, immune suppression, or injury.

The temptation to overtrain increases as recovery ability increases. One of the features of improved recovery ability is reduced post-workout muscle discomfort and pain, even as e-intensity increases. This can be deceptive because the absence of soreness leads people to believe, erroneously, that recovery is complete. Don't make this mistake; **muscle soreness is not an accurate index of recovery**.

Growth Hormone Response to Exercise: Critiquing Training Routines

Now that we have explored some major concepts relating to the hormonal response to exercise, we can return to the question of how to structure your workouts to enhance growth hormone levels. First, let's review what you have learned so far about the growth hormone response to exercise.

• Growth hormone release is determined by anabolic intensity. Specifically, growth hormone release is related to effort intensity (e-intensity), which refers to how much effort you exert while exercising, and relative intensity (r-intensity), which refers to the quantum of physical stress imposed by your workout. (Remember that stress can only be quantified with reference to the person undergoing it - a workout that is stressful to you may not be stressful to a fitter person.)

• R-intensity is related to progressivity in the following way: if you do not progressively *increase* e-intensity and/or load (or *change* your workout in other ways), r-intensity will decline and, consequently, so will growth hormone output.

Now let's see how this operates in real life. . .

HYPOTHETICAL #1

Joe is a 25-year-old couch potato who is embarking upon a resistance training program for the first time, in compliance with his New Year's resolution to get in shape. The heaviest things Joe has lifted during the preceding year are a telephone receiver and a TV remote control. On his first day in the gym, Joe, following the instructions of his $100-per-hour personal trainer, takes it easy: after an extensive warm-up on the treadmill, he begins his weight training session, performing repetitions until the set becomes difficult, at about 10 reps, then he stops, not approaching the point of failure. A few minutes later, he does another set of the same exercise and then moves on to another exercise. After a total of 10 sets of 10 reps, all performed up to the same e-intensity level, he goes home.

Let's analyze Joe's workout:

Effort Intensity: Moderate. E-intensity is moderate because Joe did not even approach the point of failure on his final repetition of any of his sets - a wise decision in view of his beginner status. However, Joe did proceed to the point at which each set became "difficult"; and since each set became difficult at about 10 reps, Joe was using a significant load. (Even though Joe is young, his previously sedentary lifestyle and his unfamiliarity with weight training would counsel a lower e-intensity level and lesser load on his first day in the gym, with emphasis on proper exercise execution.)

Relative Intensity: High. Compared with a telephone receiver and a TV remote control, the weights Joe lifted at the gym were very heavy. Furthermore, the muscular effort required to lift the weight repetitively to the point at which it became difficult constituted a substantially greater output of muscular effort than Joe is accustomed to as a couch potato who has not exercised at all during the last year.

Growth Hormone/Adaptive Response: Yes. Joe's body will perceive his experience in the gym as a threat and will "defend" against a recurrence of that stressful episode by adapting. The adaptation will be aimed at making sure that if a stressor of a similar nature and extent were to emerge in the future, it would be less stressful. Growth hormone will be released in response to the stress of Joe's workout to orchestrate the adaptive process by shifting metabolism into a fat-burning mode, which will simultaneously preserve glycogen and will make extra fuel available (from bodyfat) to fulfill the heightened energy demands of the recovery/restructuring process. Additionally, growth hormone spurs protein synthesis, the process by which distressed muscles, bones, and connective tissues are strengthened (i.e., made better able to withstand the stress imposed by a similar workout in the future). Remember, *the body hates stress* - it views it as a threat to its survival - and it will go to extraordinary lengths (including dramatically changing shape and composition) to neutralize stress.

If these workouts continue, and if Joe progressively increases e-intensity and load, Joe's body will be forced to change its shape and composition to better deal with the physical stress of lifting weights. Specifically, Joe's fat/muscle ratio will drop. This will cause a redistribution of tissue (since muscle and fat are each concentrated in different areas), accounting for a transformation in the shape of Joe's body.

HYPOTHETICAL #2

Jessica is a 22-year-old healthy woman. She has been exercising regularly for one year. She jogs two miles each day, and she trains with weights. She performs each set to the point at which it becomes difficult, at about 25 reps. She scrupulously avoids the point of failure based on advice from a friend to the effect that if she works-out too intensely she'll "get big." Fearing for her femininity, and just interested in "toning-up," Jessica adheres to her friend's advice.

First, let's analyze the weight training component of Jessica's regimen:

<u>Effort Intensity</u>: Moderate (same as Joe, above).

<u>Relative Intensity</u>: Low (very different from Joe).

<u>Growth Hormone/Adaptive Response</u>: No. Jessica is being led astray by her misinformed friend. A healthy 22-year-old woman who has been weight training regularly for one year is well-suited to higher intensity exercise than what she is doing. Because Jessica's workout routine has changed neither quantitatively nor qualitatively since she began working-out a year ago, neither will the shape and composition of her body change. Stated differently, Jessica is not applying challenging stress to her body; hence, growth hormone will not be released, and adaptation will not occur. Because her weight- training routine is fundamentally flawed, Jessica is deriving little benefit from her time spent lifting weights.

While Jessica's resistance training routine will not produce positive results, the minimal stress it imposes will maintain previously achieved fitness increments (as opposed to quitting training, which would cause r-intensity to plummet resulting in a rollback of training-induced adaptations). As a 22-year-old woman, Jessica is probably not much concerned about the degenerative aspects of aging, poised to strike like a crouching cougar lying in wait. But if she is going to offset the age-related trend of muscle loss and bone loss that will commence sometime around her 30th birthday, she is going to have to generate enhanced anabolic activity; and that means progressively increasing the e-intensity of her workouts. A modicum of added muscle and bone density secured in young adulthood pays large dividends later in life in terms of reducing the risk of osteoporosis and preserving the firm shapeliness that defines a youthful, sexy body.

With regard to load, the weight Jessica is using is too light, as evidenced by the fact that she can do 25 reps before each set becomes difficult. Inadequate resistance is problematic because, in addition to making it more difficult to generate sufficient intensity, it precludes stimulation of the full spectrum of muscle fibers. The inadequate load, as well as her low e-intensity level, probably stems from the popular notion that light weight and high reps are ideal for "toning-up." In fact, "toning-up" is an adaptive response, and Jessica's workout does not meet the standard for inducing such a response.

Now, let's analyze the aerobic component of Jessica's regimen:

Jessica deserves credit for including both resistance training and cardiovascular training in her exercise regimen, but she is making the same mistake with regard to the latter as she is with the former: no progression. Ideally, she should increase the e-intensity of her running by employing the interval format described on p. 267-268.

280

However, if she enjoys jogging, that's fine; she can rely on weight training for growth hormone release (provided she upgrades the intensity), and increase the distance rather than the intensity of her running. Low-intensity, high-duration aerobic exercise, while not ideal hormonally, is nevertheless beneficial in terms of cardiovascular fitness and fat loss. Jogging becomes hormonally problematic only when 1) it comprises your entire exercise regimen, or 2) when it "pushes you over the top" in terms of overall (aerobic + anaerobic) volume.

While increasing the distance she runs can help Jessica lose fat, it can also unfavorably shift her hormonal profile by increasing volume without a corresponding increase in intensity (thus reducing the intensity/volume ratio). Therefore, Jessica must be extra diligent in keeping her weight-training sessions brief, intense, and not too frequent in order to counter the intensity/volume reduction caused by increasing her running distance. In addition to the intensity/volume ratio, total volume must also be carefully monitored, with reference to sleep, nutrition, and emotional stress (see p. 258).

HYPOTHETICAL #3

Bill, a world-class rower, departs from his usual 60-minute workout in his boat and instead does a 60-minute workout, of equal e-intensity, consisting of calisthenics and running.

Effort Intensity: High (same as Bill's rowing workouts).

Relative Intensity: High (different from Bill's rowing workouts). Although Bill is a world-class athlete, he is a rower not a runner. And as you learned earlier, adaptations are stress specific and fitness increments obtained through one mode of exercise are not fully transferable to other modes of exercise. Therefore, although the e-intensity of his running/calisthenics workout is the same as the e-intensity of his rowing workouts, the r-intensity of his running/calisthenics workout is greater.

Growth Hormone/Adaptive Response: Yes. This hypothetical is based on a study of world-class rowers published in the *British Medical Journal* in 1973.[234] In this study, a 60-minute rowing workout did not elevate growth hormone levels, but a significant elevation was registered by the same subjects after a 60-minute running/calisthenics workout. This is an example of qualitative progression: the running/calisthenics workout represented an unaccustomed stress to the rowers and thus it triggered an adaptive response even though there was no increase in any quantitative stress factor.

The Hyperadaptive Period
(Beginner and Early Intermediate Stages)

Typically, the most dramatic results from exercise occur during the first 6-8 months. The adaptive response is greatest at this time, because the body is unaccustomed to the stress of exercise. Adaptations occur in virtually all physiological systems, including: cardiovascular, neuromuscular, respiratory, endocrine, and skeletal.

With resistance exercise, hyperadaptivity is amplified due to the centrality of the neuromuscular system in this type of training. Neuromuscular conditioning is sometimes referred to as the "mind-muscle connection." No matter how big, a muscle is useless unless the brain can effectively communicate stimulatory signals to the motor units that comprise the muscle. When you begin a weight-training program, the mind-muscle connection is not well-established for the specific task of lifting weights. If you have ever experienced "the shakes" (where your hands quiver under the strain of lifting), you have experienced what happens when the brain tries to order the muscles to do something they are not accustomed to doing - they balk like a person given an urgent command in a foreign language. With each successive workout, the brain is able to recruit more motor units (motor unit = a motor nerve + the muscle fibers it activates). In technical terms, this is called "neural facilitation" or "neural disinhibition," and it constitutes a much larger component of "strength" than most people realize.

Enhanced motor unit recruitment is the most immediate and extensive improvement that occurs in response to resistance training. In fact, most of the strength gains that occur during the early stages of this type of exercise program result from neural facilitation not from structural changes in the muscle fibers.[235,236,237] This explains how substantial increases in strength can occur absent an increase in muscle size. During the first month of resistance training, approximately 70% of strength gains are owed to adaptations within the nervous system.[238] Thereafter, neural adaptations continue at a slower rate, and muscular adaptations become the predominant contributor to strength gains.

Thus, in the beginning, as new neuromuscular pathways are being established, strength improves independently of change in muscle structure (which also occurs, but accounts for much less of the initial jump in strength). After that, the rate of neural adaptation slows and, consequently, so do strength gains which now are wholly dependent on development of muscle fibers (a much slower and more energy-intensive process than neural facilitation). The sharp increase in strength that occurs during the first few months of resistance training allows for correspondingly greater physical stress self-imposition via exercise. Accordingly, quantitative progression occurs more or less automatically, and so do adaptive responses. For this reason, weight trainees typically experience a steady onward march of progress during the first 6-8 months. But as the hyperadaptive period ends, the rate of progress slows considerably.

Why Layoffs are Often More Helpful than Harmful

Just as neuromuscular conditioning occurs rapidly upon beginning a weight-training program, so neuromuscular de-conditioning occurs rapidly upon stopping working-out, accounting for much of the depressing drop in strength that results from even a brief layoff.[239] But take heart, "muscle memory" allows you to regain your strength faster than the first time around[240] (this is *not* intended to provide a rationalization for taking unwarranted layoffs!).

One detraining effect of taking a layoff from lifting weights is a steep reduction in muscle glycogen and water storage.[241] The combination of becoming "weaker" (from neuromuscular regression) and "smaller" (from a reduction in muscle glycogen and water content) can be quite unsettling for some people. It is common to hear people bemoan their rapid loss of muscle and strength following a brief layoff. In fact, this feeds the tendency toward overtraining. "Once bitten" by the psychological trauma of witnessing his or her hard-earned gains apparently evaporate in a matter of weeks, the weight trainee becomes "twice shy" about a repetition of this unpleasant experience; and this often manifests itself as an irrational fear of losing muscle and a consequent compulsion to train too frequently. But although the weight loss, muscle shrinkage, and strength reduction associated with a brief layoff are real and not imagined, these changes are not cause for alarm or despair because they do not reflect an actual loss of muscle mass; and the pre-detraining level of muscle size and strength can be restored as rapidly, or more rapidly, as it was lost.

In fact, layoffs can often work to your advantage both mentally and physically. Mentally, trainees frequently report renewed focus and resolve upon returning to the gym following a layoff. Physically, a layoff can have a "recharging effect," especially for someone who had been overtraining. Remember, overtraining is a cumulative phenomenon; and any time you are training at a high level of relative intensity you are, in effect, "training on the edge." (By "training on the edge," I am referring to the fact that there is a fine line between optimal training and overtraining, and when you train at a high level of relative intensity you are treading this line.) For this reason, I actually recommend occasional layoffs as a sort of "insurance" against overtraining.

Oftentimes, by re-igniting the adaptive process, a layoff will jump-start new physiological improvements, propelling you beyond barriers or plateaus. As odd as it may seem, it is not uncommon for anabolic and lipolytic hormone levels to *increase* during a brief layoff. For example, in a study conducted at East Carolina University, a 14-day layoff from training in weightlifters corresponded with increases in growth hormone (58.3%) and testosterone (19.2%), and a decrease in cortisol (21.5%).[242] Naturally, the hormonal benefits of a layoff are greater the more overtrained you are at the time of the layoff, and are minimal if you are not overtrained. But the point is that, contrary to what the average compulsive exerciser may think, and contrary to what his/her body may seem to be suggesting by becoming "weaker" and "smaller" during a brief layoff, an occasional layoff is, in the final analysis, more likely to be helpful than harmful.

Once the initial "shock" of a new form of physical stress (i.e., weight training) begins to taper-off, it becomes increasingly difficult to stimulate adaptive responses. Accordingly, after the hyperadative period ends, diminishing returns become the order of the day, leading to a cessation of noticeable improvement, referred to as a "plateau." Some people assume at this point that they have maximized their genetic potential - but this is rarely the case. It is at this point where bodybuilders, despairing of their lack of progress, will often begin to flirt with the idea of taking steroids.

To avoid "plateauing," it is important to understand that physical improvements resulting from exercise do not happen at a steady rate. Consider, for example, that it is not unusual for a man's bench press to increase from 150 lbs. to 200 lbs. during the first six months of a weight-training program. Does this mean that if this guy continues training consistently for the next ten years that he will be able to bench press more than 1,000 lbs.? (1000 = 50-pound increase every 6 months for twenty 6-month periods) Or that after twenty years he will be able to bench press a small automobile? I think not. Clearly, fitness/strength does not advance along a linear upward path. Rather, the greatest increment occurs during the hyperadative period.

As you exit the hyperadaptive period, the rate of increase in strength (and therefore load) slows markedly. Similarly, once you reach 100% e-intensity on the last rep of each set, this stress factor too supplies less stress than it had previously (when it was increasing). Thus, with quantitative progression grinding to a halt, the quantum of physical stress delivered by each workout diminishes. Recall that "the quantum of physical stress" = relative intensity = hormonal release. In effect, at this point you are "boxed-in" by your own progress. If you don't want to be stuck in this box forever, you had better pay close attention to the following discussion.

Progressing Beyond
(Late Intermediate and Advanced Stages)

As explained above, completion of the first 6-8 months of resistance training generally marks the beginning of the end of visible results. By this time, you have been training at 100% final-rep e-intensity for several months and (assuming you began training as a fully grown adult) your strength gains have begun to slow considerably. *To avoid having your results stymied by these inexorable trends, you must find a way to increase r-intensity by means other than increasing e-intensity or load.* In other words, you must find new ways to self-impose challenging physical stress.

You know, based on what you have learned so far, that although increasing frequency or duration would represent additional stress, it would likely be bad stress from a hormonal standpoint. Working-out more frequently would curtail recovery and, therefore, impede desired adaptations. In addition, because increased frequency would increase volume but not e-intensity, it would decrease the intensity/volume ratio. An increase in duration is likely to have an even worse effect on the intensity/volume ratio by both increasing volume and decreasing e-intensity. (And a reduction in the intensity/volume ratio negatively shifts your hormonal profile away from growth hormone and testosterone toward cortisol, right?)

Another way to introduce new stress is to increase load. Unlike increasing duration, increasing load does not decrease e-intensity. In fact, increasing load tends to boost e-intensity, because greater intensity of effort is required to lift a greater load than a lesser load over a given period of time, see p. 251. However, you are limited in your ability to increase load after the hyperadaptive period, because of a sharp reduction in the rate of strength gains. Thus, increasing load may force your repetitions down too low, resulting in sub-optimal muscle fiber recruitment. Furthermore, increasing load will increase volume if all other training variables remain the same; and higher volume brings you closer to overtraining.

As you can see, whereas quantitative progression was your ticket to success in the beginning and early intermediate stages of your exercise career, a new strategy for generating physical stress is required if you are to maintain r-intensity and continue to elicit positive adaptive responses. This new strategy is called qualitative progression.

Qualitative Progression

Unlike increasing e-intensity, frequency, duration, or load, qualitative progression does not involve changing the degree of stress, but rather the nature of stress. We saw an example of qualitative progression in Hypothetical #3 (p. 281).

The best and worst feature of exercise is that it is habit-forming.

The saying, "habit can be the best of servants or the worst of masters" applies to exercise. While habit can work to your advantage by keeping you adhered to an exercise program, it can also work to your detriment by keeping you in a rut once you get into one. There are many veteran exercise enthusiasts who do the exact same workout week after week, month after month, year after year. Any psychologist knows that routine is a source of psychological comfort and security. However, physical discomfort and insecurity imposed by unaccustomed stress is what triggers adaptive changes in the human body. This discrepancy represents a trap that ensnares most people who work-out.

This is not to suggest that you should not have a set routine. *Especially as a novice, you should be as consistent and regimented as possible;* and this means largely disregarding qualitative progression and, instead, concentrating on 1) gradually increasing e-intensity and load (quantitative progression) and 2) practicing proper exercise execution. Only later (6-12 months after beginning training) when quantitative progression becomes unavailing, does it become imperative to employ qualitative progression. And this entails deliberate departures from your training routine.

Apollo's Creed

Our discussion of qualitative progression calls to mind a scene from one of the Rocky movies. In Rocky III, Rocky's former-adversary-turned-trainer, Apollo Creed, asked Rocky's brother-in-law, Paulie, if Rocky could swim. Paulie replied, "With a name like Rock?" Undeterred, Creed had Rocky swim laps as part of his training regimen. When Paulie protested, Creed responded to the effect that Rocky had to stretch and use muscles he never knew he had. This emphasis, not on training harder or longer, but rather on training *differently*, illustrates the concept of qualitative progression.

The effects of qualitative progression can be quite remarkable. For instance, an experienced bodybuilder, who has for years intensely trained his shoulders and lats (muscles on the outer part of the back), is likely to experience acute soreness in those muscles as a result of hitting a punching bag. Even though the muscles trained are the same, hitting the punching bag is likely to produce much more soreness than the bodybuilder's weight-lifting workouts (and vice versa if a boxer who regularly hits the bag lifts weights one day instead). The same applies to a runner who goes roller-blading for the first time, or a long-jumper who high-jumps, or an overhand pitcher who throws sidearm.

Similarly, although weightlifters tend to scoff at push-ups because it is a relatively low-resistance exercise, push-ups can be an effective adaptive stimulus. Musculoskeletal exercises that entail moving the body through space against gravity, like push-ups and pullups, involve neuromuscular activation patterns different from bench press and pulldowns, even though the movements are the same, respectively. Even a bodybuilder who can bench-press 500 pounds is likely to become very sore, indicating exposure to unaccustomed stress, if he attempts a workout of similar duration and e-intensity consisting of push-ups.

Likewise, whether you are a champion powerlifter who can squat 700 pounds or a 200-meter Olympic gold medalist, playing basketball is likely to produce soreness if your legs are not accustomed to the specific stress of jumping. Why? Because, although all three activities train the same bodypart, the stress imposed by each is *qualitatively* different. Unaccustomed physical stress is conducive to hormonal release.

$$\textbf{Unaccustomed Stress} \xrightarrow{\text{increases}} \textbf{Relative Intensity} \xrightarrow{\text{increases}} \textbf{Hormonal Release}$$

Even among advanced trainees, few make a calculated effort to introduce new stress. Instead, most people who exercise make the mistake of "sticking with what works" until it no longer works, and then continuing to stick with it. Avoid this mistake, don't stagnate. Keep your workout routine fresh and always stay one step ahead of your body by applying quantitative progression and then, when you are further along, qualitative progression as well. This will keep growth hormone flowing, and it will promote continued adaptation resulting in positive remodeling of your body.

Progression = Progress

You are limited only by your imagination in applying the principle of qualitative progression. Be creative. If you usually jog, try hiking. Or try running backwards (carefully), which shifts the emphasis from the hamstrings and calves to the quadriceps and tibialles anterior muscles. If you usually swim using the breast stroke and the crawl, try the backstroke and the butterfly. Apply qualitative progression in the gym by tinkering with: rest intervals between sets, exercise selection, repetition speed, or the sequence in which you perform exercises.

As elaborated below, you can also employ qualitative progression by means of short-term manipulations in volume. In other words, short-term alterations in *quantitative* factors - frequency, duration, e-intensity, and load - can act as a means of *qualitative* progression. Forced reps, a technique in which a spotter assists the lifter past the point of failure, thereby enabling the lifter to transcend 100% e-intensity, can be an effective means of introducing new stress. Other techniques like supersets and weighted negatives also can be used to vary the stress. However, these advanced techniques should be used sparingly and followed by added recovery time. Another caveat: do not go overboard with qualitative progression such that your exercise regimen loses all continuity and becomes haphazard. Maintain a foundational routine and work within those confines most of the time with only occasional, calculated departures.

Qualitative Progression is Good for the Brain

New and exciting research suggests that qualitative progression techniques not only benefit the body, but the brain too. Scientists have long known that exercise can elevate mood and foster feelings of well-being by means of its effect on neurotransmitters and endorphins. Now it is becoming evident that exercise can improve cognitive function, as well.[243,244,245,246,247]

Evidence suggests that establishing new neuromuscular pathways causes positive neurological changes in the structure of the brain,[248,249] which may be helpful in preventing Alzheimer's disease[250] and improving intelligence.[251,252] The key to obtaining these benefits is to challenge your brain and muscles to interact to produce new and different movements. Striving to master new motor skills by taking up new sports or physically demanding, technique-oriented hobbies like dance, rock climbing, or golf are effective ways to accomplish this objective. Weight training is exceptionally well-suited for improving motor skills because of the wide variety of movements and the coordination needed to execute the exercises properly.[253] Each time you master a new motor skill, you force your brain and muscles to develop a closer relationship by means of forging new mind-muscle connections. Furthermore, reinforcement of mind-muscle communication helps maintain reaction time, hand-eye coordination, and balance in the face of advancing age. In fact, it is lack of activity, more so than aging itself, that accounts for motor skill deterioration in the elderly.[254]

If you do aerobics at your gym, look into "boxercise," "aqua-aerobics," "jazzercise," "spinning," and "step aerobics." Rope skipping is an excellent form of exercise from a neuromuscular standpoint because of the cooperation it requires between the arms and legs. In short, seek out and pursue new neuromuscular challenges!

Testosterone Response to Exercise

The effect of exercise on androgen levels has been the subject of much study and debate for many years. The scientific evidence appears to be contradictory with studies showing exercise increases testosterone levels, others showing it decreases testosterone levels, and still others showing no effect. We can reconcile the seemingly conflicting evidence in view of our present understanding that the effect of exercise on testosterone status depends on the exercise variables that we have been discussing throughout this chapter (frequency, intensity, duration, volume, load, and exercise selection).

At the most basic level, exercise is physical activity and, in general, men who are active and fit have higher testosterone levels than men who are inactive and unfit. Exercise can lower testosterone levels too, however. As is the case with growth hormone, proper modulation of exercise variables is the key to testosterone enhancement. In particular, excessive volume is associated with reduced testosterone levels and elevated cortisol levels. Remember, too, that anything that supports growth hormone production indirectly enhances testosterone production due to the mutually-reinforcing relationship between these two hormones (see Chapter 4).

If you overtrain, your testosterone levels will fall, period. Subject to that important qualification, resistance exercise is less likely to lower testosterone levels and more likely to raise them than endurance exercise. Endurance exercise, by increasing overall fitness, can increase testosterone levels;[255] however, this type of physical stress (low e-ntensity) does not evoke substantial positive testosterone or growth hormone responses.

287

Unchecked by a countervailing anabolic stimulus, low-intensity/volume-ratio exercise produces a substantial catabolic effect when volume is high. Especially where sleep, nutrition, and emotional stress are sub-optimal, endurance training is hormonally problematic.

The effect of endurance training on testosterone status can be summarized as follows. Moderate-volume endurance exercise may increase testosterone levels as compared with being sedentary, and it generally will not lower testosterone levels. However, a training regimen that consists of high-volume, aerobic-only exercise is likely to reduce testosterone levels. This may not be welcome news to avid joggers, but the scientific evidence leaves no doubt regarding the potentially suppressive effect of high-volume, low-intensity exercise on testosterone levels in men.[256,257,258,259,260,261,262]

Unlike endurance training, resistance training, with its higher intensity/volume ratio, positively impacts upon the pituitary-testicular axis.[263,264,265] Whereas the stimulus for testosterone enhancement - intensity - is the same as for growth hormone enhancement, the testosterone response to exercise is more complex. Specifically, testosterone enhancement resulting from resistance training is a net result produced by the enhancing effect outweighing an associated suppressive effect (see diagram p. 265). The growth hormone response, by contrast, is more immediate and one-directional. The delayed and dualistic nature of the testosterone response to resistance training creates an opportunity to either magnify or negate the hormonal benefits of such exercise depending on how adeptly you manipulate recovery periods and other variables. Where exercise variables are properly modulated, resistance training increases testosterone levels in men.[266,267,268]

Whereas the pituitary/adrenocortical (growth hormone and cortisol) response to exercise is rapid and occurs during exercise, the gonadal (testosterone) response is largely delayed and occurs mainly during the recovery period. For a period of time after an intense workout, testosterone levels are suppressed and cortisol levels are elevated. If, *and only if*, adequate recovery time follows, testosterone will rebound beyond initial levels to drive the anabolic process, and cortisol levels will fall (see diagram p. 265). **This flip-flop in the testosterone/cortisol ratio is the pivotal event in the muscle-building process.** If you train too frequently, testosterone never gets a chance to rebound fully, and cortisol remains elevated. In this catabolic hormonal state, muscle growth cannot occur. If you chronically make this mistake, you become overtrained, a condition marked by the predominance of cortisol over testosterone.[269,270,271]

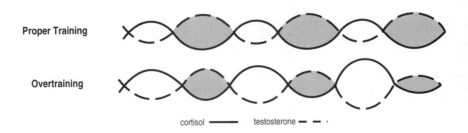

Let's examine testosterone kinetics more closely. Shortly after a workout ends, or during a workout if it runs too long, testosterone levels fall.[272,273,274] Where intensity is high, testosterone can begin its descent as early as 30 minutes after you begin exercising.[275] Continuing to hammer-away at the weights after testosterone has begun to fall exacerbates the decline, forcing testosterone levels even lower while elevating cortisol levels. If like so many enthusiastic and dedicated weight trainees you are doing 2-hour marathon workout sessions - WAKE-UP - you are sabotaging muscle growth and undermining your hormonal health. Train intensely and get out of the gym within one hour, preferably within 30-45 minutes.

You will be amazed at how focus and intensity can more than compensate for duration; and a time limit promotes focus and intensity. By contrast, not having a time limit fosters a leisurely attitude inconsistent with the burning sense of purpose that is the quintessence of great workouts. Thus, you will find that self-imposed time urgency serves not only to constrain your workout to hormonally correct duration, but it also helps you cultivate a more focused workout mindset.

Remember, from the time you begin your workout, the hormonal clock is ticking.

The amount of time after an intense workout ends before testosterone rebounds can range from a few hours to several days.[276] There are several factors that influence the timing of the testosterone rebound, all of which have appeared repetitively throughout this chapter. The better your status in terms of *fitness level, nutrition, emotional stress*, and *sleep*, the shallower the exercise-induced testosterone drop will be and the quicker and stronger the rebound will be.

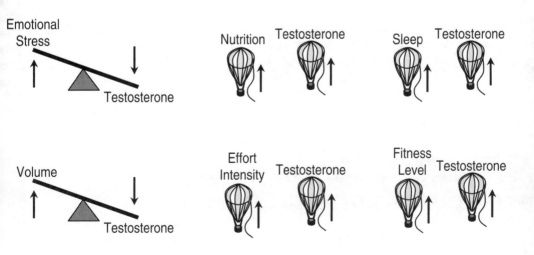

The greater the volume of a workout, the deeper testosterone will drop[277] and the longer it will take to make its comeback. E-Intensity modifies this dynamic,[278] with higher e-intensity propelling testosterone higher on the rebound and increasing the potential differential between the catabolic period and the ensuing anabolic period (see discussion of "anabolic potential" on p. 253).

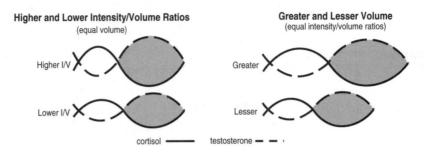

Where a man exercises at an intensity level greatly in excess of his fitness level, testosterone can remain depressed for several days. Conversely, an insufficiently intense workout is likely to produce a minimal post-exercise drop in testosterone (or none at all). This may, on the surface, appear desirable. But no drop means no rebound, and no rebound means no enhancement. *The strategy for testosterone enhancement is to exercise at an intensity level sufficient to cause a **temporary post-exercise drop** in testosterone and then use optimal nutrition and rest to cause a **rapid and exaggerated rebound**.*

When testosterone consistently rises higher than it falls and stays high longer than it stays low, the net result is a higher overall testosterone level (hormonal enhancement).

Anabolic intensity (see p. 254) is the decisive variable in testosterone enhancement, but even where a-intensity is low, men will derive testosterone-boosting benefits from exercise due to increased blood flow to the testicles. Leg presses and squats, in particular, channel blood flow to this area. This serves to illustrate how, in terms of testosterone status (and all other physiological parameters, for that matter), *although more exercise is not necessarily better, some exercise is better than no exercise.*

Beyond the fact that testosterone levels dip in the post-intense-exercise hours and then rebound later, it is difficult to generalize about the schedule of exercise-induced testosterone fluctuations because of the multitude of variables that affect it. This makes determining optimal recovery periods an inexact science. Even so, the factors discussed on p. 289 will give you meaningful guidance regarding how to structure your training program for optimal testosterone response.

In addition to the factors discussed on p. 289, genetics bear on testosterone levels and on hormonal status in general. Like all biological parameters, testosterone levels reflect a continuum, ranging from low-normal to high-normal. For a man with naturally high testosterone levels, the lows will be higher and the highs will also be higher than for a man with a lower baseline testosterone level. Nonetheless, no matter where you are on the testosterone continuum, optimizing nutrition, fitness, exercise volume and the intensity/volume ratio, sleep, and emotional stress, will translate to higher testosterone levels and improved hormonal status across the board.

Steroids and Testosterone Levels

Steroids block cortisol and unnaturally enhance testosterone, thereby blunting the exercise-induced fall in testosterone and hastening and heightening the testosterone rebound. This accounts for the enhanced recovery ability of steroid-users *and it exposes the folly of adopting the training routines of professional bodybuilders* (since virtually all pro bodybuilders take steroids, see Appendix A). The powerful anabolic and anti-catabolic effects of steroids explain why steroids are so effective at building muscle. While there is no doubt that steroids facilitate muscle growth, there is also no doubt that they can cause serious health problems. We have discussed the dangers of exogenous hormones at various points in this book, and I would recommend closely re-reading those sections if you are considering taking steroids (see also "Yuppie Steroids - The Testosterone Revolution," in Chapter 22).

Given the vagaries of testosterone dynamics, it would be of great help to be able to monitor changes in testosterone levels (and growth hormone and cortisol levels, too, for that matter). In fact, daily blood sampling has reportedly been employed by Eastern European athletes for decades; and this practice has likely been instrumental in the training innovations that have emanated from that part of the world. I predict that blood sampling will become an increasingly common practice among world-class athletes, as it takes much of the guesswork out of designing a training program. For the average person, regular blood sampling is impractical. One highly inexact but easy way for men to gauge their testosterone status is to monitor sex drive and potency, which tend to track testosterone fluctuations.

Testosterone Dynamics and the Effect on Muscle Growth and Sex Drive

The sweaty aftermath of an appropriately brief and intense workout session is typically characterized by a transient increase in sex drive owing to a lingering elevation in the "excitatory" neurotransmitter dopamine.[279] (In addition to conducting mind-muscle impulse traffic during exercise,[280] dopamine facilitates sexual arousal and orgasm.[281,282]) Shortly thereafter, conditions change.

Around the time when perspiration ceases and blood flow to the muscles normalizes after an intense training session, dopamine levels fall and serotonin levels rise.[283] Serotonin has the opposite effect of dopamine on alertness[284] and sex drive[285,286] (explaining why diminished libido is a common side effect of serotonin-re-uptake-inhibitor anti-depressant drugs). This pro-serotonin shift in your neurotransmitter profile accounts for why you feel tired after an intense workout (not because of physical exhaustion per se, as most people logically assume, but because of a shift in brain chemistry occasioned by intense physical activity). The concomitant rise and fall of serotonin and dopamine, respectively, coincides with post-intense-workout testosterone suppression.*

The post-intense-workout, low-testosterone period is marked by relatively diminished sex drive and sexual potency. During this period, the body is in a catabolic state, with the testosterone/cortisol ratio tipped sharply in favor of cortisol. Acidic conditions prevail inside the muscles at this time, and muscle tissue may still be getting broken-down even though the workout has ended (the post-workout meal is an extremely important factor here). I call this the "pre-recovery" stage. During "pre-recovery," the body struggles to neutralize the trauma caused by the workout and re-establish homeostasis. Specifically, biological toxic wastes produced by intense exercise are cleared away and pH balance is restored. Until your biochemistry (which is significantly altered by an intense workout) stabilizes, the beneficial restructuring process cannot proceed.

At about ten hours post-intense-exercise (maybe sooner, maybe later, depending on nutrition [better = sooner], fitness level [higher = sooner], emotional stress [more = later], and workout volume [greater = later]), testosterone will begin its resurgence, culminating in the all-important "exaggerated rebound." In most cases, testosterone will peak sometime between 24 and 48 hours post-exercise, rising above baseline levels and staying there for 1-3 days.[287] During this anabolic period, the muscles are "remodeled" in accordance with the physical stress imposed by the workout; and additional calories are burned to fuel this energy-intensive restructuring process.

During the time when the testosterone/cortisol ratio is high, libido and sexual potency are high. This is also when muscle growth occurs. Assuming adequate recovery time and sound nutrition, the net effect of this cycle will be positive, with the testosterone peak more pronounced and longer-lasting than the valley; and the opposite true of cortisol.

Missing your post-workout meal - don't - in the wake of an intense weight training session will retard pre-recovery thereby postponing recovery, deepen the post-workout testosterone fall, and delay the testosterone rebound. **The post-workout meal provides the nutritional raw materials needed by the body to turn the tide from catabolism to anabolism**. By neglecting to eat soon after working-out (ideally within 40 minutes), you are ensuring that you will remain mired in a catabolic state for longer than is

---

* The decline in dopamine relative to serotonin probably influences the post-exercise drop in testosterone, and perhaps vice versa, given the close relationship between dopamine and testosterone.[287a,287b,287c] The subsequent rebound in dopamine levels probably helps drive the testosterone rebound, and perhaps vice versa. This is another illustration of the intimate interrelationship between neurotransmitters and hormones, which we explored earlier in connection with food cravings, energy levels, mental productivity, and emotional well-being (see Chapters 10, 11, 17). The hormone/neurotransmitter nexus is a frontier with profound implications for health and human performance. Together, neurotransmitters and hormones influence everything that goes on inside our body and our mind. I believe that the hormone/neurotransmitter connection, exceedingly complicated and marginally understood though it is at this juncture, holds the key to unlocking human potential. The new millennium will, hopefully, witness great strides in this area.

necessary. Because an intense workout temporarily suppresses digestion,[288,289] a protein shake (see p. 243) is the most effective way to deliver nutrients to muscles immediately after training. This should be followed, 2-3 hours later, by a medium-sized meal. By employing this strategy, you get two smaller feedings into the critical first three hours post-workout, rather than one large feeding; hence, higher protein absorption (which promotes a speedy transition from catabolism to anabolism) and more stable insulin levels (which maximizes post-workout fat burning).

For a fit athlete training in a hormonally intelligent fashion and practicing good nutrition, the post-workout low-testosterone sexual symptoms are likely to be mild and fleeting; therefore, they may be imperceptible. Even so, where one trains at a high level of intensity, sexual desire and performance will be greater during the anabolic "rebound" period than during the post-exercise catabolic period. Chronic sexual apathy is suggestive of overtraining, whereas consistently powerful sex drive indicates a low probability of overtraining (but does not necessarily mean you are training optimally).

Guidelines for Structuring a Hormonally Intelligent Weight Training Routine

Don't Lift Weights Every Day

It should be obvious to men from the foregoing discussion that in order to reap the benefits of the "testosterone/cortisol flip-flop," which generally occurs 24-48 hours post-exercise, you cannot weight train every day. The cumulative effect of weight training every day is a decrease in testosterone levels. For women, too, training with weights every day is inadvisable.

Like men, women experience a hormonal "flip-flop" in which catabolism yields to anabolism. But with women, testosterone is not the major player in this process that it is with men, anabolism in women does not produce large muscles, and menstrual cycles modify the hormonal response to exercise.[290] Notwithstanding these differences, the basic principles of hormonally intelligent training apply to both sexes. In both men and women, cortisol levels rise and growth hormone levels fall if volume is excessive. This catabolic hormonal profile, if it persists, will inhibit, bar, or cause a reversal of, progress in both men and women. *

Recovery Requires Energy

Remember, the adaptive remodeling process occurs mainly during rest not during work. In other words, the physical improvements you seek, though they are prompted by what you do *during your workouts*, are brought to fruition during the period of time *between workouts*. Moreover, the beneficial restructuring of the body - a function of

* Because women have less muscle, less ability to regain lost muscle, smaller bones, and less ability to regain lost bone, catabolic hormonal shifts are arguably more damaging to them.

recovery* - requires energy. **The more energy you expend exercising, the less energy is available to fuel the recovery process and, consequently, the slower recovery will proceed**. Therefore, the greater the volume of exercise you do, the more time you must allow for recovery. One practical implication of this is that moderate-volume aerobic exercise performed on days when you do not lift weights is generally okay and will not interfere with recovery. However, a greater volume of aerobic exercise necessitates a reduction in frequency, *not intensity*, of your weight-training workouts.

> **EXAMPLE**: Four days per week of weight training might be okay (depending on nutrition, sleep, and emotional stress) if you are either not exercising at all on the other three days of the week or if you are doing moderate-volume cardiovascular exercise on those days. If, however, on your three weight-training "off days," you are engaging in high-volume cardiovascular exercise, your hormonal profile is likely to shift unfavorably, leading to overtraining syndrome. Note that the adverse effects of this training regimen may not be immediately apparent. As explained earlier, *overtraining syndrome is a cumulative phenomenon*. In other words, if you consistently overtax your body's recovery abilities, eventually you will pay the price.

Men who are concerned solely with building maximum muscle mass are advised to minimize aerobic exercise or eliminate it, to allow for the fastest possible recovery. Faster recovery means you can train more frequently. Extrapolated over time, *and assuming full recovery after each workout*, more workouts translates to more muscle growth in a given period of time.

The Body Must be Viewed Both as the Sum of its Parts and as an Integrated System

One of the more popular, and more pernicious, misconceptions is that weight training every day is okay provided that you do not train the same muscles two days in a row. The flaw in this thinking is that it envisions the human body as merely the sum of its parts, failing to appreciate its identity as an integrated system. You must view the body from both perspectives in order to avoid the pitfalls of overtraining. There are two such pitfalls:

Localized Overtraining: Refers to overtraining individual bodyparts

Systemic Overtraining: Refers to overtraining the body as a system
(and is associated with elevated cortisol levels)

---

* Technically, recovery refers to the restoration of the body to the level it was at before the workout. This is called *restitution* or *compensation*. But the adaptive response generally "overshoots" the stress by a narrow margin. The extra increment is called *supercompensation*; it represents the adaptive element, and it accounts for the improvements wrought by exercise. In the case of weight training, supercompensation manifests itself as stronger muscles. For the sake of simplicity, I am employing the generic usage of "recovery," which encompasses both compensation and supercompensation. Take note of the fact that because compensation must occur before supercompensation can occur, if you train too frequently you may be permitting sufficient time for compensation but insufficient time for supercompensation. When this happens, you make no progress. If you train more frequently than this, you may curtail compensation. When this happens, you regress.

What about Weight Training Two Days in a Row?

The rule against weight training every day should not be construed as a prohibition against weight training two days in a row. In general, it is preferable to allow an "off" day between weight-training sessions when you do either moderate-volume aerobics or no exercise. However, there are two bases upon which you should depart from this general rule and weight train two, or sometimes even three days in a row. First, necessity (created by work schedule or other obligations); second, as a means of qualitative progression.

Recall from our discussion of qualitative progression that once you master the fundamentals and become stronger and fitter, you should occasionally change your workout routine, in a calculated fashion, to increase r-intensity. Short-term manipulation of volume represents new stress and therefore increases r-intensity. For example, switching from a one-day-on, two-days-off weight training routine to a two-days-on, four-days-off routine, or vice versa, then back again, is an effective application of qualitative progression, which will stimulate renewed hormonal responsiveness and spur the adaptive process.

When weight training two days in a row, be sure to compensate by allowing extra recovery time. For instance, whereas two days may be a sufficient recovery period following one weight-training session, at least three days off the weights is advisable after two consecutive days of weight training. (Note - this does not mean that three days is sufficient recovery time for a *bodypart*, rather it is a guideline for avoiding systemic overtraining when different bodyparts are trained.) This adds-up to about three days of weight training per week, which is the right amount for most people under most circumstances. Four days per week is okay occasionally, as a means of qualitative progression, provided that extra recovery time follows; and two days per week is more appropriate for individuals engaged in high-volume cardiovascular exercise on their weight-training "off days."

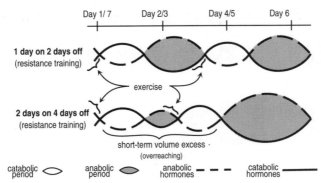

Note that two weight-training sessions performed on consecutive days constitutes short-term volume excess (short-term volume excess results in short-term catabolic predominance). However, do not confuse short-term volume excess (overreaching) with long-term volume excess (overtraining). The former is a potentially advantageous manipulation of physical stress, whereas the latter is unequivocally bad. Provided that extra recovery time follows, short-term catabolic predominance caused by short-term weight-lifting-volume-excess will generate a compensatory anabolic response.

295

Four days of weight training per week is the *maximum*. For the vast majority of non-steroid-users, regularly weight training more than four days per week will lead to a catabolic hormonal state. (This will come as a real shocker to the millions of gung-ho weight trainees who lift five or six days per week. If you are among this group, now you know why you haven't seen any positive results in the last few months or years.)

Bodypart Groupings and the Split Routine

Another way to apply qualitative progression is to change bodypart groupings. For example, it is advisable for advanced weight trainees to split bodyparts into narrower groupings to enable him/her to focus more intensely on each bodypart. Even after you have graduated from the standard upper-body/lower-body split (which I recommend for beginners) to a more advanced split (in which you do three different workouts instead of two), you should periodically revert. Training muscles in different combinations changes the nature of the stress imposed. For example, although a 3-day split is more "advanced" than the beginner's 2-day upper-body/lower-body split, training the entire upper body in one workout represents "new stress" (translating to higher relative intensity) to someone who is not accustomed to doing so. Bodybuilders who consider themselves too advanced to periodically revert to a more rudimentary training routine are also too advanced to get optimal results from training.

Review: Guidelines for Structuring a Hormonally Intelligent Weight-Training Routine

- Don't directly train the same muscles two days in a row. (Because muscles work in overlapping patterns of cooperation, you may train a muscle group directly one day and indirectly the next day. For example, in some split routines "upper back and chest" are trained on one day and "arms and shoulders" are trained on another day. In this scenario, shoulders are being trained two days in a row: indirectly as complementary or "helper" muscles on the first day and then directly on the second day.)

- Where weight-training "off" days consist of high-volume aerobic exercise or a large volume of other physical activity, additional recovery time is needed between weight-training workouts. However, low-volume aerobic exercise on weight-training "off" days does not impede recovery, and may even facilitate it (see below).

- *Don't regularly weight train three days in a row*, unless one of the three workouts is limited to any, or at most two, of the following bodyparts: calves, abdominals, forearms, or lower back. (The reason for this exception is that these are comparatively small muscles and, therefore, training them taxes the neuroendocrine system to a much lesser extent than training major muscle groups, i.e., upper back, chest, and legs.)

- *Don't regularly weight train more than three days per week.*

NOTE - The reason for the modifier "regularly" in the previous two rules is that, as discussed on p. 295, occasionally doing an excessive volume of exercise can be an effective means of qualitative progression for advanced weight trainees, *provided* that an extended recovery period follows.

One additional point - If you opt for a routine that has you weight training two days in a row, try to allow at least 20 hours between workouts. Obviously, training the same time each day would put you in compliance with this recommendation. What should be avoided is training late in the evening on Day 1 and then early in the morning on Day 2 - this is hormonally incorrect. To understand why, let's consider the following hypothetical:

Day 1, weight-training workout at 8 p.m.

Day 2, weight-training workout at 9 a.m.

The timing of these two workouts relative to each other maximizes cortisol output and promotes systemic overtraining. To appreciate why, remember from our discussion of the post-workout meal that food offsets catabolism. The better your nutrition, the faster your recovery because food provides the energy (calories), building material (protein), and catalysts and cofactors (vitamins, minerals, and electrolytes) necessary for recovery.

With the nutrition/recovery relationship in mind, let's analyze the hypothetical above. Unless this person wakes-up in the middle of the night to eat, he or she will, at most, consume two meals between workouts: dinner on Day 1 and breakfast on Day 2. This translates to two meals during the 13-hour period between workouts. Essentially, this amounts to a fast (hence break*fast*); and fasting retards recovery. **Fasting in the wake of a weight-training session amplifies the catabolic response**. By way of clarification, I am not implying that occasional fasting is a bad idea - I am stating that fasting *after an intense workout* is a bad idea.

Let's analyze three hypothetical workout routines. This will provide practical insight into how the principles we have been discussing apply in real life.

Practical Applications

HYPOTHETICAL #1

Jerry has a biceps obsession. His entire exercise program consists of doing five sets to failure of curls every day.

Analysis: Jerry is violating three rules with this routine by 1) not training all muscles, 2) directly training the same muscles two days in a row, 3) weight training every day.

Beginning with the first of these transgressions, this is an ill-conceived routine because you should not train only one muscle or muscle group. To have a proportional physique you must train all muscles. Developmental imbalances detract from your body not only aesthetically, but functionally as well. Especially where imbalances exist between antagonistic muscles (like biceps and triceps, hamstrings and quadriceps, chest and upper back), the likelihood of injury increases. Except where one is rehabilitating a specific muscle after disproportionate disuse, all muscles should be treated equally.

Pounding-away at the same muscles every day is Jerry's second mistake. This leads to *localized overtraining* of the biceps, resulting in cessation or undoing of positive results, and a heightened likelihood of injuring his biceps.

Jerry is also breaking the rule prohibiting weight training every day. However, in this instance, because of the brevity of his workouts and because the biceps are relatively small muscles, the hormonal effects are not nearly as bad as they would be if he were training a major muscle group every day. Therefore, *systemic overtraining* is not an inevitable consequence of this routine. Similarly, because curls are one of the less taxing exercises (again - because the biceps comprise a very small percentage of human musculature), Jerry's routine does not severely deplete energy resources needed for recovery.

Nonetheless, with Jerry's routine, the chronic trauma to the muscle tissues of the biceps, caused by localized overtraining, disrupts recovery and development of the biceps in the same way that constantly picking at a scab disrupts the healing of a wound. In addition, the risk of injury to the biceps muscles and the surrounding tendons and ligaments is heightened considerably by this training regimen. Therefore, although Jerry's workout routine will not necessarily have an adverse impact on his hormonal status, there are other problems that essentially make this routine, at best, a waste of time.

298

HYPOTHETICAL #2

Steven has adopted the weight-training routine – called the "Get Thick Quick Program" - endorsed by Mr. Olympia and featured in one of the bodybuilding magazines he reads religiously. Steven, however, does not take anabolic drugs (unlike the pros). He trains at a high level of intensity, five days per week, resting on Saturday and Sunday. Despite his determined efforts, Steven has not been making satisfactory progress and therefore he has set-up an appointment with Leo "The Exercise Master," to have Leo troubleshoot his training routine. Leo has recently earned his nickname and a great deal of admiration due to the astonishing improvements in his physique that occurred after applying the principles and techniques contained in *Natural Hormonal Enhancement* and *Hormonally Intelligent Exercise.*

Steven shows Leo his routine, which looks like this:

Mon	Tues	Wed
chest	triceps and shoulders	back and biceps
Thurs	**Fri**	**Sat/Sun**
abdominals and quadriceps	hamstrings and calves	off

Leo tells Steven that although he is directly training each bodypart only once per week, he is overtraining his body *as a system*, with consequent depletion of energy resources needed for recovery and an unfavorable anabolic to catabolic hormonal ratio. Leo recommends that Steven change his routine so he is lifting three days per week rather than five days. Steven listens politely, thanks Leo for his advice, and walks-out, convinced that Leo doesn't know what he's talking about. It is impossible for Steven to believe that *less* working-out will produce more and better results. Besides, he reasons, the pros know more than Leo does about working-out and many of them train five days per week. If the "Get Thick Quick Program" worked for Mr. Olympia, it will work for him too, Steven concludes. Ironically, Steven, not knowing Leo's secret (NHE/HIE) assumes that Leo must be taking steroids or some other muscle-building/fat-burning drug in light of Leo's recent burst of progress despite such "flawed" thinking about how to work-out.

Desperate to look like the guys in the bodybuilding magazines, but seeing no progress in that direction six months after spurning Leo's advice, Steven decides that the solution is to work out *more*. Accordingly, he increases exercise frequency to six days per week. In addition, Steven starts spending $100 per month on dietary supplements, most of which don't work, that are supposed to build muscle and burn fat. Leo "The Exercise Master" meanwhile, a regular visitor to the Extique website where objective and unbiased information regarding supplements can be found, spends less than $50 per month on supplements and takes only those supplements that are proven to be effective, none of which Steven takes.

299

One year later, Leo appears on the cover of a local fitness magazine after placing 1st in a statewide "natural" (drug-tested) physique competition. Steven, on the other hand, is now spending close to $200 per month on supplements and has defaulted on his last car payment. In addition, Steven is finding himself unable to shake a cold that has been lingering for the past month. He has not lost any bodyfat, but his weight has dropped by five pounds due to muscle loss. His relationship with his girlfriend, Sara, is in serious trouble because he has become irritable and grouchy and spends virtually all his free time at the gym, convinced that longer, harder workouts are the answer to his problems. Sara was further offended recently when Steven asked to borrow money to buy a new bodybuilding supplement that promised to build "rock-hard granite slabs of Godzilla-like muscle mass practically overnight." Adding insult to injury is the fact that, in the minimal amount of time they do spend together, Steven, formerly a competent and enthusiastic lover, shows no interest in sex and his occasional efforts at performance are lame despite his girlfriend's patient and supportive coaxing.

Depressed, frustrated, and desperate for answers, Steven begins taking anabolic steroids. Finally, he begins seeing results despite working-out six days per week. After three months on " 'roids," Steven quits taking them, prompted by concern for his long-term health. Consequently, despite continuing the exact same training routine, he begins rapidly losing muscle mass, and his sex drive, which had returned, plummets. Unable to bear watching his hard-earned muscle mass evaporate like a puddle in the desert, Steven resumes taking steroids. Five years later, Steven is still taking steroids. Sarah meanwhile has found a new boyfriend, named Leo.

Analysis: The story of Steven is common and some version of it is playing itself out in gyms across America. *The path of Steven or Leo is your choice.*

Leo's critique of Steven's workout routine is basically correct. There is, however, an additional mistake that Steven is making. Leo's evaluation of Steven's training regimen was that it promotes systemic overtraining. True. But it will likely lead to localized overtraining of the shoulders, too. A great many people overtrain their shoulders, because they do not appreciate that some combination of the shoulder muscles (anterior, posterior, and/or medial deltoids) are involved in practically every upper-body exercise. Even though Tuesday is the only day on which Steven directly trains his shoulders, they are engaged as complementary or "helper" muscles on Monday and Wednesday as well. Training the same muscles three days in a row is not advisable, even where on two of the three days the muscles are trained indirectly.

This general rule applies especially to the shoulders. Like the knee, the shoulder joint is highly susceptible to overuse injuries. And like the knee, a shoulder injury can be debilitating. Bodybuilders don't realize that although they may have massive shoulder muscles, their shoulder joint is delicate. In fact, the disparity between the high developmental capacity of the shoulder muscles and the low developmental capacity (or, in many cases, cumulative degeneration) of the shoulder joint, causes the risk of shoulder injury to increase with advancing strength and years of lifting. Furthermore, the shoulder joint is subject not only to forces generated by the deltoid muscles, but is also caught in the crossfire of the much larger pushing (chest) and pulling (upper back)

300

muscles of the upper body. These facts about the shoulders, along with the widespread lack of appreciation of the extensive "helper" role they play in exercises not denominated as "shoulder exercises," explain why shoulder problems are so common among veteran weight trainees.

Another reason for the prevalence of shoulder problems among weight lifters is poor *exercise selection* and poor *exercise execution.* An example of faulty exercise selection is doing behind-the-neck barbell presses with heavy weight. The behind-the-neck press, a popular exercise, is murder on your rotator cuffs. Weighted dips is another extremely hazardous exercise. Exercise execution (biomechanics) is discussed below.

HYPOTHETICAL #3

Lauren, like most women, would like to get her hips, legs, and butt into better shape. With this objective in mind, Lauren adopts a weight-training routine in which she does squats every day, having been told that squats are a great exercise for the glutes (i.e., gluteus maximus) and thigh muscles. She does no other exercises, and trains at a high level of intensity.

<u>Analysis:</u> Lauren's routine is analogous to Jerry's (Hypothetical 1) insofar as they both perform only one exercise targeted at the bodypart each is interested in improving. Whereas Jerry trains only a small fraction of his musculature, Lauren trains a much larger percentage of hers. Still, Lauren's routine, like Jerry's, is flawed because it selectively works certain muscles while neglecting other muscles. Her choice of squats, though, is a good one.

The squat, provided it is properly executed (which it usually is not, see p. 309), is an outstanding exercise. In fact, the squat is the best exercise one can do for the lower body. Besides being a terrific exercise for the glutes, the squat works the quadriceps (front upper leg), hamstrings (back upper leg), hip flexors, lower back, and, to a modest degree, the calves. The squat is also a powerful growth hormone releaser, and that spells fat loss. Furthermore, squats heavily engage the heart and lungs, thus imparting a training effect beyond the musculoskeletal system. However, the principal virtue of the squat is also its principal drawback.

In addition to being a highly technique-oriented exercise (meaning it requires practice and instruction to execute it properly), squats are an inherently high-volume (due to high load) exercise. The squat engages a larger percentage of the human musculature than any other weight-lifting exercise, except for deadlifts. The gluteus maximus and the muscles of the upper leg are the largest muscles in the body; throw in the hip flexors, lower back, and calves, and you have an exceptionally taxing exercise. Consequently, doing squats every day at a high level of intensity will result not only in localized overtraining of the leg muscles, but it will also rapidly lead to systemic overtraining. Stated differently, the same characteristics that make the squat potentially a powerful anabolic stimulus also make it potentially a powerful catabolic stimulus. In Lauren's case, because she trains every day, the catabolic potential, not the anabolic potential, will be actualized.

Natural Hormonal Enhancement

Overtraining vs. Undertraining

I have devoted much space to discussing overtraining, and particularly systemic overtraining, which directly impacts on hormone levels by causing an unfavorable shift away from anabolism toward catabolism. The extensive treatment is warranted because systemic overtraining is the negation of your efforts in the gym and the undoing of your hormonal health. One study examining the effects of overtraining in endurance athletes found that a reduction in both the testosterone/cortisol ratio and sperm count caused by overtraining persisted for three months after resumption of normal training volume.[291]

Other research confirms that recovery from overtraining can take weeks, or in severe cases, months.[292] And as the foregoing study demonstrates, unless you stop training altogether (which no fitness enthusiast wants to do), hormonal imbalance can linger for a considerable period of time after you have reduced volume. In other words, overtraining syndrome, once it sets in, is an albatross not easily dispossessed. Therefore, to make continuous, uninterrupted gains you must avoid overtraining. However, to progress we must impose physical stress on our bodies. Thus, we are forever compelled to flirt with overtraining, while diligently guarding against traversing the blurry line that separates "optimal" from "over."

On the other hand, undertraining is not good either; and it will surely hold you back from achieving your potential. If it seems like you are treading a fine line here, you are. But overtraining does not happen overnight. Rather, it is a cumulative syndrome caused not by one lapse in judgment, but by a consistent misapplication of energy and effort. If you study NHE/HIE, you should be able to spend your life in the optimal exercise zone, where the benefits keep accruing and the detriments are avoided.

While both overtraining and undertraining are problematic, overtraining is more insidious because it results from a misapplication of the most admirable qualities: commitment, self-discipline, and determination. In most other endeavors, these traits, like a well-trained seeing-eye dog, will unfailingly lead you in the right direction. When it comes to exercise, however, these traits can betray you if they are not tempered by an understanding of the hormonal dynamics of exercise.

Undertraining, by contrast, generally results from a lack of will not of knowledge. As a practical matter, where there is a will there is not always a way. But where there is no will there is no way. Therefore, undertraining is an obvious and conspicuous enemy and is simple to defeat - intensify your commitment and redouble your resolve, and you will not undertrain.

Where there is a will, there is not always a way.
But where there is no will, there is no way.

Remember that sleep deprivation, nutritional inadequacies, and emotional stress each impede recovery and promote a catabolic hormonal state. The same exercise routine that

302

will produce overtraining syndrome in a stressed-out, sleep-deprived, poorly fed person may be ideal for someone without these deficits. Pay attention to these variables, and get in touch with your body. If you were up late cramming for an exam or trying to beat a work deadline, you might be better off skipping your workout the next day.

RULE: No matter how good you feel, *don't* train sooner than you are supposed to; however, if you are sick or run-down due to lack of sleep, poor nutrition since your last workout, an infection, or extreme emotional stress, *do* postpone your workout.

Do not invent excuses to miss workouts, but do not be so rigid that you feel obligated to workout in a compromised physical state. And if you find yourself slipping into overtraining, you should scrutinize your training routine with reference to your emotional, sleep, and nutritional status. This raises the question: how do you know when you are overtraining?

I have made reference at various points in this book to becoming attuned to your body. This is generally good advice that I am sure you have heard before, but it has special significance and applicability to Natural Hormonal Enhancement. Hormonal changes manifest themselves in ways discernible to those attuned to their body. Earlier, we discussed how diminished sex drive can be a signal to men that their testosterone/cortisol ratio is low and consequently their "muscle axis" (see Chapter 4) is out-of-whack in favor of catabolism. A chronically low testosterone/cortisol ratio is indicative of systemic overtraining. In women, too, diminished sex drive can be symptomatic of overtraining, because cortisol is antagonistic to female sex hormones (see p. 256).

While sex drive should be monitored for insight into hormonal state, do not put too much stock in it; psychological factors play a big role here. Rather, use sex drive as an alarm system: if your sexual desire slumps for no apparent reason, you should inquire further into your hormonal state. Less ambiguous than sex drive in signaling the onset of overtraining is **immunity, waking heart rate**, **exercise performance,** and **sleep quality**.

Becoming Attuned to Your Body

Immunity: There is good news to report: exercise can bolster the immune system. And there is bad news: exercise can weaken the immune system - if you overtrain. Our immune system stands between us and death. Immune deficiency disorders, like AIDS, illustrate this fact all too graphically. Without a functioning immune system, you would fall prey to the bacteria, viruses, molds, yeasts, and toxins that attack you each day, and are routinely repelled each day by your immune system. Even cancer is increasingly being viewed as a failure of the immune system.[293,294,295,296] Among its multitude of defensive tasks, the immune system destroys aberrant cells before they become established. Newly acquired insights into the immune/cancer connection has led to the development of promising experimental vaccines designed to enhance cellular immunity against tumors.[297,298]

Tumor biologist P. B. Medewar has said that every person develops cancer thousands, perhaps millions, of times. The immune system nips the problem in the bud almost every time, and you are no worse for wear. It's the "almost" part that gives rise to life-threatening malignancies. When you come to appreciate that your immune system performs lifesaving acts for you every day, you realize that supporting your immune system should be at the top of your list of priorities.

To understand how exercise can affect immunity we need only remember that growth hormone enhances immunity (see p. 5); whereas cortisol, associated with overtraining, is poison to the immune system, impairing its functioning and in some cases destroying disease-fighting cells (see p. 92). In this connection, you may find it interesting that no one ever dies of starvation. Before a starving person gets down to zero bodyfat, he/she dies of disease. The disease results from an immune system compromised by nutritional deficiency and assaulted by catabolic hormones. Under the extreme stress of starvation, ultra-high levels of cortisol and glucagon literally eat-away at the immune system. (Remember, catabolic hormones break-down protein; most of the immune system is made-up of protein.) The increasing predominance of catabolism over anabolism with advancing age[299] is a major reason why deadly diseases afflict older people at a much higher rate than younger people.

By enhancing growth hormone and suppressing cortisol, hormonally intelligent exercise can strengthen immunity and combat the immunosuppressive age-related increase in the catabolic/anabolic ratio. The immune consequences of exercise are volume-dependent and divide along the fault-line marked by overtraining: the right amount of exercise improves immunity, whereas too much of it suppresses immunity.[300,301,302,303] Reflective of the immune-boosting potential of exercise, a study published in the *International Journal of Sports Medicine* shows higher levels of natural killer cell activity in trained athletes than in sedentary people.[306] Similarly, animal studies show superior resistance to infection[304,305] and cancer[307,308] in trained subjects as compared with controls. The cancer/exercise linkage is further supported by studies consistently finding lower cancer rates among active people than inactive people, with the strongest associations found for cancers of the prostate, colon, and breast.[309,310,311,312,313,314] One study estimates that adopting an active lifestyle can reduce all-cause cancer rate by as much as 46%.[315]

The other side of this coin is represented by studies showing overtrained athletes with ravaged immune systems, characterized by reduced immune cell counts and increased incidence of infection.[316,317,318,319,320,321] With these facts in mind, you should monitor your infection rate and duration. If you find yourself getting sick often and find that colds have a tendency to linger for an undue period of time, you should carefully evaluate your workout routine and be on the look-out for other telltale signs of overtraining.

304

Waking Heart Rate: Checking your pulse rate immediately upon waking in the morning is a good practice to adopt. Do it before you get out of bed. Later, emotions, activity, and digestion will confound the analysis. Also, take your pulse in the same position each time; standing heart rate is slightly higher than seated heart rate which is slightly higher than lying-down heart rate.[322] If your waking heart rate on a given day is elevated by more than seven beats per minute over your average for the preceding week, be on notice that you may be developing overtraining syndrome. When assessing your heart rate, keep in mind that there is likely to be a downward trend in your resting heart rate correlating with increasing cardiovascular fitness. This can mask an elevated waking heart rate if you do not keep track of changes in your resting heart rate over time.

Another test performed upon waking is what I call the "Three-Second Test." It involves monitoring how you feel during the first three seconds after awakening in the morning. The instant you wake-up you should feel either a bit drowsy or refreshed but relaxed. If, instead, upon opening your eyes you are consumed with nervous energy - an uncomfortable jittery feeling - there is a good chance that your pulse is elevated and you have dipped into an overtrained, catabolic state. The "waking jitters" reflects neurotransmitter disturbances associated with overstimulation of the sympathoadrenal system (adrenal glands + nervous system). This is an early-stage indicator of overtraining.

If overtraining persists, jitteriness yields to lethargy; and chronic fatigue and inability to emotionally "get up" for training or competition (known as "staleness" in the sports world) become the dominant symptoms. At this point, you are suffering from adrenal exhaustion (see p. 250) in which the neuroendocrine system is incapable of mounting a full response to exercise. Specifically, catecholamines (adrenaline and norepinephrine) levels become depressed as a result of overtraining.[323] The catecholamines are the "biological juice" that drives exercise. They regulate virtually every aspect of exercise, including: blood flow distribution, cardiac contractility, energy mobilization, and mind-muscle communication.[324] A blunted catecholamine response to exercise can severely hamper performance.

Exercise Performance: Decrements in exercise performance are a telling symptom of overtraining.[325,326,327] If you are becoming weaker rather than stronger or are experiencing decreases in endurance rather than increases, you are obviously doing something wrong; and overtraining is very likely the cause of these reversals. Becoming weaker and feeling listless in the gym are warning signs that should not be ignored.

Sleep Quality: Overtrained people do not sleep well,[328] and they often wake-up with the uncomfortable jittery feeling (described above) in the morning, and sometimes in the middle of the night as well. Because sleep is a buffer against overtraining, sleep disturbances aggravate overtraining.

Natural Hormonal Enhancement

Mood: Overtraining is reliably linked to mood alterations.[329,330] Most commonly, these changes are manifested as depression and loss of motivation to train. The depressive effect of excessive exercise on mood contrasts sharply with the elevating effect that moderate exercise has on mood, outlook, and self-esteem.[331,332] If you find that your enthusiasm for life and specifically for exercise, has diminished, you should suspect overtraining.

Warm-Up

Warming-up before exercising is imperative. Warming-up facilitates improved subsequent performance and reduces risk of injury. **Whether you are doing aerobic or resistance exercise, the session should begin with a relatively brief, low-/moderate-intensity aerobic warm-up**.

A common mistake is to begin a workout by stretching, prompted by conventional wisdom which holds that this reduces the risk of injury. In fact, this practice promotes injury.[333] If you are going to stretch, do so after the aerobic warm-up. *Never stretch a cold muscle* - doing so is the most effective way to pull a muscle.

The aerobic warm-up serves to prepare your body for the demands of higher intensity work. This includes slightly raising body temperature and increasing oxygen transport to the muscles via enhanced blood flow. A brief, moderate-intensity warm-up also allows the cardiovascular system to gear-up, thereby offsetting the risk of irregular heartbeats or other abnormal electrocardiographic changes. The low-/moderate-intensity aerobic warm-up need only last 5 minutes; it is designed to shepherd your body past the "sweat threshold."

The importance of warming-up cannot be overstated in light of the fact that while exercise can reduce the risk of heart attack (including the risk of heart attack resulting from sudden exertion) sudden exertion can trigger a heart attack.[334] Warming-up is the way to obtain the cardioprotective benefits of exercise while avoiding the risk. In one study, 44 men free of overt symptoms of coronary disease ran on a treadmill at a high level of intensity for 10-15 seconds without prior warm-up. Electrocardiogram tracings indicated that 70% of the subjects displayed abnormal electrocardiographic changes. Significantly, when 22 of the men with abnormal ECGs during the treadmill test were again tested, this time after a 2-minute warm-up, 20 of the men exhibited improved electrocardiographic responses.[335] Another study found similarly beneficial effects of warming-up in relation to blood pressure changes attendant with sudden physical exertion.[336] These observations underscore the fact that coronary blood flow response to a sudden increase in cardiac work is not instantaneous, and momentary heart oxygen starvation (called transient myocardial ischemia) can occur in apparently healthy individuals. Warming-up prior to exercise helps even-out the supply and demand of cardiac oxygen, thereby substantially reducing the risk of sparking adverse coronary events at the onset of exercise.

306

In addition to safety considerations, warming-up can improve subsequent exercise performance.[337,338] Your warm-up should be gradual and of sufficient volume slightly to increase body temperature without causing fatigue or depleting energy stores; and the actual workout should commence promptly thereafter. If you are going to be doing a resistance workout, you should perform an additional specific warm-up directed at the muscles you will be training. But remember, never touch a weight until you have broken a sweat. The specific warm-up, which immediately follows the aerobic warm-up, can be accomplished by preceding each exercise with a "warm-up set" in which you use relatively light weight to "pump" or channel blood flow to the particular muscles you intend to train.

By beginning a resistance workout with a low- to moderate-intensity aerobic warm-up followed by warm-up sets, you increase the elasticity of the muscles and tendons. This reduces significantly the likelihood of muscle/connective tissue injury, which, though largely preventable, is widely prevalent among weight trainees.[339] In addition, you will get a better workout because "pumped" muscles perform better than cold muscles.[340]

Organizing Your Workout: The Order of Operations

Should You Do Aerobic Exercise on the Same Day You Weight Train?

There are a couple of reasons why it is better to do weight training and cardiovascular exercise on separate days than to do them in the same workout. For one, low-/moderate-intensity aerobic exercise performed on your weight training "off" days serves as a form of "active recovery." Active recovery facilitates recovery by increasing blood flow and transport of oxygen and nutrients to the muscles. In addition, with workouts on successive days, the potential exists to get two exercise-induced growth hormone surges instead of just one. The next best option, if your schedule does not permit you to do weight training and aerobic training on separate days, is to do one in the morning and the other in the afternoon. However, this is often inconvenient or impractical; and psychologically, "two-a-days" can be a real drag.

How to Structure a Workout to Include Both Weight Training and Aerobic Exercise

If your schedule is such that on certain days of the week you cannot exercise at all, you will be forced to do resistance exercise and aerobic exercise on the same day. Remember, though, the laws of human biochemistry do not bend to accommodate your schedule. Therefore, the duration rule still applies (see p. 263).

Conforming a workout which includes both weight lifting and cardiovascular exercise to the one-hour time limit may seem impossible to someone accustomed to long, leisurely, unfocused, or excessive-volume workouts - but it's not. With a well-designed routine (which would likely include "splitting" your bodyparts in this case, see p. 296), a proper amount of time between sets, and focused intensity, you can get an excellent weight-lifting workout in 20-30 minutes. This leaves 30 minutes for the aerobic component of your workout. (The warm-up does not count toward the one-hour limit.)

If you do interval training as recommended in this book, 30 minutes is more than enough time for a cardiovascular workout. Even if you do not do interval training, recall that as your cardiovascular fitness level increases, you should increase the intensity, not the duration, of your cardiovascular workouts. Therefore, 30 minutes is sufficient for a cardiovascular workout regardless of your fitness level.* As you can see, it is easy to keep your workouts under one hour if you properly organize your workouts - and your mindset.

Which Should You Do First in a Dual Workout, Weight Training or Aerobic Exercise?

When doing resistance exercise and aerobic exercise in the same workout, do resistance exercise first (but after the 5-minute aerobic warm-up). It is more important to preserve your strength and energy for the weight-training component of the workout, because intensity is more critical to weight training than to cardiovascular training. With this in mind, and because you are more capable of generating intensity at the beginning of your workout than at the end of it, it is advantageous to structure your workout such that weight training precedes aerobic training.

Moreover, structuring a dual workout in this way can help you burn more fat than if you did the aerobic part first. Here's how: recall that weight training is the most effective form of exercise for stimulating growth hormone release, and growth hormone increases the percentage of fat burned for energy. Recall also that if your workout is sufficiently intense, growth hormone can increase within minutes. Therefore, the earlier in your workout you stimulate growth hormone release, the better; because it maximizes the amount of fat burned to fuel your workout.

Review - Organizing Your Workout: The Order of Operations

Best – Resistance exercise one day, aerobic exercise the next day. [Allows for highest intensity and lowest duration per workout (thus increasing the intensity/volume ratio), allows for two growth hormone surges, and enhances recovery.]

Next Best - Same day: part 1 in the morning, part 2 in the afternoon. [Allows for two growth hormone surges, but intensity and enthusiasm are likely to flag during the second

---

* Although 30 minutes is sufficient for a cardiovascular workout regardless of fitness level, it is to your benefit occasionally to alter your workout such that intensity is decreased and duration is increased, even though this would reduce the intensity/volume ratio. If you have any question about why such a manipulation of exercise variables would be advantageous, please refer to the preceding discussion of *qualitative progression*.

workout; and it is often inconvenient, impractical, or psychologically draining to train twice in one day.]

Third Best - Same day, same workout: first resistance exercise, then aerobic exercise. [Reduces overall intensity, requires more focus and efficiency to stay within the one-hour time limit, and allows for only one exercise-induced growth hormone surge.]

Biomechanics

Biomechanics refers to the way you execute exercises. It is often referred to as "form" or "technique"; and it is exceedingly important for avoiding injury and achieving full benefit from weight lifting. I have trained in gyms across the United States, and I am consistently dismayed at the prevalence of faulty exercise execution. Based on my observations, *I have no hesitation in saying that in any given gym in America, at any given moment in time, there are more people doing exercises incorrectly than there are people doing exercises correctly.* Along with overtraining, undertraining, and poor exercise selection, flawed biomechanics deprives millions of people of the results from exercise they seek - and often produces negative results, including injury. Here are a couple of examples.

EXAMPLE 1 (Bench Press)

Bench press is one of the more popular exercises, and it is one of the more effective exercises for stimulating growth hormone release. However, the difference between executing the bench press correctly and incorrectly is literally a matter of inches, and relates to the "touchpoint" (where the barbell touches the chest). The touchpoint should be at approximately nipple level. Next time you are in a gym, take note of how many people bring the bar down to a touchpoint high on the chest; or simply take my word for it - a lot.

By lowering the barbell to a touchpoint closer to the collarbone than to the nipples, these individuals are de-emphasizing their chest in favor of their anterior deltoids. What is worse, because bench press entails greater load than any other upper-body exercise (due to the many muscles that assist in this movement) and because a high touchpoint requires the shoulders to exert force from a biomechanically compromised position, performing this exercise with incorrect form invites rotator cuff problems. Anyone who has experienced a rotator cuff injury knows that it is a sharply painful, partially disabling, never-ending nuisance. Just a few inches makes the difference between an exceptionally effective growth-hormone-releasing chest exercise, and a minimally effective chest exercise hazardous to your rotator cuffs.

EXAMPLE 2 (Squat)

In Hypothetical 3 on p. 301, you saw that the squat can be a superb exercise for the lower body. And like the bench press, the squat is an excellent growth-hormone releaser.

One of the many virtues of the squat is that it works the glutes (butt). Like the abdominals, the glutes are generally regarded as one of the more significant "cosmetic" muscle groups. But unlike the abs, the glutes are difficult to target. There is an endless variety of exercises that work the abdominals, but very few that work the glutes. This fact makes the squat an exercise of exceptional importance for individuals seeking to firm and shape this area. However, while many people do squats for their glutes, a large percentage commit a biomechanical error that essentially takes the glutes out of the exercise.

The biomechanics of the squat are such that from the bottom position to the point where your upper leg is parallel to the ground, the glutes and hamstrings are primarily engaged. From the parallel point up to the standing position, the emphasis shifts to the quadriceps muscles of the front thigh. In light of these facts, it should be obvious that if you go down only halfway, your glutes and hamstrings are largely excluded from the exercise.

Most people do not appreciate that half squats produce half results. In addition, there is a popular idea being passed along from the misinformed to the uninformed that full squats are bad for your knees. In fact, the opposite is true.

Before I go any further, let me make this clear: if you have a lower back problem, a knee problem, or any other musculoskeletal deficiency in your lower body, you should not do any type of weighted squat: half, full, or otherwise. Doing weighted squats requires a sound lower body, so if you have old war injuries - forget it. Having said that, I believe, based on anatomical considerations and my own practical experience, that half squats are bad for your knees, not full squats. If I am right, then there is a perverse situation prevailing in gyms across America: people are doing the right exercise (squats) the wrong way (half-way down) for the right reason (to protect their knees). The net result is that they are putting their knees at risk while greatly diminishing the effectiveness of the exercise.

When doing a half squat, the knees absorb most of the stress of decelerating (stopping) the weight midway through the movement. By contrast, in the deep position, the movement reaches its natural termination point, and in rising from the bottom position the knees get assistance, not only from the quadriceps but also from the hamstrings and glutes. I have been doing full squats with heavy weight for many years without any problem (and I know many other people who have been, too). The one time I tried half squats with heavy weight, I felt a shooting pain that caused my athletic career to flash before my eyes (if there's "good pain" and "bad pain," shooting knee pain is definitely in the latter category). One final point on the knee issue: if you execute the squat properly, not only is it not bad for your knees but, in fact, it is good for your knees because it strengthens the surrounding tendons, ligaments, and muscles, thereby stabilizing the joint.

There are other important biomechanical features of the squat that are crucial to avoiding injury and maximizing the effectiveness of the exercise. First, never, ever, bounce out of the bottom position - this is a prescription for disaster. Instead, *ease* into the bottom position, then rise from the bottom position in a forceful but fully controlled manner. I believe that the prevalence of this technical flaw - bouncing out of the bottom position - and the resulting injuries, is what gave rise to the myth that full squats are dangerous and should be avoided in favor of half squats. Secondly, it is crucial that you keep your back flat, as opposed to rounded, when doing squats. Performing squats with a rounded back is highly conducive to lower back injury (in the same way that a high touchpoint when doing bench press is highly conducive to rotator cuff injury). As is the case with knees, if you perform the squat improperly you can injure your lower back; but if you perform the squat properly (with a flat back), it will strengthen your lower back.

A good tip to remember when doing squats is to keep your head up - focus your eyes on the spot directly in front of you where the wall meets the ceiling. This will help you keep your back flat. Also, if you have never done squats or if you are new to weight training, I strongly recommend doing squats without weight the first few times. Graduation to weighted squats is not appropriate until you are certain that your biomechanics are correct. And remember that the bar itself weighs a significant amount (about 45 lbs.); so the bar only is your next step up from non-weighted squats. One more point - squats, like bench press, *should not* be performed without a spotter (i.e., someone ready to assist you if necessary). In fact, anytime you are training intensely with weights, you should have a spotter.

You see how important proper biomechanics is for avoiding injury and getting the most out of your workouts. Other Extique products provide a wealth of biomechanical tips and techniques along the lines of that presented here. If you can afford it, I also recommend that you hire a personal trainer for at least one session to demonstrate how properly to execute exercises and to critique your biomechanics. As noted on p. 249, there is vast disparity in quality among personal trainers. And, in many ways, you will be far ahead of those trainers who have not yet read this book. Having said that, the general knowledge level among personal trainers on the subject of exercise execution is fairly high, so listen to what the trainers have to say on this subject.

While personal trainers can be helpful, be wary of vocal self-proclaimed experts at your gym. There appears to be a direct correlation between the readiness with which a person gives unsolicited training advice and the likelihood that the advice given is inaccurate. I hope you will take advantage of other Extique resources to help you progress in your journey to achieving your utmost potential and realizing all the benefits that Natural Hormonal Enhancement has to offer.

References

1. Hultman E. Studies on Muscle Metabolism of Glycogen and Active Phosphate in Man with Special Reference to Exercise and Diet. *Scand J Clin Lab Invest* 1967;94S.

2. McArdle WD, Katch FI, Katch VL. *Exercise Physiology*. Baltimore, MD: Williams and Wilkins 1996, p. 102.

3. Id. at 102-103.

4. Id. at 122.

5. Hogan MC, et al. Increased Lactate in Working Dog Muscle Reduces Tension Development Independent of pH. *Med Sci Sports Exerc* 1995;27:371.

6. Mainwood GW, Renaud JM. The Effect of Acid-Base Fatigue of Skeletal Muscle. *Can J Physiol Pharmacol* 1985;63:403.

7.   Hermansen L, Stevensvold I. Production and Removal of Lactate during Exercise in Man. *Acta Physiol Scand* 1972;86:191.

8.   Margarita R, et al. The Possible Mechanisms of Contracting and Paying the Oxygen Debt and the Role of Lactic Acid in Muscular Contraction. *Am J Physiol* 1933;106:689.

9.   Sahlin K, et al. Resynthesis of Creatine Phosphate in Human Muscle after Exercise in Relation to Intramuscular pH and Availability of Oxygen. *Scand J Clin Lab Invest* 1979;39:551.

10. Id.

11. MacRae HS-H, et al. Effects of Training on Lactate Production and Removal During Progressive Exercise. *J Appl Physiol* 1992;72:1649.

12. Seip RL, et al. Perceptual Responses and Blood Lactate Concentration: Effect of Training State. *Med Sci Sports Exerc* 1991;23:80.

13. Bonadonna RC, et al. Dose-Dependent Effect of Insulin on Plasma Free Fatty Acid Turnover and Oxidation in Humans. *Am J Physiol* 1990;259:E736.

14. Groop LC, et al. Role of Free Fatty Acids and Insulin in Determining Free Fatty Acid and Lipid Oxidation in Man. *J Clin Invest* 1991;87:83.

15. Sidossis LS, et al. Glucose and Insulin-Induced Inhibition of Fatty Acid Oxidation: The Glucose-Fatty Acid Cycle Reversed. *Am J Physiol* 1996;270:E733.

16. Muller-Hess R, et al. Interactions of Insulin and Epinephrine in Human Metabolism: Their Influence on Carbohydrate and Lipid Oxidation Rate. *Diabete Metab* 1975;1:151.

17. Glisezinski I, et al. Effect of Carbohydrate Ingestion on Adipose Tissue Lipolysis during Long-Lasting Exercise in Trained Men. *J Appl Physiol* 1998;84:1627.

18. Rauch LH, et al. Fuel Utilisation during Prolonged Low-to-Moderate Intensity Exercise when Ingesting Water or Carbohydrate. *Pflugers Arch* 1995;430:971.

19. Horowitz JF, et al. Lipolytic Suppression following Carbohydrate Ingestion Limits Fat Oxidation during Exercise. *Am J Physiol* 1997;273:E768.

20. Ahlorg G, et al. Carbohydrate Utilization by Exercising Muscle following Pre-Exercise Glucose Ingestion. *Clin Physiol* 1987;7:181.

21. MacLaren DP, et al. Hormonal and Metabolic Responses to Maintained Hyperglycemia during Prolonged Exercise. *J Appl Physiol* 1999;87:124.

22. Paul GL, et al. Oat, Wheat or Corn Cereal Ingestion before Exercise Alters Metabolism in Humans. *J Nutr* 1996;126:1372.

23. Wee SL, et al. Influence of High and Low Glycemic Index Meals on Endurance Running Capacity. *Med Sci Sports Exerc* 1999;31:393.

24. Sparks MJ, et al. Pre-Exercise Carbohydrate Ingestion: Effect of the Glycemic Index on Endurance Exercise Performance. *Med Sci Sports Exerc* 1998;30:844.

25. MacLean DA, Graham TE, Saltin B. Branched-Chain Amino Acids Augment Ammonia Metabolism while Attenuating Protein Breakdown during Exercise. *Am J Physiol* 1994;267:E1010

26. MacLean DA, et al. Plasma and Muscle Amino Acid and Ammonia Responses during Prolonged Exercise in Humans. *J Appl Physiol* 1991;70:2095.

27. Henriksson J. Effect of Exercise on Amino Acid Concentration in Skeletal Muscle and Plasma. *J Exp Biol* 1991;160:149.

28. Tipton KD, et al. Exercise-Induced Changes in Protein Metabolism. *Acta Physiol Scand* 1998;162:377.

29. Crist DM. "Arginine's New Growth Potential." *Muscle and Fitness,* August 1997, p. 142.

30. Bonen A, et al Hormonal Responses during Intense Exercise Preceded by Glucose Ingestion. *Can J Appl Sport Sci* 1980;5:85.

31. Hansen AP. The Effect of Intraveneous Glucose Infusion on the Exercise-Induced Serum Growth Hormone Rise in Normals and Juvenile Diabetics. *Scand J Clin Lab Invest* 1971;28:195.

32. Bonen A, et al. Hormonal Responses during Rest and Exercise with Glucose. *Med Sci Sports* 1977;9:64.

33. Galbo H, Holst JJ, Christenson NJ. The Effect of Different Diets and of Insulin on Hormonal Response during Prolonged Exercise. *Acta Physiol Scand* 1979;19:107.

34. MacLaren DP, et al. Hormonal and Metabolic Responses to Maintained Hyperglycemia during Prolonged Exercise. *J Appl Physiol* 1999;87:124.

35. Vist GE, Maughan RJ. Gastric Emptying of Ingested Solutions in Man: Effect of Beverage Glucose Concentration. *Med Sci Sports Exerc* 1994;26:1269.

36. Davis JM, Bailey SP. Possible Mechanisms of Central Nervous System Fatigue during Exercise. *Med Sci Sports Exerc* 1997;29:45.

37. Newsholme EA, Blomstrand E. Tryptophan, 5-Hydroxytryptamine and a Possible Explanation for Central Fatigue. *Adv Exp Med Biol* 1995;384:315.

38. Newsholme EA, Blomstrand E. The Plasma Level of Some Amino Acids and Physical and Mental Fatigue. *Experientia* 1996;52:413.

39. Balsom PD, et al. High-Intensity Exercise and Muscle Glycogen Availability in Humans. *Acta Physiol Scand* 1999;165:337.

40. Langfort J, et al. The Effect of a Low-Carbohydrate Diet on Performance, Hormonal and Metabolic Responses to a 30-S Bout of Supramaximal Exercise. *Eur J Appl Physiol* 1997;76:128.

41. Conlee RK, et al. Glycogen Repletion and Exercise Endurance in Rats Adapted to a High Fat Diet. *Metabolism* 1990;39:289.

312

42. Saitoh S, et al. Effects of Short-Term Dietary Change from High Fat to High Carbohydrate Diets on the Storage and Utilization of Glycogen and Triacylglycerol in Untrained Rats. *Eur J Appl Physiol* 1996;74:13

43. Miller WC, Bryce GR, Conlee RK Adaptations to a High-Fat Diet that Increase Exercise Endurance in Male Rats. *J Appl Physiol* 1984;56:78.

44. Nakamura M, Brown J, Miller WC. Glycogen Depletion Patterns in Trained Rats Adapted to a High-Fat or High-Carbohydrate Diet. *Int J Sports Med* 1998;19:419.

45. Helge JW, et al. Impact of a Fat-Rich Diet on Endurance in Man: Role of the Dietary Period. *Med Sci Sports Exerc* 1998;30:456.

46. Lambert EV, et al. Enhanced Endurance in Trained Cyclists during Moderate Intensity Exercise following 2 Weeks Adaptation to a High Fat Diet. *Eur J Appl Physiol* 1994;69:287.

47. Muoio DM, et al. Effect of Dietary Fat on Metabolic Adjustments to Maximal VO2 and Endurance in Runners. *Med Sci Sports Exerc* 1994 Jan;26:81.

48. Boyadjiev N. Increase of Aerobic Capacity by Submaximal Training and High-Fat Diets. *Folia Med (Plovdiv)* 1996;38:49.

49. Simi B, et al. Additive Effects of Training and High-Fat Diet on Energy Metabolism during Exercise. *J Appl Physiol* 199;71:197.

50. Kiens B, et al. Lipoprotein Lipase Activity and Intramuscular Triglyceride Stores after Long-Term High-Fat and High-Carbohydrate Diets in Physically Trained Men. *Clin Physiol* 1987;7:1.

51. Pendergast DR, et al. The Role of Dietary Fat on Performance, Metabolism, and Health. *Am J Sports Med* 1996;24(Suppl):S53.

52. Coyle EF. Substrate Utilization during Exercise in Active People. *Am J Clin Nutr* 1995;61(Suppl):968S.

53. Lambert EV, et al. Nutritional Strategies for Promoting Fat Utilization and Delaying the Onset of Fatigue during Prolonged Exercise. *J Sports Sci* 1997;15:315.

54. Id.

55. Biolo G, et al. An Abundant Supply of Amino Acids Enhances the Metabolic Effect of Exercise on Muscle Protein. *Am J Physiol* 1997;273:E122.

56. Tipton KD, et al. Postexercise Net Protein Synthesis in Human Muscle from Orally Administered Amino Acids. *Am J Physiol* 1999;276:E628

57. Melby C, et al. Effect of Acute Resistance Exercise on Postexercise Energy Expenditure and Resting Metabolic Rate. *J Appl Physiol* 1993;75:1847.

58. Gillette CA, et al. Postexercise Energy Expenditure in Response to Acute Aerobic or Resistive Exercise. *Int J Sport Nutr* 1994;4:347.

59. Maehlum S, et al. Magnitude and Duration of Excess Postexercise Oxygen Consumption in Healthy Young Subjects. *Metabolism* 1986;35:425.

60. Lefavi B. "Answer to Your Questions from the American College of Sports Medicine Meeting," *Muscular Development Fitness and Health*, October 1996, p. 104.

61. Bahr R, et al. Effect of Duration of Exercise on Excess Postexercise O2 Consumption. *J Appl Physiol* 1987;62:485

62. Bahr R, Sejersted OM. Effect of Intensity of Exercise on Excess Postexercise O2 Consumption. *Metabolism* 1991;40:836

63. Sedlock DA, Fissinger JA, Melby CL. Effect of Exercise Intensity and Duration on Postexercise Energy Expenditure. *Med Sci Sports Exerc* 1989;21:662.

64. Short KR, Wiest JM, Sedlock DA. The Effect of Upper Body Exercise Intensity and Duration on Post-Exercise Oxygen Consumption. *Int J Sports Med* 1996;17:559.

65. Gore CJ, Withers RT. The Effect of Exercise Intensity and Duration on the Oxygen Deficit and Excess Post-Exercise Oxygen Consumption. *Eur J Appl Physiol* 1990;60:169.

66. Almuzaini KS, et al. Effects of Split Exercise Sessions on Excess Postexercise Oxygen Consumption and Resting Metabolic Rate. *Can J Appl Physiol* 1998;23:433.

67. Kaminsky LA, et al. Effect of Split Exercise Sessions on Excess Post-Exercise Oxygen Consumption. *Br J Sports Med* 1990;24:95.

68. Giesecke K, et al. Protein and Amino Acid Metabolism during Early Starvation as Reflected by Excretion of Urea and Methylhistidines. *Metabolism* 1989;38:1196.

69. Fryburg DA, et al. Effect of Starvation on Human Muscle Protein Metabolism and its Response to Insulin. *Am J Physiol* 1990;259:E477.

70. Pozefsky T, et al. Effects of Brief Starvation on Muscle Amino Acid Metabolism in Nonobese Man. *J Clin Invest* 1976;57:444.

71. Sherwin RS, Hendler RG, Felig P. Effect of Ketone Infusions on Amino Acid and Nitrogen Metabolism in Man. *J Clin Invest* 1975;55:1382.

72. Owen OE, et al. Energy Metabolism in Feasting and Fasting. *Adv Exp Med Biol* 1979;111:169.

73. Cahill GF Jr. Starvation in Man. *Clin Endocrinol Metab* 1976;5:397.

74. See Chapter 9, p. 66.

75. Newmark ST, et al. Adrenocortical Response to Marathon Running. *J Clin Endocrinol Metab* 1976;42:393.

76. Cook NJ, et al. Salivary Cortisol for Monitoring Adrenal Activity during Marathon Runs. *Horm Res* 1987;25:18.

313

77. Lindholm C, et al. Altered Adrenal Steroid Metabolism Underlying Hypercortisolism in Female Endurance Athletes. *Fertil Steril* 1995;63:1190.

78. Maron MB, Horvath SM, Wilkerson JE. Acute Blood Biochemical Alterations in Response to Marathon Running. *Eur J Physiol* 1975;34:173.

79. Morville R, et al. Plasma Variations in Testicular and Adrenal Androgens during Prolonged Physical Exercise in Man. *Ann Endocrin* 1979;40:501.

80. Dohm GL, Tapscott EB, Kasperek GJ. Protein Degradation during Endurance Exercise and Recovery. *Med Sci Sports Exerc* 1987;19(Suppl):S166.

81. Tsai L, et al. Cortisol and Androgen Concentrations in Female and Male Elite Endurance Athletes in Relation to Physical Activity. *Eur J Appl Physiol* 1991;63:308.

82. Tegelman R, et al. Endogenous Anabolic and Catabolic Steroid Hormones in Male and Female Athletes during Off Season. *Int J Sports Med* 1990;11:103.

83. ABC News transcript, "Lifting for Life," May 10, 1991.

84. Colgan M. *Optimum Sports Nutrition*. NY: Advanced Research Press 1993, p. 138.

85. Pratley R, et al. Strength Training Increases Resting Metabolic Rate and Norepinephrine Levels in Healthy 50-to 65-yr-old Men. *J Appl Physiol* 1994;73:133.

86. Campbell WW, et al. Increased Energy Requirements and Changes in Body Composition with Resistance Training in Older Adults. *Am J Clin Nutr* 1994;60:167.

87. Id.

88. Pratley R, et al. Strength Training Increases Resting Metabolic Rate and Norepinephrine Levels in Healthy 50-to 65-yr-old Men. *J Appl Physiol* 1994;73:133.

89. Nelson ME, et al. Analysis of Body-Composition Techniques and Models for Detecting Change in Soft Tissue with Strength Training. *Am J Clin Nutr* 1996;63:678.

90. Treuth MS, et al. Effects of Strength Training on Total and Regional Body Composition in Older Men. *J Appl Physiol* 1994;77:614.

91. Ryan AS. Resistive Training Increases Fat-Free Mass and Maintains RMR Despite Weight Loss in Postmenopausal Women. *J Appl Physiol* 1995;79:818.

92. Van Etten LM, Verstappen FT, Westerterp KR. Effect of Body Build on Weight-Training-Induced Adaptations in Body Composition and Muscular Strength. *Med Sci Sports Exerc* 1994;26:515.

93. Riviere D, et al. Lipolytic Response of Fat Cells to Catecholamines in Sedentary and Exercise-Trained Women. *J Appl Physiol* 1989;66:330.

94. Hurley BF, et al. Muscle Triglyceride Utilization during Exercise: Effect of Training. *J Appl Physiol* 1986;5:62.

95. Klein S, Coyle EF, Wolfe RR. Fat Metabolism during Low-Intensity Exercise in Endurance-Trained and Untrained Men. *Am J Physiol* 1994;267:E934.

96. Coggan AR, et al. Fat Metabolism during High-Intensity Exercise in Endurance-Trained and Untrained Men. *Metabolism* 2000;49:122.

97. Romijn JA, et a. Strenuous Endurance Training Increases Lipolysis and Triglyceride-Fatty Acid Cycling at Rest. *J Appl Physiol* 1993;75:108.

98. Langfort J, et al. Hormone-Sensitive Lipase (HSL) Expression and Regulation in Skeletal Muscle. *Adv Exp Med Biol* 1998;441:219.

99. Oscai LB, Essig DA, Palmer WK. Lipase Regulation of Muscle Triglyceride Hydrolysis. *J Appl Physiol* 1990;69:1571.

100. Svedenhag J, et al. Increase in Skeletal Muscle Lipoprotein Lipase following Endurance Training in Man. *Atherosclerosis* 1983;49:203.

101. Podl TR, et al. Lipoprotein Lipase Activity and Plasma Triglyceride Clearance are Elevated in Endurance-Trained Women. *Metabolism* 1994;43:808.

102. Askew EW, et al. Adipose Tissue Cellularity and Lipolysis. Response to Exercise and Cortisol Treatment. *J Clin Invest* 1975;56:521.

103. Rambaut PC, Goode AW. Skeletal Changes during Space Flight. *Lancet* 1985;2:1050.

104. Id.

105. Hetland ML, Haarbo J, Christiansen C. Low Bone Mass and High Bone Turnover in Male Long Distance Runners. *J Clin Endocrinol Metab* 1993;77:770.

106. Bilanin JE, Blanchard MS, Russek-Cohen E. Lower Vertebral Bone Density in Male Long Distance Runners. *Med Sci Sports Exerc* 1989;21:66.

107. Kirk S, et al. Effect of Long-Distance Running on Bone Mass in Women. *J Bone Miner Res* 1989;4:515.

108. Woodhead GA, Moss MM. Osteoporosis: Diagnosis and Prevention *Nurse Pract* 1998;23:18, 23

109. Hurley DL, Khosla S. Update on Primary Osteoporosis. *Mayo Clin Proc* 1997;72:943.

110. Tucci JR. Osteoporosis Update. *Med Health R I* 1998;81:169.

111. Center JR, et al. Mortality after All Major Types of Osteoporotic Fracture in Men and Women: An Observational Study. *Lancet* 1999;353:878.

112. Riggs BL, Melton LJ 3rd. The Worldwide Problem of Osteoporosis: Insights Afforded by Epidemiology. *Bone* 1995;17(Suppl):505S.

314

113. Smith EL, Gilligan C Physical Activity Effects on Bone Metabolism. *Calcif Tissue Int* 1991;49(Suppl):S50

114. Johannsson G, et al. Two Years of Growth Hormone Treatment Increases Bone Mineral Content and Density in Hypopituitary Patients with Adult-Onset Growth Hormone Deficiency. *J Endocrinol Metab* 1996;81:2865.

115. Inzucchi SE, Robbins RJ. Effects of Growth Hormone on Human Bone Biology. *J Clin Endocrinol Metab* 1994;79:691.

116. Degerblad M, et al. Reduced Bone Mineral Density in Adults with Growth Hormone Deficiency: Increased Bone Turnover during 12 Months of GH Substitution Therapy. *Eur J Endocrinol* 1995;133:180.

117. Layne JE, Nelson ME. The Effects of Progressive Resistance Training on Bone Density: A Review. *Med Sci Sports Exerc* 1999;31:25.

118. Ryan AS. Effects of Strength Training on Bone Mineral Density: Hormonal and Bone Turnover Relationships. *J Appl Physiol* 1994;77:1678.

119. Dornemann TM, et al. Effects of High-Intensity Resistance Exercise on Bone Mineral Density and Muscle Strength of 40-50-Year-Old Women. *J Sports Med Phys Fitness* 1997;37:246.

120. Uusitalo AL, et al. Hormonal Responses to Endurance Training and Overtraining in Female Athletes. *Clin J Sport Med* 1998;8:178.

121. Lehmann M, et al. Autonomic Imbalance Hypothesis and Overtraining Syndrome. *Med Sci Sports Exerc* 1998;30:1140.

122. Kibler WB, Chandler TJ, Stracener ES. Musculoskeletal Adaptations and Injuries Due to Overtraining. *Exerc Sport Sci Rev* 1992;20:99.

123. Prior JC. Physical Exercise and the Neuroendocrine Control of Reproduction. *Baillieres Clin Endocrinol Metab* 1987;1:299.

124. De Souza MJ, et al. Gonadal Hormones and Semen Quality in Male Runners. A Volume Threshold Effect of Endurance Training. *Int J Sports Med* 1994;15:383.

125. Roberts AC, et al. Overtraining Affects Male Reproductive Status. *Fertil Steril* 1993;60:686.

126. Cumming DC, Wheeler GD, McColl EM. The Effects of Exercise on Reproductive Function in Men. *Sports Med* 1989;7:1

127. Arce JC, De Souza MJ. Exercise and Male Factor Infertility. *Sports Med* 1993;15:146.

128. MacConnie SE, et al. Decreased Hypothalamic Gonadotrophin Releasing Hormone Secretion in Male Marathon Runners. *N Engl J Med* 1986;315:411.

129. Arce JC, et al. Subclinical Alterations in Hormone and Semen Profile in Athletes. *Fertil Steril* 1993;59:398.

130. Fry AC, Kraemer WJ, Ramsey LT. Pituitary-Adrenal-Gonadal Responses to High-Intensity Resistance Exercise Overtraining. *J Appl Physiol* 1998;85:2352.

131. See p. 287-288, discussing the disparate effects of resistance training and endurance training on testosterone levels.

132. Loucks AB. Effects of Exercise Training on the Menstrual Cycle: Existence and Mechanisms. *Med Sci Sports Exerc* 1990;22:275.

133. Dale E, Gerlach DH, Wilhite AL. Menstrual Dysfunction in Distance Runners. *Obstet Gynecol* 1979;54:47.

134. Baker ER. Menstrual Dysfunction and Hormonal Status in Athletic Women: A Review. *Fertil Steril* 1981;36:691.

135. Nesheim BI, Bergsjo P. Physical Activity and Reproductive Function in Women. *Scand J Soc Med Suppl* 1982;29:77.

136. Boyden TW, et al. Prolactin Responses, Menstrual Cycles, and Body Composition of Women Runners. *J Clin Endocrinol Metab* 1982;54:711.

137. Boyden TW, et al. Sex Steroids and Endurance Running in Women. *Fertil Steril* 1983;39:629.

138. Bonen A, et al. Profiles of Selected Hormones during Menstrual Cycles of Teenage Athletes. *J Appl Physiol* 1981;50:545.

139. Shangold M, et al. The Relationship between Long-Distance Running, Plasma Progesterone, and Luteal Phase Length. *Fertil Steril.* 1979;31:130.

140. Mesaki N, et al. [Hormonal Changes during Incremental Exercise in Athletic Women]. *Nippon Sanka Fujinka Gakkai Zasshi* 1986;38:45. Japanese.

141. Cumming DC, et al. The Effect of Acute Exercise on Pulsatile Release of Luteinizing Hormone in Women Runners. *Am J Obstet Gynecol* 1985;153:482.

142. Barrow GW, Saha S. Menstrual Irregularity and Stress Fractures in Collegiate Female Distance Runners. *Am J Sports Med* 1988;16:209.

143. Lloyd T, et al. Women Athletes with Menstrual Irregularity have Increased Musculoskeletal Injuries. *Med Sci Sports Exerc* 1986;18:374.

144. Myburgh KH, et al. Low Bone Mineral Density at Axial and Appendicular Sites in Amenorrheic Athletes. *Med Sci Sports Exerc* 1993;25:1197.

145. Rencken ML, Chesnut CH 3rd, Drinkwater BL. Bone Density at Multiple Skeletal Sites in Amenorrheic Athletes. *JAMA* 1996;276:238.

146. Pettersson U, et al. Low Bone Mass Density at Multiple Skeletal Sites, Including the Appendicular Skeleton in Amenorrheic Runners. *Calcif Tissue Int* 1999;64:117.

147. Berga SL, Daniels TL, Giles DE. Women with Functional Hypothalamic Amenorrhea But Not Other Forms of Anovulation Display Amplified Cortisol Concentrations. *Fertil Steril* 1997;67:1024.

148. Hesse V, et al. Thyroid Hormone Metabolism under Extreme Body Exercises. *Exp Clin Endocrinol* 1989;94:82.

149. Jahreis G, et al. Influence of Intensive Exercise on Insulin-Like Growth Factor I, Thyroid and Steroid Hormones in Female Gymnasts. *Growth Regul* 1991;1:95.

150. Boyden TW, et al. Thyroidal Changes Associated with Endurance Training in Women. *Med Sci Sports Exerc* 1984;16:243

315

151. Pritzlaff CJ, et al. Impact of Acute Exercise Intensity on Pulsatile Growth Hormone Release in Men. *J Appl Physiol* 1999;87:498.

152. Chwalbinska-Montera J, et al. Threshold Increases in Plasma Growth Hormone in Relation to Plasma Catecholamine and Blood Lactate Concentrations during Progressive Exercise in Endurance-Trained Athletes. *Eur J Appl Physiol* 1996;73:117.

153. Luger A, et al. Hormonal Responses to the Stress of Exercise. *Adv Exp Med Biol* 1988;245:273.

154. Felsing NE, Brasel JA, Cooper DM. Effect of Low and High Intensity Exercise on Circulating Growth Hormone in Men. *J Clin Endocrinol Metab* 1992;75:157.

155. Viru A. *Hormonal Ensemble in Exercise.* Hormones in Muscular Activity, Volume I. Boca Raton, FL: CRC Press 1985, p. 67-69.

156. Rennie MJ, Johnson RH. Alteration of Metabolic and Hormonal Responses to Exercise by Physical Training. *Eur J Appl Physiol* 1974;33:215.

157. Bloom SR, et al. Differences in the Metabolic and Hormonal Response to Exercise between Racing Cyclists and Untrained Individuals. *J Physiol* (Lond) 1976;258:1.

158. Weltman A, et al. Exercise Training Decreases the Growth Hormone (GH) Response to Acute Constant-Load Exercise. *Med Sci Sports Exerc* 1997;29:669.

159. Luger A, et al. Plasma Growth Hormone and Prolactin Responses to Graded Levels of Acute Exercise and to a Lactate Infusion. *Neuroendocrinology* 1992;56:112.

160. Vasankari TJ, et al. Effects of Endurance Training on Hormonal Responses to Prolonged Physical Exercise in Males. *Acta Endocrinol* (Copenh) 1993;129:109.

161. Urhausen A, Gabriel H, Kindermann. Blood Hormones as Markers of Training Stress and Overtraining. *Sports Med* 1995;20:251.

162. Urhausen A, Gabriel HH, Kindermann W. Impaired Pituitary Hormonal Response to Exhaustive Exercise in Overtrained Endurance Athletes. *Med Sci Sports Exerc* 1998;30:407.

163. Barron JL, et al. Hypothalamic Dysfunction in Overtrained Athletes. *J Clin Endocrinol Metab* 1985;60:803.

164. Lehmann M, et al. Training-Overtraining: Performance, and Hormone Levels, after a Defined Increase in Training Volume versus Intensity in Experienced Middle- and Long-Distance Runners. *Br J Sports Med* 1992;26:233.

165. Lehmann M, Wieland H, Gastmann U. Influence of an Unaccustomed Increase in Training Volume vs Intensity on Performance, Hematological and Blood-Chemical Parameters in Distance Runners. *J Sports Med Phys Fitness* 1997;37:110

166. Lehmann M, et al. Unaccustomed High Mileage Compared to Intensity Training-Related Neuromuscular Excitability in Distance Runners. *Eur J Appl Physiol* 1995;70:457.

167. Gotshalk LA, et al. Hormonal Responses of Multiset versus Single-Set Heavy-Resistance Exercise Protocols. *Can J Appl Physiol* 1997;22:244.

168. Elias AN, et al. Effects of Blood pH and Blood Lactate on Growth Hormone, Prolactin, and Gonadotropin Release after Acute Exercise in Male Volunteers. *Proc Soc Exp Biol Med* 1997;214:156.

169. Luger A, et al. Plasma Growth Hormone and Prolactin Responses to Graded Levels of Acute Exercise and to a Lactate Infusion. *Neuroendocrinology* 1992;56:112.

170. Borer KT, Nicoski DR, Owens V. Alteration of Pulsatile Growth Hormone Secretion by Growth-Inducing Exercise: Involvement of Endogenous Opiates and Somatostatin. *Endocrinology* 1986;118:844.

171. Harber VJ, Sutton JR. Endorphins and Exercise. *Sports Med* 1984;1:154.

172. Buckler JM. The Effect of Age, Sex, and Exercise on the Secretion of Growth Hormone. *Clin Sci* 1969;37:765.

173. Buckler JM. Exercise as a Screening Test for Growth Hormone Release. *Acta Endocrinol* 1972;69:219.

174. Viru A. *Hormonal Ensemble in Exercise.* Hormones in Muscular Activity, Volume I. Boca Raton, FL: CRC Press 1985, p. 69.

175. Felsing NE, Brasel JA, Cooper DM. Effect of Low and High Intensity Exercise on Circulating Growth Hormone in Men. *J Clin Endocrinol Metab* 1992;75:157.

176. Nevill ME, et al. Growth Hormone Responses to Treadmill Sprinting in Sprint- and Endurance-Trained Athletes. *Eur J Appl Physiol* 1996;72:460.

177. Schwarz F, et al. Response of Growth Hormone (GH), FFA, Blood Sugar and Insulin to Exercise in Obese Patients and Normal Subjects. *Metabolism* 1969;18:1013.

178. Viru A. *Hormonal Ensemble in Exercise.* Hormones in Muscular Activity, Volume I. Boca Raton, FL: CRC Press 1985, p. 69 (citing, Rychlowski T, et al. Zmiany Poziomu Niektorych Lipidow I Hormonu-Wzrostu W Sorowicy Pod Wplywem Wysilku Maksymalnego Monogr., Podr., Sur. *AWF-Poznaniu SerMonogr* 1978;115:113).

179. Gordon SE, et al. Effect of Acid-Base Balance on the Growth Hormone Response to Acute High-Intensity Cycle Exercise. *J Appl Physiol* 1994;76:821.

180. Viru A. *Hormonal Ensemble in Exercise.* Hormones in Muscular Activity, Volume I. Boca Raton FL: CRC Press 1985, p. 69.

181. Few JD. The Effect of Exercise on the Secretion and Metabolism of Cortisol. *J Endocrinol* 1971;51:10.

182. Davies CTM, Few JD. Effect of Exercise on Adrenocortical Function. *J Appl Physiol* 1973;35:887.

183. Hartley LH, et al. Multiple Hormonal Responses to Prolonged Exercise in Relation to Physical Training. *J Appl Physiol* 1972;33:607.

316

184. Tipton KD, Wolfe RR. Exercise-Induced Changes in Protein Metabolism. *Acta Physiol Scand* 1998;162:377

185. Devlin JT, et al. Amino Acid Metabolism after Intense Exercise. *Am J Physiol* 1990;258:E249.

186. Chilibeck PD, et al. Higher Mitochondrial Fatty Acid Oxidation following Intermittent versus Continuous Endurance Exercise Training. *Can J Physiol Pharmacol* 1998;76:891.

187. Gray AB, Telford RD, Weidemann MJ. Endocrine Response to Intense Interval Exercise. *Eur J Appl Physiol* 1993;66:366.

188. Karagiorgos A, Garcia JF, Brooks GA. Growth Hormone Response to Continuous and Intermittent Exercise. *Med Sci Sports* 1979;11:302.

189. Vanhelder WP, Goode RC, Radomski MW. Effect of Anaerobic and Aerobic Exercise of Equal Duration and Work Expenditure on Plasma Growth Hormone Levels. *Eur J Appl Physiol* 1984;52:255.

190. Christenson EH, et al. Intermittent and Continuous Running. *Acta Physiol Scand* 1960;50:269.

191. Gorostiaga EM, et al. Uniqueness of Interval and Continuous Training at the Same Maintained Exercise Intensity. *Eur J Appl Physiol* 1991;63:101.

192. Tabata I, et al. Effects of Moderate-Intensity Endurance and High-Intensity Intermittent Training on Anaerobic Capacity and VO2max. *Med Sci Sports Exerc* 1996;28:1327.

193. Hickson RC, Rosenkoetter MA. Reduced Training Frequencies and Maintenance of Increased Aerobic Power. *Med Sci Sports Exerc* 1981;13:13.

194. Hickson RC, et al. Reduced Training Duration Effects on Aerobic Power, Endurance, and Cardiac Growth. *J Appl Physiol* 1982;53:225.

195. Hickson RC, et al. Reduced Training Intensities and Loss of Aerobic Power, Endurance, and Cardiac Growth. *J Appl Physiol* 1985;58:492.

196. Charette SL, et al. Muscle Hypertrophy Response to Resistance Training in Older Women. *J Appl Physiol* 1991;70:1912.

197. Singh NA, Clements KM, Fiatarone MA. A Randomized Controlled Trial of Progressive Resistance Training in Depressed Elders. *J Gerontol A Biol Sci Med Sci* 1997;52:M27.

198. Harridge SD, Kryger A, Stensgaard A. Knee Extensor Strength, Activation, and Size in Very Elderly People following Strength Training. *Muscle Nerve* 1999;22:831.

199. McCartney N, et al. Long-term Resistance Training in the Elderly: Effects on Dynamic Strength, Exercise Capacity, Muscle, and Bone. *J Gerontol A Biol Sci Med Sci* 1995;50:B97.

200. Pyka G, et al. Muscle Strength and Fiber Adaptations to a Year-Long Resistance Training Program in Elderly Men and Women. *J Gerontol* 1994;49:M22.

201. Fiatarone MA, et al. Exercise Training and Nutritional Supplementation for Physical Frailty in Very Elderly People. *N Engl J Med* 1994;330:1769.

202. Fiatarone MA, et al. High-Intensity Strength Training in Nonagenarians. Effects on Skeletal Muscle. *JAMA* 1990;263:3029.

203. Sipila S, Suominen H. Effects of Strength and Endurance Training on Thigh and Leg Muscle Mass and Composition in Elderly Women. *J Appl Physiol* 1995;78:334.

204. McArdle WD, Katch FI, Katch VL. *Exercise Physiology*. Baltimore, MD: Williams and Wilkins 1996, p. 642.

205. Hagberg JM. Physiologic Adaptations to Prolonged High-Intensity Exercise Training in Patients with Coronary Artery Disease. *Med Sci Sports Exerc* 1991;23:661.

206. Kavanagh T, Shephard RJ, Kennedy J. Characteristics of Postcoronary Marathon Runners. *Ann NY Acad Sci* 1977;301:455.

207. Kavanagh T, Shephard RH, Pandit V. Marathon Running after Mycardial Infarction. *JAMA* 1974;229:1602.

208. Jackson CG, Dickinson AL, Ringel SP. Skeletal Muscle Fiber Area Alterations in Two Opposing Modes of Resistance-Exercise Training in the Same Individual. *Eur J Appl Physiol* 1990;61:37.

209. Kraemer, WJ, et al Compatibility of High-Intensity Strength and Endurance Training on Hormonal and Skeletal Muscle Adaptations. *J Appl Physiol* 1995;78:976.

210. Pechar GS, et al. Specificity of Cardiorespiratory Adaptation to Bicycle and Treadmill Training. *J Appl Physiol* 1974;36:753.

211. McArdle WD, et al. Specificity of Run Training on Vo2max and Heart Rate Changes during Running and Swimming. *Med Sci Sports* 1978;10:16.

212. Fernhall B, Kohrt W. The Effect of Training Specificity on Maximal and Submaximal Physiological Responses to Treadmill and Cycle Ergometry. *J Sports Med Phys Fitness* 1990;30:268.

213. Boutcher SH, et al. The Effects of Specificity of Training on Rating of Perceived Exertion at the Lactate Threshold. *Eur J Appl Physiol* 1989;59:365.

214. Pierce EF, et al. Effects of Training Specificity on the Lactate Threshold and VO2 Peak. *Int J Sports Med* 1990;11:267.

215. Magel JR, et al. Specificity of Swim Training on Maximum Oxygen Uptake. *J Appl Physiol* 1975;38:151.

216. Schneider DA, Pollack J. Ventilatory Threshold and Maximal Oxygen Uptake during Cycling and Running in Female Triathletes. *Int J Sports Med* 1991;12:379.

217. Bunc V, Leso J. Ventilatory Threshold and Work Efficiency during Exercise on a Cycle and Rowing Ergometer. *J Sports Sci* 1993;11:43.

218. Hill DW, et al. Temporal Specificity in Adaptations to High-Intensity Exercise Training. *Med Sci Sports Exerc* 1998;30:450.

317

219. Hill DW, Cureton KJ, Collins MA. Circadian Specificity in Exercise Training. *Ergonomics* 1989;32:79.

220. Donaldson HH. On the Effects of Exercise Carried through Seven Generations on the Weight of the Musculature and on the Composition and Weight of Several Organs of the Albino Rat. *Am J Anat* 1932;50:359.

221. Donaldson HH. On the Effect of Exercise Beginning at Different Ages on the Weight of the Musculature and of Several Organs of the Albino Rat. *Am J Anat* 1933;53:403.

222. Donaldson HH. Effects of Prolonged Rest following Exercise on the Weights of the Organs of the Albino Rat. *Am J Anat* 1935;56:46.

223. Rosfors S, et al. Longterm Neuroendocrine and Metabolic Effects of Physical Training in Intermittent Claudication. *Scand J Rehabil Med* 1989;21:7.

224. Kraemer WJ, et al. The Effects of Short-Term Resistance Training on Endocrine Function in Men and Women. *Eur J Appl Physiol* 1998;78:69.

225. Viru A. *Adaptive Effect of Hormones in Exercise*. Hormones in Muscular Activity, Volume II. Boca Raton, FL: CRC Press 1985.

226. Poehlman ET, Copeland KC. Influence of Physical Activity on Insulin-like Growth Factor-1 in Healthy Younger and Older Men. *J Clin Endocrinol Metab* 1990;71:1468.

227. Nagasawa J, Sato Y, Ishiko T. Effect of Training and Detraining on In Vivo Insulin Sensitivity. *Int J Sports Med* 1990;11:107.

228. Remes K, Kuoppasalmi K, Adlercreutz H. Effect of Long-Term Physical Training on Plasma Testosterone, Androstenedione, Luteinizing Hormone and Sex-Hormone-Binding Globulin Capacity. *Scand J Clin Lab Invest* 1979;39:743

229. Colgan M. *Hormonal Health*. BC, Canada: Apple Publishing 1996, p. 247-248.

230. Winder WW, et al. Time Course of Sympathoadrenal Adaptation to Endurance Exercise Training in Man. *J Appl Physiol* 1978;45:370.

231. Wittert GA, et al. Adaptation of the Hypothalamopituitary Adrenal Axis to Chronic Exercise Stress in Humans. *Med Sci Sports Exerc* 1996:1015.

232. Winder WW, et al. Training-Induced Changes in Hormonal and Metabolic Responses to Submaximal Exercise. *J Appl Physiol* 1979;46:766.

233. Sutton JR. Hormonal and Metabolic Responses to Exercise in Subjects with High and Low Work Capacities. *Med Sci Sports* 1978;10:1.

234. Sutton JR, et al. Androgen Responses during Physical Exercise. *Br Med J* 1973;1:520.

235. Hakkinen K, Komi PV. Electromyographic Changes during Strength Training and Detraining. *Med Sci Sports Exerc* 1983;15:455.

236. Moratini T, Devries H. Neural Factors versus Hypertrophy in the Time Course of Muscle Strength Gain. *Am J Phys Med* 1979;58:115.

237. Sale DG, et al. Neural Adaptation to Resistance Training. *Med Sci Sports Exerc* 1988;20:135S.

238. McArdle WD, Katch FI, Katch VL. *Exercise Physiology*. Baltimore, MD: Williams and Wilkins 1996, p. 348.

239. Hakkinen K, Komi PV. Electromyographic Changes during Strength Training and Detraining. *Med Sci Sports Exerc* 1983;15:455.

240. Taaffe DR, Marcus. Dynamic Muscle Strength Alterations to Detraining and Retraining in Elderly Men. *Clin Physiol* 1997;17:311.

241. Costill DL, et al. Metabolic Characteristics of Skeletal Muscle during Detraining from Competitive Swimming. *Med Sci Sports Exerc* 1985;17:339.

242. Hortobagyi T, et al. The Effects of Detraining on Power Athletes. *Med Sci Sports Exerc* 1993;25:929.

243. Clarkson-Smith L, Hartley AA. Structural Equation Models of Relationships between Exercise and Cognitive Abilities. *Psychol Aging* 1990;5:437.

244. Rikli RE, Edwards DJ. Effects of a Three-Year Exercise Program on Motor Function and Cognitive Processing Speed in Older Women. *Res Q Exerc Sport* 1991;62:61.

245. Lichtman S, Poser EG. The Effects of Exercise on Mood and Cognitive Functioning. *J Psychosom Res* 1983;27:43

246. Clarkson-Smith L, Hartley A. A Structural Equation Models of Relationships between Exercise and Cognitive Abilities. *Psychol Aging* 1990;5:437.

247. Lupinacci NS, et al. Age and Physical Activity Effects on Reaction Time and Digit Symbol Substitution Performance in Cognitively Active Adults. *Res Q Exerc Sport* 1993;64:144.

248. van Praag H, Kempermann G, Gage FH. Running Increases Cell Proliferation and Neurogenesis in the Adult Mouse Dentate Gyrus. *Nat Neurosci* 1999;2:266.

249. van Praag H, et al. Running Enhances Neurogenesis, Learning, and Long-Term Potentiation in Mice. *Proc Natl Acad Sci U S A* 1999;96:13427.

250. No authors listed. Too Soon to Link Exercise to Alzheimer's Disease Prevention. *Mayo Clin Health Lett* 1998;16:4.

251. Young RJ. The Effect of Regular Exercise on Cognitive Functioning and Personality. *Br J Sports Med* 1979;13:110.

252. Elsayed M, Ismail AH, Young RJ. Intellectual Differences of Adult Men Related to Age and Physical Fitness Before and After an Exercise Program. *J Gerontol* 1980;35:383.

253. Rutherford OM, Jones DA. The Role of Learning and Coordination in Strength Training. *Eur J Appl Physiol* 1986;55:100.

254. Rikli R, Busch S. Motor Performance of Women as a Function of Age and Physical Activity Level. *J Gerontol* 1986;41:645.

255. Remes K, Kuoppasalmi K, Adlercreutz H. Effect of Long-Term Physical Training on Plasma Testosterone, Androstenedione, Luteinizing Hormone and Sex-Hormone-Binding Globulin Capacity. *Scand J Clin Lab Invest* 1979;39:743

318

256. McColl EM, et al. The Effects of Acute Exercise on Pulsatile LH Release in High-Mileage Male Runners. *Clin Endocrinol* (Oxf) 1989;31:617.

257. Wheeler GD, et al. Endurance Training Decreases Serum Testosterone Levels in Men without Change in Luteinizing Hormone Pulsatile Release. *J Clin Endocrinol Metab* 1991;72:422.

258. Houmard JA, et. Testosterone, Cortisol, and Creatine Kinase Levels in Male Distance Runners during Reduced Training. *Int J Sports Med* 1990;11:41.

259. Hackney AC, Sinning WE, Bruot BC. Reproductive Hormonal Profiles of Endurance-Trained and Untrained Males. *Med Sci Sports Exerc* 1988;20:60.

260. Hackney AC, Fahrner CL, Gulledge TP. Basal Reproductive Hormonal Profiles are Altered in Endurance Trained Men. *J Sports Med Phys Fitness* 1998;38:138.

261. Gulledge TP, Hackney AC. Reproducibility of Low Resting Testosterone Concentrations in Endurance Trained Men. *Eur J Appl Physiol* 1996;73:582.

262. Wheeler GD, et al. Reduced Serum Testosterone and Prolactin Levels in Male Distance Runners. *JAMA* 1984;252:514.

263. Kraemer WJ, et al. Endogenous Anabolic Hormonal and Growth Factor Responses to Heavy Resistance Exercise in Males and Females. *Int J Sports Med* 1991;12:228.

264. Kraemer WJ, et al. Acute Hormonal Responses to Heavy Resistance Exercise in Younger and Older Men. *Eur J Appl Physiol* 1998;77:206.

265. Hakkinen K, et al. Daily Hormonal and Neuromuscular Responses to Intensive Strength Training in 1 Week. *Int J Sports Med* 1988;9:422.

266. Kraemer WJ, et al. Effects of Heavy-Resistance Training on Hormonal Response Patterns in Younger vs. Older Men. *J Appl Physiol* 1999;87:982.

267. Kraemer WJ, et al. The Effects of Short-Term Resistance Training on Endocrine Function in Men and Women. *Eur J Appl Physiol* 1998;78:69.

268. Hakkinen K, et al. Neuromuscular and Hormonal Adaptations in Athletes to Strength Training in Two Years. *J Appl Physiol* 1988;65:2406.

269. Vervoorn C, et al. The Behaviour of the Plasma Free Testosterone/Cortisol Ratio during a Season of Elite Rowing Training. *Int J Sports Med* 1991;12:257.

270. Hoogeveen AR, Zonderland ML. Relationships between Testosterone, Cortisol and Performance in Professional Cyclists. *Int J Sports Med* 1996;17:423.

271. Marinelli M, et al. Cortisol, Testosterone, and Free Testosterone in Athletes Performing a Marathon at 4,000 M Altitude. *Horm Res* 1994;41:225.

272. de Lignieres B, et al. [Testicular Secretions of Androgens after Prolonged Physical Effort in Man]. *Nouv Presse Med* 1976;5:2060. French.

273. Harkonen M, et al. Pituitary and Gonadal Function during Physical Exercise in the Male Rat. *J Steroid Biochem* 1990;35:127.

274. Kuoppasalmi K. Plasma Testosterone and Sex-Hormone-Binding Globulin Capacity in Physical Exercise. *Scand J Clin Lab Invest* 1980;40:411.

275. Kuoppasalmi K, et al. Plasma Cortisol, Androstenedione, Testosterone and Luteinizing Hormone in Running Exercise of Different Intensities. *Scand J Clin Lab Invest* 1980;40:403.

276. Viru A. *Hormonal Ensemble in Exercise.* Hormones in Muscular Activity, Volume I. Boca Raton, FL: CRC Press 1985, p. 116.

277. Lutoslawska G, et al. Plasma Cortisol and Testosterone following 19-km and 42-km Kayak Races. *J Sports Med Phys Fitness* 1991;31:538.

278. Jezova D, et al. Plasma Testosterone and Catecholamine Responses to Physical Exercise of Different Intensities in Men. *Eur J Appl Physiol* 1985;54:62.

279. Dimsdale JE, et al. Postexercise Peril. Plasma Catecholamines and Exercise. *JAMA* 1984;251:630.

280. Gilbert C. Optimal Physical Performance in Athletes: Key Roles of Dopamine in a Specific Neurotransmitter/Hormonal Mechanism. *Mech Ageing Dev* 1995;84:83.

281. Wiedeking C, et al. Plasma Noradrenaline and Dopamine-Beta-Hydroxylase during Sexual Activity. *Psychosom Med* 1977;39:143.

282. Pomerantz SM. Dopaminergic Influences on Male Sexual Behavior of Rhesus Monkeys: Effects of Dopamine Agonists. *Pharmacol Biochem Behav* 1992;41:511.

283. Chaouloff F. Effects of Acute Physical Exercise on Central Serotonergic Systems. *Med Sci Sports Exerc* 1997;29:58.

284. See Chapter 10, p. 83.

285. Alcantara AG. A Possible Dopaminergic Mechanism in the Serotonergic Antidepressant-Induced Sexual Dysfunctions. *J Sex Marital Ther* 1999;25:125.

286. Hull EM, et al. Hormone-Neurotransmitter Interactions in the Control of Sexual Behavior. *Behav Brain Res* 1999;105:105.

287. MacDougall JD, et al. The Time Course for Elevated Muscle Protein Synthesis following Heavy Resistance Exercise. *Can J Appl Physiol* 1995;20:480.

287a. Szczypka MS, Zhou QY, Palmiter RD. Dopamine-Stimulated Sexual Behavior is Testosterone Dependent in Mice. *Behav Neurosci* 1998;112:1229.

287b. Hull EM, et al. Testosterone, Preoptic Dopamine, and Copulation in Male Rats. *Brain Res Bull* 1997;44:327.

287c. Vermes I, Toth EK, Telegdy G. Effects of Drugs on Brain Neurotransmitter and Pituitary-Testicular Function in Male Rats. *Horm Res* 1979;10:222.

288. Moses FM. The Effect of Exercise on the Gastrointestinal Tract. *Sports Med* 1990;9:159.

289. Brouns F, Beckers E. Is the Gut an Athletic Organ? Digestion, Absorption and Exercise. *Sports Med* 1993;15:242.

290. Viru A. *Hormonal Ensemble in Exercise.* Hormones in Muscular Activity, Volume I. Boca Raton, FL: CRC Press 1985, p. 89-92.

291. Roberts AC, et al. Overtraining Affects Male Reproductive Status. *Fertil Steril* 1993;60:686.

292. Fry AC, Kraemer WJ. Resistance Exercise Overtraining and Overreaching. Neuroendocrine Responses. *Sports Med* 1997;23:106.

293. de Visser KE, Kast WM. Effects of TGF-Beta on the Immune System: Implications for Cancer Immunotherapy. *Leukemia* 1999;13:1188.

294. Kuriyami S, et al. Cancer Gene Therapy with HSV-Tk/GCV System Depends on T-Cell-Mediated Immune Responses and Causes Apoptotic Death of Tumor Cells In Vivo. *Int J Cancer* 1999;83:374.

295. Boermeester MA, Butzelaar RM. [Interaction between Breast Cancer, Psychosocial Stress and the Immune Response]. *Ned Tijdschr Geneeskd* 1999;143:838. Dutch.

296. von Bernstorff W, et al. Pancreatic Cancer Cells Can Evade Immune Surveillance via Nonfunctional Fas (APO-1/CD95) Receptors and Aberrant Expression of Functional Fas Ligand. *Surgery* 1999;125:73.

297. Chen CH, Wu TC. Experimental Vaccine Strategies for Cancer Immunotherapy. *J Biomed Sci* 1998;5:231.

298. Ressing ME, et al. Immunotherapy of Cancer by Peptide-Based Vaccines for the Induction of Tumor-Specific T Cell Immunity. *Immunotechnology* 1996;2:241.

299. See Chapter 20, notes 127-128.

300. Baum M, Liesen H. [Sports and the Immune System]. *Orthopade* 1997;26:976. German.

301. Shephard RJ, Shek PN. Infectious Diseases in Athletes: New Interest for an Old Problem. *J Sports Med Phys Fitness* 1994;34:11.

302. Nieman DC. Exercise, Upper Respiratory Tract Infection, and the Immune System. *Med Sci Sports Exerc* 1994;26:128.

303. Shephard RJ, Shek PN. Potential Impact of Physical Activity and Sport on the Immune System – A Brief Review. *Br J Sports Med* 1994;28:247.

304. Pedersen BK, et al. Natural Killer Cell Activity in Peripheral Blood of Highly Trained and Untrained Persons. *Int J Sports Med* 1989;10:129.

305. Liu YG, Wang SY. The Enhancing Effect of Exercise on the Production of Antibody to Salmonella Typhi in Mice. *Immunol Lett* 1987;14:117.

306. Cannon JG, Kluger MJ. Exercise Enhances Survival Rate in Mice Infected with Salmonella Typhimurium. *Proc Soc Exp Biol Med* 1984;175:518.

307. Lu Q, et al. Chronic Exercise Increases Macrophage-Mediated Tumor Cytolysis in Young and Old Mice. *Am J Physiol* 1999;276:R482.

308. Jadeski L, Hoffman-Goetz L. Exercise and In Vivo Natural Cytotoxicity against Tumour Cells of Varying Metastatic Capacity. *Clin Exp Metastasis* 1996;14:138.

309. McTiernan A, et al. Physical Activity and Cancer Etiology: Associations and Mechanisms. *Cancer Causes Control* 1998;9:487.

310. Kohl HW, Laporte RE, Blair SN. Physical Activity and Cancer. An Epidemiological Perspective. *Sports Med* 1988;6:222.

311. Oliveria SA, Christos PJ. The Epidemiology of Physical Activity and Cancer. *Ann N Y Acad Sci* 1997;833:79.

312. Sternfeld B. Cancer and the Protective Effect of Physical Activity: The Epidemiological Evidence. *Med Sci Sports Exerc* 1992;24:1195.

313. Friedenreich CM, et al. Epidemiologic Issues Related to the Association between Physical Activity and Breast Cancer. *Cancer* 1998;83(Suppl):600S.

314. Shephard RJ. Physical Activity and Cancer. *Int J Sports Med* 1990;11:413.

315. Shephard RJ, Futcher R. Physical Activity and Cancer: How May Protection be Maximized? *Crit Rev Oncog* 1997;8:219.

316. Sharp NC, Koutedakis Y. Sport and the Overtraining Syndrome: Immunological Aspects. *Br Med Bull* 1992;48:518.

317. Fitzgerald L. Overtraining Increases the Susceptibility to Infection. *Int J Sports Med* 1991;12(Suppl):S5.

318. Fry RW, et al. Psychological and Immunological Correlates of Acute Overtraining. *Br J Sports Med* 1994;28:241.

319. Peters EM. Exercise, Immunology and Upper Respiratory Tract Infections. *Int J Sports Med* 1997;18 (Suppl):S69.

320. Peters EM, Bateman ED. Ultramarathon Running and Upper Respiratory Tract Infections. An Epidemiological Survey. *S Afr Med J* 1983;64:582.

321. Pizza FX, et al. Run Training Versus Cross-Training: Effect of Increased Training on Circulating Leukocyte Subsets. *Med Sci Sports Exerc* 1995;27:355.

322. Tulen JH, et al. Cardiovascular Control and Plasma Catecholamines during Rest and Mental Stress: Effects of Posture. *Clin Sci* (Colch) 1999;96:567.

323. Lehmann M, et al. Decreased Nocturnal Catecholamine Excretion: Parameter for an Overtraining Syndrome in Athletes? *Int J Sports Med* 1992;13:236.

324. McArdle WD, Katch FI, Katch VL. *Exercise Physiology.* Baltimore, MD: Williams and Wilkins 1996, p. 367-368.

320

325.   Callister R, et al. Physiological and Performance Responses to Overtraining in Elite Judo Athletes. *Med Sci Sports Exerc* 1990;22:816.

326.   Lehmann M, et al. Training-Overtraining. A Prospective, Experimental Study with Experienced Middle- and Long-Distance Runners. *Int J Sports Med* 1991;12:444.

327.   Budgett R. Fatigue and Underperformance in Athletes: The Overtraining Syndrome. *Br J Sports Med* 1998;32:107.

328.   Fry RW, et al. Psychological and Immunological Correlates of Acute Overtraining. *Br J Sports Med* 1994;28:241.

329.   Urhausen A, et al. Ergometric and Psychological Findings during Overtraining: A Long-Term Follow-Up Study in Endurance Athletes. *Int J Sports Med* 1998;19:114.

330.   O'Connor PJ, et al. Mood State and Salivary Cortisol Levels following Overtraining in Female Swimmers. *Psychoneuroendocrinology* 1989;14:303.

331.   Taylor CB, Sallis JF, Needle R. The Relation of Physical Activity and Exercise to Mental Health. *Public Health Rep* 1985;100:195.

332.   Byrne A, Byrne DG. The Effect of Exercise on Depression, Anxiety and other Mood States: A Review. *J Psychosom Res* 1993;37:565.

333.   Safran MR, et al. The Role of Warmup in Muscular Injury Prevention. *Am J Sports Med* 1988;16:123.

334.   Mittleman MA, Siscovick DS. Physical Exertion as a Trigger of Myocardial Infarction and Sudden Cardiac Death. *Cardiol Clin* 1996;14:263.

335.   Barnard RJ, et al. Cardiovascular Responses to Sudden Strenuous Exercise—Heart Rate, Blood Pressure, and ECG. *J Appl Physiol* 1973;34:833.

336.   Barnard RJ, et al. Ischemic Response to Sudden Strenuous Exercise in Healthy Men. *Circulation* 1973;48:936.

337.   De Bruyn-Prevost P, Lefebvre F. The Effects of Various Warming Up Intensities and Durations during a Short Maximal Anaerobic Exercise. *Eur J Appl Physiol* 1980;43:101.

338.   Ingjer F, Stromme SB. Effects of Active, Passive or No Warm-Up on the Physiological Response to Heavy Exercise. *Eur J Appl Physiol* 1979;40:273.

339.   Safran MR, Seaber AV, Garrett WE Jr. Warm-Up and Muscular Injury Prevention. An Update. *Sports Med* 1989;8:239.

340.   Bergh U, Ekblom B. Influence of Muscle Temperature on Maximal Muscle Strength and Power Output in Human Skeletal Muscles. *Acta Physiol Scand* 1979;107:33.

Chapter 22

Testosterone: The Man-Maker

For most of the century, endocrinologists insisted that there is no age-related decline in testosterone, and only within the past decade has the fact that testosterone levels actually decline as we age been proven conclusively. Moreover, science has only recently come to understand that testosterone is not merely a male hormone but is a superhormone that plays a profound role in our ability to maintain a strong body and a well-functioning mind - in essence, in when and how we age.

William Regelson, M.D., The Super-Hormone Promise

Don't let your testosterone levels peter-out to an impotent dribble.
Rob Faigin

Testosterone is a metaphor for all that is male, and everything that defines "manliness" is at least partly owed to testosterone. In terms of body composition, testosterone is a powerful fat-burning (lipolytic) and muscle-building (anabolic) hormone. Testosterone is also *androgenic*, which means that it is responsible for sexual characteristics. Women, too, have testosterone, but only a fraction as much as men, produced mainly in the ovaries and adrenal glands.[1] It is because of their vastly differing testosterone/estrogen ratio that women cannot build large muscles like men.

It's easy to see testosterone in action. At puberty, testosterone levels rise sharply; and it is escalating testosterone that literally turns boys into men. Of particular significance is the way boys become leaner and more muscular during puberty - and this happens regardless of whether they exercise. A study published in the *New England Journal of Medicine* demonstrates that testosterone injections can grow muscle even in men who do not exercise.[2]

Unfortunately, as is the case with growth hormone, testosterone levels tend to decline with advancing age.[3,4,5,6] More significant than total serum testosterone is bioavailable or "free testosterone," which excludes testosterone bound to sex-hormone-binding gobulin (SHBG). Free testosterone is a more sensitive indicator of tissue-available androgens than total serum testosterone; and measurement of the latter, although more common, tends to understate testosterone decline in men.[7,8,9]

The rate of testosterone reduction varies with the individual, but for most men the descent begins at about the age of forty. From that point on, testosterone drops slowly but steadily with each passing year.[10] As testosterone levels decline, so does the man. Just as an upsurge in testosterone transforms boys into men, a downturn in testosterone turns men into feeble, frail, old men.

The age-related decline in testosterone has been called "male menopause." But because it is gradual, not sudden and dramatic like female menopause, it has not received much attention until about ten years ago. The debilitating effects of low testosterone include decreased muscle and bone mass, increased bodyfat, weakness, depression, cognitive impairment[11] - and the drop-off can turn a stallion into a gelding. As if the age-related decline weren't bad enough, *many men are systematically lowering their testosterone levels with hormonally incorrect dietary, exercise, and lifestyle practices.*

Impotence: The Hard Facts are Very Troubling

In the U.S., it is estimated that between 10-20 million American males are impotent.[12] (The laws of political correctness now dictate that impotence be referred to as erectile dysfunction - or if you really want to sound culturally sophisticated, then "E.D.") Thus, approximately a quarter of the male population of the U.S. is at least partially impotent, a 100% increase from the 1940's.[13] Childless couples, once rare, have become common, with over five million couples being treated for inability to have children.[14] As much as men hate to have the blame for this problem dropped in their lap, that's exactly where much of the problem originates.

The causes of the impotency epidemic are varied and include certain prescription drugs and circulatory insufficiency from clogged arteries. With respect to the vascular problem, a study published in the *American Journal of Epidemiology* found that erectile dysfunction correlates with high total serum cholesterol and low HDL relative to LDL[15] (atherosclerotic plaque accumulates on penile arteries just like other arteries). One way to treat this condition is with penile bypass surgery in which, like heart bypass, blood flow is rerouted. The take-home message here is to keep your arteries clean or else you may wind-up with both a bum ticker and a lame sex life.

"Pharmaceutical impotence" is another threat to sexual performance, and it is a very serious one in our drug-happy society. Among the assortment of adverse side effects that they cause, anti-hypertensives, anti-depressants, diuretics, and tranquilizers impact deleteriously upon sexual potency in both men and women; and many of these drugs hit testosterone directly.[16]

Sexuality is far too complex a human activity to be reduced to a few micrograms of any chemical, testosterone included. Furthermore, as Dr. Fran Kaiser points-out, "we know more about sending a rocket to the moon than we actually understand about the physiology of erections."[17] Nevertheless, you don't have to be a rocket scientist to appreciate the connection between testosterone and reproductive drive.

For those men who experience most acutely the age-related decline in testosterone, reproductive drive is no longer a pressing desire, but rather a fond memory. Low testosterone is characterized by any or all of the following: inability to achieve an erection, inability to maintain an erection, diminished libido, and reduced ejaculate volume.[18] The impotency problem has gotten so bad that in 1995 the FDA approved *alprostadil* (Caverject) for injection into the penis to create artificial erections. This is only the latest on the list of anti-impotency treatments that includes implants, vacuum pumps, and other similar devices designed to uplift mens' sex lives mechanically.

323

Erection injections and Viagra notwithstanding, men are unlikely to get the impotency problem straightened-out if prevailing dietary, exercise, and lifestyle practices persist. Additionally, because testosterone is a fat-burning and muscle-building hormone, a reduction in testosterone levels tends to increase bodyfat percentage in men and makes it more difficult to build muscle.[19,20] Generally speaking, men today are fatter, weaker, and less virile than at any time in the past. In the scathingly blunt words of Dr. Michael Colgan, "the average modern man is a wimp compared with his forefathers."[21] This fact, coupled with society's anti-aging obsession, has created a wave of interest in testosterone injections.

Yuppie Steroids - The Testosterone Revolution

Like growth hormone, testosterone injections have been used for many years as a medical treatment for people with abnormally low endogenous production (abnormally low levels of testosterone is a medical condition called *hypogonadism*). While few people question the wisdom of using testosterone to treat hypogonadism, recent discoveries concerning the relationship between aging and testosterone have raised a more controversial question: given that testosterone decline can be counteracted, why tolerate *any* fall-off in testosterone, even within the normal range? With aging increasingly being viewed as a disease rather than a normal, acceptable process, why not consider a reduction in testosterone to be a "disease" (since it promotes aging) and treat it accordingly?

This philosophy has sparked an explosion of interest in testosterone that is parallel, in many respects, to what is happening with growth hormone (but with an added twist, discussed below). Testosterone replacement therapy clinics are appearing across the U.S. and Europe and sales have jumped by the hundreds of millions of dollars, fueled by reports of restored vitality and virility. While the short-term results of testosterone injections are indeed impressive, it appears that we may be sliding down a slippery slope toward a health disaster.

The problem with exogenous testosterone enhancement is fundamental and applies to all exogenous hormones, except the names are different in each case. The testes are the final step or "end-organ" in the process of testosterone production. Shooting-up testosterone ignores all the other critical points in the testosterone production line. This process begins at the hypothalamus, which secretes *gonadotropin-releasing hormone*, which, in turn, stimulates the pituitary gland to produce *luteinizing hormone*, which signals the testes to produce testosterone. Even this is a grossly oversimplified model of testosterone production, as it ignores the involvement of intermediate hormones, such as: *adrenocorticotropic hormone*, *dehydroepiandrosterone*, *progesterone*, and *pregnenolone*. Targeting only the last point in this process is not a solution, because it does nothing to support testosterone production. In fact, it *impairs* testosterone production, as you will see in a moment.

As noted above, testosterone has two functions: *anabolic* and *androgenic*. Most of the adverse side effects of exogenous testosterone are associated with the androgenic properties. So wouldn't it be a great scientific advance if we could chemically alter testosterone to make it more anabolic and less androgenic? That way, if men want to roll the dice with their health, at least their odds would be more favorable. The fact of the matter is that such substances already exist: they are called "anabolic steroids." Anabolic steroids are synthetic derivatives of testosterone and were developed to be more effective and safer than testosterone.

Hence, the anti-aging wonder drug being prescribed to baby boomers is a crude, unrefined, anabolic/androgenic *steroid*. Why isn't this term ever used? For the same reason that a nuclear bomb is sometimes referred to by politicians as a "radiation device"; truth often takes a back seat to political correctness. The fact that the more dangerous version of the drug widely demonized as a "killer drug" in the 1980's is now being prescribed as a "miracle drug" is, in the words of Dr. Michael Colgan, a "sick joke."[22]

324

Interestingly, the anti-anabolic-steroid movement is of relatively recent origin. In fact, it was not long ago that steroids were popularized and widely prescribed by doctors to athletes. But steroids were abused, people died, and popular sentiment turned negative on steroids - and rightfully so. Arnold Schwarzenegger personifies this turnaround. Schwarzenegger, who became chairman of the President's Council on Physical Fitness in the Bush (senior) administration, and is now passionately opposed to anabolic steroids, used them throughout his career (when they were legal). As the saying goes: there is no prude so zealous as the reformed prostitute.

Now steroids are back. But with all the less dangerous forms still blacklisted by law and public opinion, the harsh, fully androgenic "testosterone" forms have become the steroids of choice. This time, however, athletes are not the ones taking them because it is difficult and expensive to obtain a prescription. Besides, they would rather use anabolic steroids like *deca-durabolin* and *primobolan*, which offer better results with fewer side effects, from the black market. Rather, it is the upper-class, middle-aged and older male population who are on the testosterone kick.

Anabolic steroids, too, are making a comeback, but not among athletes - they never stopped taking them and never will stop as long as "winning at all costs" remains in currency. Rather, anabolic steroids are gaining favor in medical circles based on recent studies showing that they serve valuable medical purposes. Specifically, anabolic steroids have proven effective at counteracting muscle-wasting and improving well-being and quality of life in AIDS patients.[23,24,25,26,27] Anabolic steroids have also shown considerable promise in treating osteoporosis,[28,29,30] chronic obstructive pulmonary disease,[31,32] and in patients receiving dialysis.[33] Given that anabolic steroids are politically incorrect, and given that helping the sick is politically and otherwise correct, it will be interesting to see how this issue shakes-out. If the winds of political correctness shift once again and anabolic steroids regain a measure of respectability, might anabolic steroids replace testosterone as the anti-aging drug of preference for the congressmen, judges, and other respected professionals who are currently using testosterone? And might the concurrent rise in popularity of resistance training and anabolic steroids foreshadow an era in which pumping iron and shooting 'roids is the prevailing anti-aging strategy employed by the more genteel elements of the American bourgeoisie?

It bears emphasis that while many types of "steroids" are inherently less dangerous than "testosterone" they are usually *more* dangerous as a practical matter, because they are sold by ignorant black-market dealers who are unqualified to give advice as to dosage. Whereas doctors administering testosterone attempt to keep the dosage within the normal range (which, to make matters more difficult, varies with the individual), steroid dealers and users are typically imbued with the "more is better" mentality. And at supraphysiological dosages, the dangers of steroids are greatly increased.

Furthermore, anabolic steroids can be infinitely worse than doctor-administered testosterone because there is no quality assurance or enforced standards of purity in the streets and gyms of America; and steroids laced with amphetamines, heroin, or other addicting or toxic substances are not uncommon. In addition to the health hazards they convey, anabolic steroids should be avoided for the simple reason that they are illegal under the Anabolic Steroids Control Act of 1990. But, in any event, the distinction between "testosterone" and "steroids" is scientifically untenable and yet another example of health-industry hypocrisy.

Both "yuppie steroids" (testosterone) and anabolic steroids are exogenous hormones. As such, they are physiologically problematic. In particular, as we discussed in Chapter 3, the brain responds to exogenous hormones by reducing endogenous (natural) production. In effect, taking hormones "trains" your body to produce less of its own hormones via a counterregulatory "feedback loop." This is why, when men stop taking steroids they rapidly lose the muscle they gained, and are left with little or nothing to show for months of effort except for the psychological scars associated with this form of drug abuse. Moreover, hormone levels ebb and flow naturally throughout the day. Injected hormones cannot precisely match these subtle daily hormonal rhythms, and the consequences of such disruption are not fully known. Regardless of whether you are a bodybuilder striving to build muscle or a middle-aged man seeking restored youthfulness, you should be aware that introducing hormones into your body has serious consequences attached, some known and some unknown. Natural Hormonal Enhancement avoids these problems by operating within the parameters of your physiological system.

325

Natural Testosterone Enhancement: An Overview

At the outset, I must make clear that I do not universally advocate testosterone enhancement. For some men, like those with prostate problems, even natural testosterone enhancement may not be appropriate. To enhance or not to enhance is a personal decision. Having said that, there are substantial benefits to testosterone enhancement for men in terms of health, physique, and emotional well-being.

If one concludes that testosterone enhancement is worthwhile and personally suitable, the next question is how to accomplish it. For the average person, natural enhancement is a far better course to pursue than the costly, inconvenient, physiologically disruptive, and potentially dangerous methods of exogenous testosterone enhancement that have become a fast-growing, multi-million-dollar business. But whether you are naturally enhancing it, or injecting it, there are some health issues that should first be addressed in relation to testosterone.

The Heart of the Issue: Testosterone and Cardiovascular Disease

A recent study indicates that men who suffer heart attacks usually have low testosterone and that higher testosterone levels are correlated with higher levels of "good" HDL cholesterol.[34] This research contradicts the popular notion of heart attack as a "masculine" condition. This myth is captured by Dr. Gerald B. Phillips, Professor of Medicine at Columbia University: "When I went to medical school. . . I was told that it was the robust man who was most prone to get a heart attack, the most 'masculine' man, whatever that meant, the man who had the highest levels of testosterone."[35] Dr. Phillips, through his research on the relationship between hormones and heart disease, is credited with helping to overturn this intellectual regime and showing that among the risk factors for heart disease in men is low, not high, testosterone.* Other studies reinforce this finding and show that the age-related decline in testosterone fosters an internal environment hospitable to cardiovascular disease.[36,37,38]

In Europe, exogenous testosterone has been used for more than fifty years to treat a wide range of circulatory problems, including atherosclerosis. In the last few years, a spate of research has emerged supporting the use of exogenous testosterone in coronary patients.[39,40,41,42] Unfortunately, evidence indicating the benefits of testosterone as a treatment for cardiovascular disease has been largely ignored by cardiologists in the United States ever since the 1960's, when they decided upon the surgeon's knife as the treatment of choice.

---

* The tip-off that there was more to the testosterone/heart disease connection than meets the eye came when Dr. Phillips discovered a distinct hormonal abnormality in men who were victims of the relatively rare occurrence of a heart attack in young adulthood: significantly higher than normal levels of *estrogen*.[42a] Further research confirmed that estrogen does not exert the cardioprotective influence in men that it does in women, and may even promote heart disease in men.[42b] In addition to discrediting the widely held belief that testosterone contributes to heart disease in men, Dr. Phillips's findings expose the pitfall of drawing inferences about sex hormones across the sexual divide. This gender dichotomy is further highlighted by studies showing a direct correlation between testosterone levels and insulin levels in women; and an inverse correlation between testosterone levels and insulin levels in men.[42c,42d,42e] The take-home message is that *a given sex hormone does not necessarily have the same effect in men as in women.*

There is no disputing that bypass surgery has saved and improved many lives. But the real question is: has open heart surgery, an exceedingly expensive and traumatic procedure, saved and improved more lives than promising treatments, like testosterone, *would have* had they been explored? We'll never know. A broader question that arises in this connection is whether a standing ovation is merited where a disease (heart disease in this case) is successfully treated, which very likely could have been prevented had the orientation of the medical community been different. I have great difficulty answering this question in the affirmative. Hopefully, the progressive research of Dr. Phillips and others will spur a reevaluation of the use of testosterone enhancement in the United States as a non-invasive, less expensive, less traumatic, treatment for heart disease than what we have currently.

There is still much to be learned about the hormonal factors involved in heart disease. Chapter 8 elucidates the relationship between insulin and cardiovascular disease. While the insulin/heart disease connection is well-established, the role of other hormones, including testosterone, in heart disease is less clear. Future research promises to expand our knowledge in this area.

Testosterone and Prostate Cancer

While testosterone is generally a "good" hormone for men, there may be unfavorable implications as well. The prostate is an androgen-regulated organ, meaning that testosterone is one of the hormones that controls the growth and functioning of the prostate.[43,44] This fact has stirred interest in the role of testosterone in prostate cancer, the most common malignancy and the second leading cause of cancer death among men in Western nations.[45,46] Although evidence of a hormonal etiology for prostate cancer exists, it is circumstantial and inconsistent.

The widely held belief that high testosterone levels is a predisposing factor in prostate cancer is riddled with contrary evidence.[47,48,49,50,51,52,53,54] These studies command the conclusion that prostate carcinogenesis is related to more factors than merely how much testosterone you have coursing through your body. Accordingly, this simplistic notion should be discarded in favor of a multi-factorial view that includes hereditary predisposition, environmentally mediated oxidative stress, and the action of two hormones that the body makes from testosterone: dihydrotestosterone and estrogen.

Dihydrotestosterone (DHT) and estrogen are testosterone metabolites, both of which are commonly found to be elevated in men with benign prostatic hyperplasia (prostate growth associated with subsequent development of cancer[55]).[55,56,57,58,59,60] The correlations observed for DHT and estradiol (a form of estrogen) and benign prostatic hyperplasia are much stronger than for testosterone and this condition. This suggests that changes in the rate at which testosterone is converted to other hormones, rather than testosterone itself, is implicated in the development of prostate cancer.

Conversion of testosterone to DHT is a function of the enzyme *5-alpha reductase*,[61] while the enzyme *aromatase* converts testosterone to estrogen.[62] Beyond that, and the fact that estrogen and DHT levels increase with age, the intricacies of testosterone metabolism are elusive. In particular, determining the factors that govern testosterone/DHT and testosterone/estrogen ratios will likely yield important leads in the investigation of prostate pathology, and may disclose viable avenues of treatment and prevention. Bear in mind the prevailing uncertainty about the hormonal dynamics influencing prostate cancer when deciding whether or not to enhance testosterone. And if you currently have prostate problems, testosterone enhancement of any kind is not recommended.

Diet is a salient factor in prostate cancer as it is in most cancers,[63] and cancer risk is inversely correlated with dietary antioxidant intake.[64] With regard to prostate cancer in particular, vitamins E and C,[65,66,67,68] the carotenoid lycopene,[69,70] vitamin D,[71,72] and soy isoflavones[73,74,75,76] have been identified as protective.

On the subject of diet, recall the connection between trans fatty acids and cancer highlighted in Chapter 18. Ann Gittleman, author of *Super Nutrition for Men* assigns culpability to trans fat as a cause of prostate cancer in particular. She further asserts that essential fatty acids "are absolutely critical to the health of the prostate gland," and she contends that processed foods and a diet high in carbohydrate, not meat and animal fat, are the principal dietary culprits responsible for this type of cancer.[77] If this view, supported on all counts by recent clinical studies,[78,79,80,81] is correct, it would mean that the NHE Eating Plan, with carbohydrate, trans fat, and processed foods, restricted, and essential fatty acid and dietary antioxidant consumption encouraged, is exceptionally well-tailored to prostate health.

On a final note, the plant extracts *pygeum* and *saw palmetto* have been used successfully in Europe for many years to combat prostate enlargement, and for centuries before that by primitive cultures to treat urinary disorders. Recent studies have confirmed the efficacy of both pygeum[82,83] and saw palmetto.[84,85] And unlike the prostate drug Proscar, which garners close to one billion dollars in annual sales, saw palmetto and pygeum do not produce undesirable side effects. Similarly, garlic, the closest thing to a cure-all existing in nature, with anti-microbial and blood-lipid-lowering effects, has shown promise as a treatment for prostate cancer.[86,87]

The Enemy of My Friend is My Enemy:
Enhancing Testosterone By Suppressing Cortisol

Natural testosterone enhancement should be approached from two angles: 1) directly enhancing testosterone, and 2) suppressing cortisol, an adrenal hormone antagonistic to testosterone. If insulin and glucagon are "double-edged swords," and growth hormone and testosterone are "good" hormones, cortisol is a "bad" hormone (see Chapter 4). Of course, no hormone is truly bad since all hormones serve important functions. You would not want to eliminate cortisol entirely from your hormonal ensemble. But as it is impossible to do so through natural means, this is a moot point. Undue cortisol elevation, however, is a different matter given that cortisol can increase drastically in response to natural factors; and at high levels this hormone can sabotage your efforts to build a strong, healthy, attractive body. Cortisol is catabolic, which means it breaks-down muscle; and it is indirectly lipogenic (fat-producing), because it reduces insulin sensitivity (see p. 92).

Not only does cortisol block the anabolic action of testosterone, but it also reduces testosterone production.[88] To understand how cortisol suppresses testosterone requires a quick plunge into human biochemistry. Testosterone is made through a complex sequence of steps, which can be simplified as follows: cholesterol to pregnenolone to progesterone/dehydroepiandrosterone to androstenedione to testosterone. Cortisol, too, is made from pregnenolone, and because of cortisol's evolutionary superiority as a fight-or-flight hormone (see p. 198) it takes precedence over testosterone in the production process.[89] Therefore, the more cortisol production you stimulate, the more pregnenolone gets siphoned-off, unavailable for conversion into androstenedione and then testosterone.

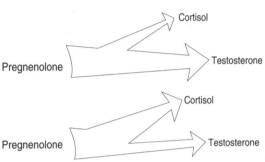

In addition to opposing the anabolic action of testosterone and competitively reducing testosterone production, chronically elevated cortisol reduces growth hormone output.[90,91,92,93] Not only is this an undesirable effect in itself, but it also indirectly bears ill for testosterone given the mutually supporting relationship between growth hormone and testosterone (see Chapter 4). Finally, there is also evidence indicating that cortisol, and stress in general, suppresses luteinizing hormone and interferes with production of testosterone at the testicular level (see p. 197).

Dietary Influences on Testosterone

The NHE Eating Plan is growth-hormone-enhancing and, in men, testosterone-enhancing. I will explain why and suggest additional dietary measures that can be employed to enhance testosterone.

Recent research has revealed a number of important facts about the influence of diet on hormone levels. For one, studies have established that a positive correlation exists between dietary fat and testosterone levels in men.[94,95] This does not mean that eating a super-high-fat diet will result in super-high testosterone levels, but it is clear that a low-fat can lower testosterone levels. A study conducted at Penn State University, published in 1997 in the *Journal of Applied Physiology*,[96] has helped clarify the relationship between dietary fat and testosterone.

In the Penn State study, the subjects eating moderate fat exhibited higher testosterone levels than the subjects eating low fat - this finding merely confirmed previous studies demonstrating that dietary fat is positively linked with testosterone levels. More impressively, the Penn State researchers showed that the effect of dietary fat on testosterone levels depended on *the kind of fat* consumed. Specifically, they found that monounsaturated and saturated fat raise testosterone levels, but polyunsaturated fat does not. Two previous studies had hinted at this conclusion,[97,98] but both had altered total fat in the same direction as the saturated/polyunsaturated fat ratio (making it impossible to ascertain whether lower total fat or a lower saturated/polyunsaturated ratio was responsible for lowering testosterone levels). The stunning implication of this research is that, in addition to the other problems associated with polyunsaturated fat (see Chapter 18), restricting total fat intake <u>and</u> replacing saturated fat with polyunsaturated fat (exactly what the "experts" are telling you to do) would appear to be the perfect prescription for *lowering* testosterone levels!

Review: The Effect of Carbohydrate and Protein on Growth Hormone, IGF-1, and Cortisol

Like fat, carbohydrate and protein, too, influence hormones. A high-carbohydrate diet, especially when compounded by infrequent or irregular eating, can adversely impact upon testosterone, growth hormone, and IGF-1 levels. Recall from Chapter 11 that insulin and growth hormone levels are inversely related, such that higher insulin corresponds with lower growth hormone. A diet high in carbohydrate stimulates excessive insulin secretion. And this undesirable hormonal effect is exacerbated where high carbohydrate consumption is coupled with fat restriction, because of fat's blunting effect on insulin. Moreover, protein, which supports production of both growth hormone and IGF-1, often takes a backseat to carbohydrate or is intentionally restricted on the high-carbohydrate diet, thus ensuring sub-optimal levels of these two important hormones as well. Finally, also recall from Chapter 11 that when a sugar-burner is deprived of sugar (by missing meals) the catabolic, "anti-testosterone hormone," cortisol, is secreted. In this way, a high-carbohydrate diet locks you into a sugar-burning state and thus keeps you perpetually on the verge of cortisol release, while at the same time suppressing your "good" hormones. As you can see, **macronutrients are like buttons on your hormonal control center - each time you eat, you push buttons that trigger hormonal activity**.

The dietary fat/testosterone connection has resounding ramifications for athletes given that they are the group most likely to practice extreme dietary fat restriction, while possibly suppressing their testosterone levels by overtraining as well (see Chapter 21). If your muscular development has stalled, scrutinize your diet. In many cases, the dreaded "plateau" that bodybuilders experience is owed to depressed testosterone levels resulting from overtraining coupled with overzealous dietary fat restriction.

While a diet high in carbohydrate is potentially suppressive of testosterone (via the cortisol escalations it can cause[99] and by promoting insulin resistance[100]), the dietary practice most damaging to testosterone status is extreme fat restriction. **While a high-fat diet does not necessarily translate to high testosterone levels, an extremely low-fat diet is likely to lower testosterone levels**.

The NHE Eating Plan bolsters testosterone by advocating the exact opposite of all the testosterone-depressing dietary practices outlined above. Protein, not carbohydrate, is the centerpiece of the Eating Plan; fat consumption in moderation is encouraged, not restricted; and specific emphasis is placed on essential fatty acids and monounsaturated fat, both of which facilitate optimal testosterone production. While chronically elevated insulin levels can lower testosterone levels, continuously low insulin levels (characteristic of "Atkins"-type diets) are not optimal for testosterone enhancement, either (see p. 139). Rather, the soundest dietary strategy for enhancing testosterone is to punctuate a low-carb diet with periodic, high-carbohydrate, insulin-stimulating meals; consume ample "good" fats; and limit trans fat consumption which, among its litany of misdeeds, may lower testosterone levels.[101]

If you wish to go beyond the basic NHE Eating Plan and take additional dietary measures to enhance testosterone levels, you can increase fat consumption. However, while monounsaturated/saturated fat is positively correlated with testosterone, you are not likely to experience an equal increment of benefit going from moderate fat intake to high fat intake as you would going from low fat to moderate fat. Even so, a high-fat diet may confer additional testosterone-enhancing benefits.

Should you opt for a high-fat diet, it is important to remember that you must not eat high fat *and* high carbohydrate. This is an unhealthy combination, and it is the perfect recipe for maximum fat storage. (This hearkens back to the "conveyor belt problem," described in Chapter 10, in which the insulin spike engendered by the carbs turns-on the "conveyor belt" which, in turn, transports the ingested fat to adipose tissue for storage.) Accordingly, if you wish to experiment with a higher-fat diet, I recommend doing it within the framework of the NHE Eating Plan. As you would suspect, fat loss will be slowed or halted by the additional calories, so assess your priorities before embarking on a higher-fat diet. Additionally, be sure to heed the cautionary instructions on p. 131 before altering your diet in this fashion. If you are engaged in a weight-training program and muscle growth is your top priority, then the Bodybuilders' NHE Eating Plan - a cyclical high-fat diet - is your best choice: it incorporates a high-fat, testosterone-enhancing element along with several other anabolic features (see Chapter 14).

References

1. Longcope C. Adrenal and Gonadal Androgen Secretion in Normal Females. *J Clin Endocrinol Metab* 1986;15:213.

2. Bhasin S, et al. The Effects of Supraphysiological Doses of Testosterone on Muscle Size and Strength in Normal Men. *N Engl J Med* 1996;335:1.

3. Morley JE, et al. Longitudinal Changes in Testosterone, Luteinizing Hormone, and Follicle-Stimulating Hormone in Healthy Older Men. *Metabolism* 1997;46:410.

4. Roshan S, Nader S, Orlander P. Review: Ageing and Hormones. *Eur J Clin Invest* 1999;29:210.

5. Gooren LJ. Endocrine Aspects of Ageing in the Male. *Mol Cell Endocrinol* 1998;145:153.

6. Mitchell R, et al. Age Related Changes in the Pituitary-Testicular Axis in Normal Men; Lower Serum Testosterone Results from Decreased Bioactive LH Drive. *Clin Endocrinol* (Oxf) 1995;42:501.

7. Itoh N, et al. The Assessment of Bioavailable Androgen Levels from the Serum Free Testosterone Level. *Nippon Naibunpi Gakkai Zasshi* 1991;67:23

8. Nankin HR, Calkins JH. Decreased Bioavailable Testosterone in Aging Normal and Impotent Men. *J Clin Endocrinol Metab* 1986;63:1418.

9.   Magoha GA. Effect of Ageing on Androgen Levels in Elderly Males. *East Afr Med J* 1997;74:642.

10. Lund BC, Bever-Stille KA, Perry PJ. Testosterone and Andropause: The Feasibility of Testosterone Replacement Therapy in Elderly Men. *Pharmacotherapy* 1999;19:951.

11. Sternbach H. Age-Associated Testosterone Decline in Men: Clinical Issues for Psychiatry. *Am J Psychiatry* 1998;155:1310.

12. Impotence: NIH Consensus Conference. *JAMA* 1993;270:83.

13. Id

14. Colgan M. *Hormonal Health*. BC, Canada: Apple Publishing 1996, p. 3

15. Ming W, et al. Total Cholesterol and High Density Lipoprotein Cholesterol as Important Predictors of Erectile Dysfunction. *Am J Epidemiol* 1994;140:930.

16. Colgan M. *Hormonal Health*. BC, Canada: Apple Publishing 1996, p. 55-60.

17. Regelson W. *The Super-Hormone Promise*. NY: Simon and Schuster 1996, p. 103

18. Id. at 101.

19. Vermeulen A, et al. Testosterone, Body Composition and Aging. *J Endocrinol Invest* 1999;22:110.

20. Snyder PJ, et al. Effect of Testosterone Treatment on Body Composition and Muscle Strength in Men Over 65 Years of Age. *J Clin Endocrinol Metab* 1999;84:2647.

21. Colgan M. *Hormonal Health*. BC, Canada: Apple Publishing 1996, p. 199.

22. Id. at p. 202.

23. Segal DM, Perez M, Shapshak P. Oxandrolone, Used for Treatment of Wasting Disease in HIV-1-Infected Patients, Does Not Diminish the Antiviral Activity of Deoxynucleoside Analogues in Lymphocyte and Macrophage Cell Cultures. *J Acquir Immune Defic Syndr Hum Retrovirol* 1999;20:215.

24. Strawford A, et al. Resistance Exercise and Supraphysiologic Androgen Therapy in Eugonadal Men with HIV-Related Weight Loss: A Randomized Controlled Trial. *JAMA* 1999;281:1282.

25. Strawford A, et al. Effects of Nandrolone Decanoate Therapy in Borderline Hypogonadal Men with HIV-Associated Weight Loss. *J Acquir Immune Defic Syndr Hum Retrovirol* 1999;20:137.

26. Gold J, et al. Safety and Efficacy of Nandrolone Decanoate for Treatment of Wasting in Patients with HIV Infection. *AIDS* 1996;10:745.

27. Sattler FR, et al. Effects of Pharmacological Doses of Nandrolone Decanoate and Progressive Resistance Training in Immunodeficient Patients Infected with Human Immunodeficiency Virus. *J Clin Endocrinol Metab* 1999;84:1268.

28. Flicker L, et al. Nandrolone Decanoate and Intranasal Calcitonin as Therapy in Established Osteoporosis. *Osteoporos Int* 1997;7:29.

29. Geusens P. Nandrolone Decanoate: Pharmacological Properties and Therapeutic Use in Osteoporosis. *Clin Rheumatol* 1995;14(Suppl):32S

30. Passeri M, et al. Effects of Nandrolone Decanoate on Bone Mass in Established Osteoporosis. *Maturitas* 1993;17:211.

31. Schols AM, et al. Physiologic Effects of Nutritional Support and Anabolic Steroids in Patients with Chronic Obstructive Pulmonary Disease. A Placebo-Controlled Randomized Trial. *Am J Respir Crit Care Med* 1995;152:1268.

32. Ferreira IM, et al. The Influence of 6 Months of Oral Anabolic Steroids on Body Mass and Respiratory Muscles in Undernourished COPD Patients. *Chest* 1998;114:19.

33. Johansen KL, Mulligan K, Schambelan M. Anabolic Effects of Nandrolone Decanoate in Patients Receiving Dialysis: A Randomized Controlled Trial. *JAMA* 1999;281:1275.

34. Phillips GB, Pinkernell BH. The Association of Hypotestosteronemia with Coronary Artery Disease in Men. *Arterioscler Thromb* 1994;14:701.

35. Regelson W. *The Super-Hormone Promise*. NY: Simon and Schuster 1996, p. 117.

36. Zmuda JM, et al. Longitudinal Relation between Endogenous Testosterone and Cardiovascular Disease Risk Factors in Middle-Aged Men. A 13-Year Follow-Up of Former Multiple Risk Factor Intervention Trial Participants. *Am J Epidemiol* 1997;146:609.

37. Guitai J, et al. Plasma Testosterone, High Density Lipoprotein Cholesterol and other Lipoprotein Fractions. *Am J Cardiol* 1981;48:897.

38. Simon D, et al. Association between Plasma Total Testosterone and Cardiovascular Risk Factors in Healthy Adult Men: The Telecom Study. *J Clin Endocrinol Metab* 1997;82:682.

39. Rosano GM, et al. Acute Anti-Ischemic Effect of Testosterone in Men with Coronary Artery Disease. *Circulation* 1999;99:1666.

40. Webb CM, et al. Effect of Acute Testosterone on Myocardial Ischemia in Men with Coronary Artery Disease. *Am J Cardiol* 1999;83:437.

41. Tripathy D, et al. Effect of Testosterone Replacement on Whole Body Glucose Utilisation and other Cardiovascular Risk Factors in Males with Idiopathic Hypogonadotrophic Hypogonadism. *Horm Metab Res* 1998;30:642.

42. Webb CM, et al. Effects of Testosterone on Coronary Vasomotor Regulation in Men with Coronary Heart Disease. *Circulation* 1999;100:1690.

42a. Phillips GB, et al. Association of Hyperestrogenemia and Coronary Heart Disease in Men in the Framingham Cohort. *Am J Med* 1983;74:863.

42b. Phillips GB, Pinkernell BH, Jing TY. The Association of Hyperestrogenemia with Coronary Thrombosis in Men. *Arterioscler Thromb Vasc Biol* 1996;16:1383.

42c. Haffner SM, et al. Decreased Testosterone and Dehydroepiandrosterone Sulfate Concentrations are Associated with Increased Insulin and Glucose Concentrations in Nondiabetic Men. *Metabolism* 1994;43:599.

42d. Andersson B, et al. Testosterone Concentrations in Women and Men with NIDDM. *Diabetes Care* 1994;17:405-11.

42e. Simon D, et al. Interrelation between Plasma Testosterone and Plasma Insulin in Healthy Adult Men: The Telecom Study. *Diabetologia* 1992;35:173.

43. Liu XH, Wiley HS, Meikle AW. Androgens Regulate Proliferation of Human Prostate Cancer Cells in Culture by Increasing Transforming Growth Factor-Alpha (TGF-Alpha) and Epidermal Growth Factor (EGF)/TGF-Alpha Receptor. *J Clin Endocrinol Metab* 1993;77:1472.

44. Ross RK, et al. Androgen Metabolism and Prostate Cancer: Establishing a Model of Genetic Susceptibility. *Eur Urol* 1999;35:355.

45. Fleshner NE, Klotz LH. Diet, Androgens, Oxidative Stress and Prostate Cancer Susceptibility. *Cancer Metastasis Rev* 1999;17:325.

46. Moul JW, Lipo DR. Prostate Cancer in the Late 1990s: Hormone Refractory Disease Options. *Urol Nurs* 1999;19:125.

47. Meikle AW, et al. Effects of Age and Sex Hormones on Transition and Peripheral Zone Volumes of Prostate and Benign Prostatic Hyperplasia in Twins. *J Clin Endocrinol Metab* 1997;82:571

48. Nomura AM, et al. Serum Androgens and Prostate Cancer. *Cancer Epidemiol Biomarkers Prev* 1996;5:621.

49. Carter HB, et al. Longitudinal Evaluation of Serum Androgen Levels in Men With and Without Prostate Cancer. *Prostate* 1995;27:25.

50. Vatten LJ, et al. Androgens in Serum and the Risk of Prostate Cancer: A Nested Case-Control Study from the Janus Serum Bank in Norway. *Cancer Epidemiol Biomarkers Prev* 1997;6:967.

51. Monath JR, et al. Physiologic Variations of Serum Testosterone within the Normal Range Do Not Affect Serum Prostate-Specific Antigen. *Urology* 1995;46:58.

52. de Jong FH, et al. Peripheral Hormone Levels in Controls and Patients with Prostatic Cancer or Benign Prostatic Hyperplasia: Results from the Dutch-Japanese Case-Control Study. *Cancer Res* 1991;51:3445.

53. Meikle AW, Stanish WM. Familial Prostatic Cancer Risk and Low Testosterone. *J Clin Endocrinol Metab* 1982;54:1104.

Natural Hormonal Enhancement

54. Marchetti B, et al. Castration Levels of Plasma Testosterone have Potent Stimulatory Effects on Androgen-Sensitive Parameters in the Rat Prostate. *J Steroid Biochem* 1988;31:411.

55. Bostwick DG, et al. The Association of Benign Prostatic Hyperplasia and Cancer of the Prostate. *Cancer* 1992;70(Suppl):291S

56. Suzuki K, et al. [Endocrine Environment of Benign Prostatic Hyperplasia--Relationships of Sex Steroid Hormone Levels with Age and the Size of the Prostate]. *Nippon Hinyokika Gakkai Zasshi* 1992;83:664. Japanese.

57. Suzuki K, et al. Endocrine Environment of Benign Prostatic Hyperplasia: Prostate Size and Volume are Correlated with Serum Estrogen Concentration. *Scand J Urol Nephrol* 1995;29:65.

58. Isaacs JT, Brendler CB, Walsh PC. Changes in the Metabolism of Dihydrotestosterone in the Hyperplastic Human Prostate. *J Clin Endocrinol Metab* 1983;56:139.

59. Krieg M, et al. Androgens and Estrogens: Their Interaction with Stroma and Epithelium of Human Benign Prostatic Hyperplasia and Normal Prostate. *J Steroid Biochem* 1983;19:155.

60. Bartsch W, et al. Endogenous Androgen Levels in Epithelium and Stroma of Human Benign Prostatic Hyperplasia and Normal Prostate. *Acta Endocrinol* (Copenh) 1982;100:634.

61. Lobaccaro JM, et al. [5 Alpha-Reductase and Prostate]. *Ann Endocrinol* (Paris) 1997;58:381. French.

62. Cohen PG. The Hypogonadal-Obesity Cycle: Role of Aromatase in Modulating the Testosterone-Estradiol Shunt--A Major Factor in the Genesis of Morbid Obesity. *Med Hypotheses* 1999;52:49.

63. Eichholzer M. [The Significance of Nutrition in Primary Prevention of Cancer]. *Ther Umsch* 1997;54:457. German.

64. Stahelin HB, et al. Plasma Antioxidant Vitamins and Subsequent Cancer Mortality in the 12-Year Follow-Up of the Prospective Basel Study. *Am J Epidemiol* 1991;133:766.

65. Smigel K. Vitamin E Reduces Prostate Cancer Rates in Finnish Trial: U.S. Considers Follow-Up. *J Natl Cancer Inst* 1998;90:416.

66. Eichholzer M, et al. Smoking, Plasma Vitamins C, E, Retinol, and Carotene, and Fatal Prostate Cancer: Seventeen-Year Follow-Up of the Prospective Basel Study. *Prostate* 1999;38:189.

67. Deneo-Pellegrini H, et al. Foods, Nutrients and Prostate Cancer: A Case-Control Study in Uruguay. *Br J Cancer* 1999;80:591.

68. Maramag C, et al. Effect of Vitamin C on Prostate Cancer Cells in Vitro: Effect on Cell Number, Viability, and DNA Synthesis. *Prostate* 1997;32:188.

69. Gann PH, et al. Lower Prostate Cancer Risk in Men with Elevated Plasma Lycopene Levels: Results of a Prospective Analysis. *Cancer Res* 1999;59:1225.

70. Rao AV, Fleshner N, Agarwal S. Serum and Tissue Lycopene and Biomarkers of Oxidation in Prostate Cancer Patients: A Case-Control Study. *Nutr Cancer* 1999;33:159.

71. Konety BR, et al. Vitamin D in the Prevention and Treatment of Prostate Cancer. *Semin Urol Oncol* 1999;17:77.

72. Krill D, et al. Differential Effects of Vitamin D on Normal Human Prostate Epithelial and Stromal Cells in Primary Culture. *Urology* 1999;54:171.

73. Griffiths K, Morton MS, Denis L. Certain Aspects of Molecular Endocrinology that Relate to the Influence of Dietary Factors on the Pathogenesis of Prostate Cancer. *Eur Urol* 1999;35:443.

74. Strom SS, et al. Phytoestrogen Intake and Prostate Cancer: a Case-Control Study Using a New Database. *Nutr Cancer* 1999;33:20

75. Stephens FO. Phytoestrogens and Prostate Cancer: Possible Preventive Role. *Med J Aust* 1997;167:138.

76. Zhou JR, et al. Soybean Phytochemicals Inhibit the Growth of Transplantable Human Prostate Carcinoma and Tumor Angiogenesis in Mice. *J Nutr* 1999;129:1628.

77. Gittleman AL. *Super Nutrition for Men.* NY: M. Evans and Company 1996, p. 59-77.

78. Kolonel LN, Nomura AM, Cooney RV. Dietary Fat and Prostate Cancer: Current Status. *J Natl Cancer Inst* 1999;91:414.

79. Singh G, et al. Regulation of Prostate Cancer Cell Division by Glucose. *J Cell Physiol* 1999;180:431.

334

80. Schuurman AG, et al. Animal Products, Calcium and Protein and Prostate Cancer Risk in the Netherlands Cohort Study. *Br J Cancer* 1999;80:1107.

81. Du S, et al. [Relationship Between Dietary Nutrients Intakes and Human Prostate Cancer]. *Wei Sheng Yen Chiu* 1997;26:122. Chinese.

82. Chatelain C, Autet W, Brackman F. Comparison of Once And Twice Daily Dosage Forms of Pygeum Africanum Extract in Patients with Benign Prostatic Hyperplasia: A Randomized, Double-Blind Study, with Long-Term Open Label Extension. *Urology* 1999;54:473.

83. Breza J, et al. Efficacy and Acceptability of Tadenan (Pygeum Africanum Extract) in the Treatment of Benign Prostatic Hyperplasia (BPH): a Multicentre Trial in Central Europe. *Curr Med Res Opin* 1998;14:127.

84. Wilt TJ, et al. Saw Palmetto Extracts for Treatment of Benign Prostatic Hyperplasia: A Systematic Review. *JAMA* 1998;280:1604.

85. Gerber GS, et al. Saw Palmetto (Serenoa Repens) in Men with Lower Urinary Tract Symptoms: Effects on Urodynamic Parameters and Voiding Symptoms. *Urology* 1998;51:1003.

86. Pinto JT, et al. Effects of Garlic Thioallyl Derivatives on Growth, Glutathione Concentration, and Polyamine Formation of Human Prostate Carcinoma Cells in Culture. *Am J Clin Nutr* 1997;66:398.

87. Sigounas G, et al. S-Allylmercaptocysteine Inhibits Cell Proliferation and Reduces the Viability of Erythroleukemia, Breast, and Prostate Cancer Cell Lines. *Nutr Cancer* 1997;27:186.

88. Doerr P, Pirke KM. Cortisol-Induced Suppression of Plasma Testosterone in Normal Adult Males. *J Clin Endocrinol Metab* 1976;43:622.

89. McGilvery RW. *Biochemistry: A Functional Approach.* Philadelphia, PA: W.B. Saunders Company 1983.

90. Tonshoff B, Mehls O. Interactions between Glucocorticoids and the Growth Hormone-Insulin-Like Growth Factor Axis. *Pediatr Transplant* 1997;1:183.

91. Dieguez C, et al. Role of Glucocorticoids in the Neuroregulation of Growth Hormone Secretion. *J Pediatr Endocrinol Metab* 1996;9(Suppl):255S.

92. Devesa J, et al. Regulation of Hypothalamic Somatostatin by Glucocorticoids. *J Steroid Biochem Mol Biol* 1995;53:277.

93. See Chapter 20, notes 66-68.

94. Reed MJ, et al. Dietary Lipids: An Additional Regulator of Plasma Levels of Sex Hormone Binding Globulin. *J Clin Endocrinol Metab* 1987;64:1083.

95. Dorgan JF, et al. Effects of Dietary Fat and Fiber on Plasma and Urine Androgens and Estrogens in Men: A Controlled Feeding Study. *Am J Clin Nutr* 1996;64:850.

96. Volek JS. Testosterone and Cortisol in Relationship to Dietary Nutrients and Resistance Exercise. *J App Physiol* 1997;82:49.

97. Hamalainen E, et al. Diet and Serum Sex Hormones in Healthy Men. *J Steroid Biochem* 1984;20:459.

98. Dorgan JF, et al. Effects of Dietary Fat and Fiber on Plasma and Urine Androgens and Estrogens in Men: A Controlled Feeding Study. *Am J Clin Nutr* 1996;64:850.

99. See p. 92.

100. See p. 100.

101. Hanis T, et al. Effects of Dietary Trans-Fatty Acids on Reproductive Performance of Wistar Rats. *Br J Nutr* 1989;61:519.

APPENDIX A: A Word about Women and Muscles, and a Commentary on Professional Bodybuilding

Both women and men tend to lose muscle mass and bone mass as they get older. However, this degenerative trend is more pronounced in women due to menopausal loss of estrogen, smaller bones than men, greater propensity to engage in restrictive dieting throughout life, and lesser propensity to lift weights. This is why it is less common to see a fit, attractive 60-year-old woman than a fit, attractive 60-year-old man - it's not fair, it's not politically correct, but it's true.

It is ironic and unfortunate, even sad, that women, the ones who need resistance training most, tend to shun it because of the chauvinistic myth that resistance training is appropriate only for men. Instead, women tend to rely on calorie restriction and low-intensity/high-volume aerobic exercise, both of which do nothing to help, and can exacerbate, the age-related loss of muscle and bone, thereby depriving them of their youthful shapeliness and promoting the deadly crippler - osteoporosis. As long as the idea persists that resistance training is not suitable for women, they will continue to lose their strength, their muscle, their bone, and their sex appeal earlier in life than men. Resistance training is the key to maintaining youthful anabolic hormone levels, and by extension, the shapeliness, firmness, and leanness that defines a sexy, youthful-looking body.

Womens' professional bodybuilding is largely responsible for the average woman's fear that lifting weights will make her look unfeminine. The fact of the matter is that women who compete in bodybuilding competitions are not representative of the effect of resistance training on the female body. Truth be told, practically all female professional bodybuilders take anabolic drugs. Many women who participate in amateur bodybuilding competition at the state and local level are not on drugs (and they look much different). But at the highest amateur level, anabolic steroid use is common. And at the professional level, steroid use is absolutely essential in order to attain the freaky look necessary to compete successfully.

Without high circulating levels of testosterone, a human being cannot become extremely muscular and extremely lean. Men naturally possess a substantial amount of testosterone which can be further naturally enhanced; women do not and can not, and therefore must take testosterone (i.e., steroids) in order to look like a well-built man. When you consider that hormonal makeup is one of the defining differences between men and women - exerting profound physiological, psychological, and sexual effects - you realize that while it is unhealthy for men to take steroids, for women to take them is a grossly unnatural alteration of a human being. In a real sense, steroids turn women into men; and the health dangers of steroids are greater for women. Female East German athletes learned this lesson the hard way when Olympic glory gave way to severe health problems years later. In studies of rats, steroids produce huge, muscular females that kill and eat untreated males.

What Drug Testing?

Contrary to what many people believe, most bodybuilding competitions are not drug-tested because regulation of bodybuilding is lax and drug testing is often cost-prohibitive. The promoters of bodybuilding competitions are in business to make money just like anyone else, and, absent a groundswell of interest in seeing "natural" competitors, they have little incentive to underwrite drug testing. While such a groundswell may be forming, as evidenced by fitness publications featuring more natural physiques, the majority of bodybuilding fans still want to see the biggest, most defined, freakiest bodybuilders; and there is simply no comparison between a natural bodybuilder and a "pharmaceutically enhanced" bodybuilder. The competitions that are drug-tested typically employ inexpensive and unsophisticated methods that are easily circumvented by savvy competitors. It should also be noted that by no means are female bodybuilders guiltier than male bodybuilders of taking anabolic drugs. To the contrary, the pharmacology of male bodybuilding at the highest level of competition begins with steroids and includes anabolic drugs that did not even exist in the days when Arnold Schwarzenegger competed.

Fortunately, female bodybuilding, which never achieved mainstream acceptance, is becoming even more marginalized as female "fitness competitions" (which are a combination of physique competition and athletic talent show) rapidly grow in popularity. Virtually all fitness competitors train with weights, and are drug-free. Given that many of the top fitness competitors double as swimsuit models, I think it is safe to say that weight training has not diminished their femininity. To the contrary, weight training has helped many of the leading swimsuit models attain their status, and their magnificent physiques.

I see the ascendancy of fitness competitions as a very positive development, and I applaud both the competitors and the promoters. For one, these competitions will help dispel the myth that weight training masculinizes a woman's physique. Furthermore, the athletic component of these competitions will, hopefully, lead to similar competitions for men. As it stands now, male physique competitions are exasperatingly subjective, and they involve virtually no skill or athletic ability. (Executing a choreographed posing routine to music does involve skill, but any competitive bodybuilder knows that the winners are generally determined during the prejudging line-ups; the show is just for show.)

The women are way ahead of the men on this one, and it would be great to see the "sport" of male bodybuilding take a page out of the book of female fitness competition. In so doing, male physique competition could win the appreciation and respect of a much wider segment of the public. This would attract wealthier and more respected corporate sponsors, which ultimately would mean more money in the pockets of both the promoters and the competitors. As it stands now, big business is rightfully reluctant to associate with a sport of such little substance so heavily polluted by drug use. Compared with other sports, the prize money for all but the top competitors is paltry, and the endorsement opportunities are limited. The only way this will change is if bodybuilding sheds its "freak show" image and becomes more mainstream. Rather than merely showcasing grotesque hulking beings huffing and puffing their way through uninspiring posing routines, male physique competition should be strictly drug-tested and should include an athletic component like an obstacle course or track and field events. Alternatively, or in addition, male physique competitors could put on boxing gloves and duke it out, or shoot hoops, play home-run derby, or compete at golf or tennis. Where do I sign-up!

337

APPENDIX B: Bioenergetic Pathways, the Mind-Muscle Connection, and Sports Training

Understanding bioenergetic pathways (discussed in Chapter 21) is critical to formulating an optimal sports training program. The central point is that strength and endurance improvements are specific to the bioenergetic pathway trained. For example, a powerlifter may be able to bench press 350 lbs. one time but be able to bench press 225 lbs. for only six repetitions, whereas a bodybuilder may be unable to bench press 350 lbs., but be able to bench press 225 lbs. for twelve repetitions - who's stronger?

The Overlapping Distinction between Strength and Endurance

The answer to the above question depends on how you define strength, but any definition of strength that refers to exerting maximal effort for more than a few seconds or repeated bouts of maximal effort significantly involves energy production efficiency (i.e., ATP regeneration, lactic acid clearance, and glycolysis). As you can see, the line of demarcation between "strength" and "endurance" is a blurry one.

Physical Improvements are Specific to the Form of Training

As you learned in Chapter 21, the body adapts to each stress specifically, precisely matching the adaptation to the stress. Although the activity is the same in a general sense, the stress of lifting a heavier load once is qualitatively different from the stress of lifting a lighter load repeatedly. The same is true for jogging as compared with sprinting. For one, neuromuscular activation patterns are different, with the powerlifter and sprinter better able to recruit low-oxidative Type II muscle fibers, which are better suited to explosive bursts of output and movement against heavy resistance. In addition, each chiefly engages a different bioenergetic pathway, with the bodybuilder and jogger relying more heavily on glycogen (i.e., the glycolytic bioenergetic pathway) and the powerlifter and sprinter relying almost exclusively on the ATP/CP bioenergetic pathway. Enzymatic adaptations facilitate utilization of the particular bioenergetic pathway trained.

Another training-induced adaptation that bears on performance is increased resting levels of energy substrates (ATP, CP, and glycogen). The powerlifter's enhanced capacity to store ATP and CP in his muscles coupled with neuromuscular adaptations, largely account for his ability to lift very heavy weight for a single repetition. The bodybuilder's training involves more sets, more repetitions, and less weight per lift than does the powerlifter's; hence, it primarily engages the glycolytic bioenergetic pathway. Correspondingly, the bodybuilder's capacity to store glycogen increases. Because glycogen, which is stored along with water in the muscles, takes-up much space, bodybuilders have a "pumped" look that powerlifters lack. Although the bodybuilder's muscles may not be stronger than the powerlifter's, they are typically bigger and more bulging because they serve as repositories for vast amounts of glycogen and water.

In addition to increased glycogen storage capacity, the bodybuilder's neuromuscular conditioning (i.e., mind/muscle connection) allows him efficiently to recruit high-oxidative Type I muscle fibers needed for higher repetition weight lifting. As well, the bodybuilder undergoes other adaptations that make his body more efficient at functioning in the glycolytic bioenergetic pathway and which confer "the look" of a bodybuilder. Specifically, he develops a more extensive capillary network. Enhanced capillarization (and the bulging veins or "vascularity" associated with bodybuilders) facilitates removal of lactic acid from the muscles and transport of oxygen to the muscles to regenerate ATP after each set. These are the reasons why a bodybuilder can do more reps with lighter weight than can a powerlifter, even though the powerlifter has a higher one-rep "max."

The "Holyfield Principle"

Ill-conceived sports-training programs, stemming from a misunderstanding of bioenergetic pathways and neuromuscular activation patterns, are common. For example, high school football coaches often have their players run low-speed laps around the track. This is basically a waste of the players' limited energy resources. Instead, the football player should perform repetitions of high-intensity, explosive exercises that simulate the movements performed during the game. This constitutes optimal training because it conditions both the bioenergetic pathway predominately used for the sport, and it reinforces the applicable neuromuscular activation patterns.

Football players, boxers, basketball players, and tennis players should be especially concerned with maximizing recovery ability after repeated, intense bursts of output (specifically, this entails efficient ATP regeneration and lactic acid clearance). The objective of this type of "endurance" is to be "stronger" throughout the competition at each and every point where a burst of intense power output is required. Boxing presents an instructive case study. Boxing is a sport dominated by tradition, and this is why many boxers expend lots of energy doing "roadwork" (jogging). While roadwork can be helpful for mental discipline, fat loss, and general health, in large volume it is a misallocation of the boxer's finite energy resources. Energy resources are like money - limited and valuable. The more wisely an athlete utilizes these resources in the weeks or months leading up to a competition, the greater the advantage he or she can capture over a competitor who uses his or her pre-competition energy resources less wisely.

Evander Holyfield appreciates and practices these principles, and his "high-tech" training has attracted much attention. Holyfield repeatedly executes high-intensity boxing techniques timed to boxing rounds and rest periods, and he uses an apparatus that applies resistance against his punches. This type of training trains the specific bioenergetic pathways and neuromuscular activation patterns that he will be engaging come fight-time. Should the rules of boxing change such that a boxer has to run-down his opponent over a long distance in order to punch him, jogging will become an important part of a boxer's training regimen. But as long as "going the distance" refers to time and not actual distance, Holyfield-type training will confer an advantage over a training routine that emphasizes roadwork and other non-boxing-specific training methods.

Playing Hurt, Playing Tired, and the Breakdown in Mind-Muscle Communication

Every athlete and every coach knows that form and technique deteriorate with increasing fatigue. The neuromuscular or "mind-muscle connection" breaks down as the athlete becomes distracted by his/her own fatigue: the boxer begins throwing arm punches, the halfback begins running straight-up in stead of running low to the ground, the tennis player begins hitting off his back foot inside of shifting his weight and following through, etc. Much attention is given to the ability "to play hurt" - and in sports like football and boxing, this ability is crucial. However, the ability to play tired is very similar mentally and even more important, because athletes in strenuous sports are constantly playing in varying degrees of exhaustion. Obviously, it is not feasible to simulate playing hurt, because the benefits of practicing while hurt would be outweighed by the detriment of becoming hurt. But it is feasible, and advantageous, to simulate competing while fatigued.

Athletes should engage in technique-oriented training under conditions of near-exhaustion. Running wind sprints is not enough; it won't be that easy in the game. Come game-time, football players, boxers, tennis players, basketball players, etc. will not have the luxury of mindlessly propelling their bodies forward while in a state of semi-exhaustion. To excel, "pushing yourself" in the face of exhaustion during practice may be enough, but to become a champion, you should push yourself in the face of exhaustion while simultaneously trying to maintain perfect form and technique executing the movements required by your sport. San Francisco 49er wide receiver Jerry Rice ran perfect routes all-game-long even when exhausted; boxer Sugar Ray Leonard's exquisitely precise footwork and punches never foundered late in the fight; and anyone who has observed Michael Jordan dominate the fourth quarter of a basketball game has seen the result of a player whose quality of performance was impervious to physical exhaustion. Many other players were similarly talented in a physically fresh state as were these three men; but the "the greats" have an exceptional ability to maintain peak concentration, dexterity, and composure in the face of oppressive fatigue.

Because exhaustion breeds sloppy form, keep a close eye on your form when employing this training methodology so you do not develop bad habits. As long as you avoid this pitfall, you will acquire an advantage over an opponent who does not use this methodology and instead separates "conditioning training" from "technique training." Remember, it's not just how well you can withstand exhaustion that matters, but how well you can perform when exhaustion is bearing down on you. Your fatigue is your opponent's ally, and his/hers is yours. The nexus between exhaustion and mental concentration/mind-muscle coordination, and its implications, are commonly overlooked. Avoid this oversight by remembering that your goals in training are to: 1) minimize your level of fatigue during competition, and 2) minimize the impact of fatigue on your performance.

Psyching and Visualization

Another way to improve the mind-muscle connection is through "psyching." On p. 282, you learned that muscular output is limited by the ability of the brain to communicate stimulatory signals to the muscles, and we discussed how training "disinhibits" (i.e., facilitates) neuromuscular communication. Well, the latest research in this area suggests that physical training alone does not enable full neural facilitation. In other words, in most instances, people (even highly trained athletes) operate at a level of neural inhibition that prevents them from expressing their true strength capability. This built-in limitation is believed to be a protective mechanism. However, it has been shown that this natural minimal level of neural inhibition can be transcended under certain psychological conditions.

For example, a study found that arm strength was greater in subjects under the following circumstances: 1) after a loud noise, 2) under the influence of amphetamines, 3) under hypnosis when they were told that they would be much stronger than usual and should have no fear of injury, 4) while the subject screamed loudly at the time of exertion. It is because of supernormal motor unit recruitment that supermaximal performance can be achieved amid the excitement of competition or under the influence of disinhibitory drugs or hypnotic suggestion. Supernormal motor unit recruitment also accounts for "unexplainable" feats of strength during life-threatening situations.

To the extent that this heightened state of arousal can be achieved without drugs or the presence of a life-threatening influence, the natural level of neural inhibition can be overpassed and performance can be taken to the highest level. One way to achieve this is by intensely concentrating or "psyching" oneself into a semi-hypnotic state. This technique is frequently employed at the highest level of athletic competition. It is not easy to accomplish, and there is no simple "how to" formula for psyching. But given the advantage it confers, it is a technique that serious athletes should cultivate. Combined with the related technique of visualization, psyching can significantly elevate performance by optimizing the mind-muscle connection.

A full treatment of visualization is beyond the scope of this report, but basically visualization exploits a remarkable fact about the brain: the brain has difficulty differentiating reality from that which is intensely envisioned. The most common example of this is dreaming. Even though a dream may have no basis whatsoever in reality (it may even relate to something absurd like a ferocious three-headed dragon), the brain perceives it as real. Even after you awaken you may continue to be frightened for a few moments until actual reality displaces your mentally "real" visions. Even physical parameters, like perspiration and pulse rate, may remain elevated for a while after you have arrived at the realization that the three-headed dragon is definitely not coming to get you. Visualization aims to turn this phenomenon to your advantage.

Take the example of athlete X, who enters a competition in which he is a prohibitive underdog. From the outset, X is at a disadvantage because he is aware that he will probably lose. Even if this awareness is accompanied by a hope or even a belief that he will win, the underlying awareness that this hope or belief of victory is contrary to the odds can create a self-limiting mindset. If X falls behind early in the match, it reinforces his awareness that he will probably lose. Moreover, athlete X is competing against an athlete (athlete Y) who expects to win. Unless Y becomes complacent or overconfident, this expectation will give Y an advantage that will compound X's disadvantage.

Visualization and psyching can change all this and can "level the playing field" by making X as confident, or more confident, than Y. A compelling example of this from the boxing arena was presented by Mike Tyson vs. Buster Douglas, one of the greatest upsets in sports history. While Tyson's fighting skills were indeed exceptional throughout most of his career, he also enjoyed a major psychological advantage over every opponent he faced, up until he fought Douglas.

In his heyday, Tyson's awesome mystique was so psychologically debilitating to his opponents that many of them entered the ring with a palpable sense of their impending defeat. Mystiques are self-perpetuating, and with each man he knocked-out, Tyson's power to intimidate grew. For all intents and purposes, Tyson's opponents were mentally programmed to lose. It was as if with each punch that Tyson threw, they wondered if it was the knockout punch; and if it turned-out not to be, they were surprised still to be standing upright. With such a negative mindset, it is virtually impossible to win.

Buster Douglas, a mediocre opponent who was given essentially no chance to win by the oddsmakers, won almost every round and knocked Tyson out late in their fight, forever shattering Tyson's aura of invincibility. Even though the then-undefeated Tyson's mystique and power of intimidation were at their highest coming in to that fight, Douglas was completely unintimidated and unfazed even after getting knocked down by a brutal Tyson uppercut midway through the fight. Based on his prior and subsequent outings, it is clear that Douglas's performance against Tyson was a gross aberration. A different Douglas entered the ring that night, one that we had not seen before, have not seen since, and probably will never see again. I believe that, like so many other momentous events in sports history, the explanation for Douglas's astonishing performance on that night can be explained in terms of the mind-muscle connection.

Douglas's mother died a few days before the fight. Extreme adversity can either break a person or cause a person to break records - in Douglas's case, it was the latter. Distraught over his mother's death, Douglas was in an altered state of mind. The prospect of getting knocked-out by Tyson was trivial by comparison with the death of his mother. And to the extent that Douglas was fighting for his beloved, recently deceased mother, he had a motive that transcended money, glory, fame, or personal achievement. Douglas was a different man on that night - a man on a mission of the highest calling.

Tyson's vaunted punching power, which had left so many other opponents lying semi-conscious on the floor, hardly seemed an annoyance to Douglas. The discrepancy between the effect of other fighters' less powerful punches on Douglas and the non-effect of Tyson's punches, demonstrates the overriding power of the mind in sport

342

competition. Facing the biggest challenge of his career, fighting the world's most fearsome fighter in the wake of his mother's death, propelled Douglas to a mental state that made it virtually impossible for him to lose.

There are many other instances of athletes using psyching and visualization to attain a pinnacle of confidence and concentration. Keri Strugg's Olympic heroism is one of the more dramatic recent examples: confronting the moment she had worked for and dreamed about all her life, her injured leg, which may have disabled her from competing at any lesser moment, became a non-factor during her defining moment. Because of the tremendous power of the mind and the impossibility of seeing into the mind, there will always be major upsets in sports. All the "on paper" analysis in the world cannot accurately predict the level of motivation, confidence, and readiness of an athlete at game-time. And these factors often determine who prevails, especially where physical factors are approximately equal.

The mental factor also explains why some of the greatest athletes of all-time were not nearly the most physically gifted. For example: Pete Rose (baseball), Mike Singletary and Steve Largent (football), Larry Byrd (basketball), Rocky Marciano and Evander Holyfield (boxing), Jimmy Conners (tennis). Similarly, the greatest coaches of all-time are often not the most brilliant tacticians. Rather they have the ability, like the great military generals in history, to inspire and motivate - to elevate others to their highest potential. Bill Parcells, Pat Riley, and Belle Karoli each have the ability to touch the minds of their players in extraordinary ways. Vince Lombardi, the legendary coach of the Green Bay Packers during their heyday in the 1960s, was able to instill in his players a sense of purpose that transcended the game of football. While the players on the opposing team entered the field of play to win a championship, Lombardi's players entered the field to prove their worth as men, and to reflect honor on their family and their country. More often than not, the mind dictates who wins and who attains greatness.

Index

and growth hormone, 201, 240
and insulin resistance, 100
and hormonal hunger, 99
and mental state, 83, 103
and serum cholesterol/triglyceride, 48
and serotonin, 102-104
and sunlight, 209
and testosterone, 139, 331
and the post-workout meal, 243
and the pre-workout meal, 238-242
and thermogenesis, 149, 151-153
before sleep, 201
calories per gram, 68
consumption trend in U.S., 52
during metabolic shift period, 118
energy myth, 166
"hidden carbs", 188
insulin response to, 77, 80, 239
partitioning, 143
starchy vs. sugary, 144-145
utilization, 77
cardiovascular disease (see also
"atherosclerosis")
and alcohol, 210-211
and cholesterol, 46-48
and estrogen, 13, 326
and free radicals, 174
and insulin, 47-48
and serum triglyceride, 48-49, 178
and testosterone, 326
and trans fatty acids, 175
and Type II diabetes, 49
in other cultures, 51
catabolism (defined), 17
catechin, 211
catecholamines, 305 (see also
"norepinephrine", "adrenaline")
Caverject, 323
centenarians, 53
cheese, 193
chew test, 150
chimpanzee, 25
cholecystokinin, 167
cholesterol
and alcohol, 210
and carbohydrate, 48, 49
and cardiovascular disease, 46
and growth hormone, 5
and hunter-gatherer diet, 27
and impotence, 323
and meal size/frequency, 162
and monounsaturated fat, 172
and polyunsaturated fat, 173
and saturated fat, 175

and soy, 153-154
and sugar, 145
and trans fatty acids, 175
lowering drugs, 47
oxidation of, 46-47
regulated by insulin/glucagon, 47
relation b/w intake and serum levels, 46
relation to testosterone levels, 326
cigarette, see "smoking"
circadian rhythm, 199, 202
clothes, 113
cocaine, 83, 193
coffee, see "caffeine"
Cohen, A.M., 51
Colgan, Michael, 92, 13, 7, 246
colorectal cancer, 13
Communism, 264
conveyor-belt problem, 82
cool-down, 270
Cooper, Kenneth, 248
corticotropin-releasing hormone, 195
cortisol
and aerobic exercise, 246
and alcohol, 212
and Alzheimer's disease, 197
and blood sugar, 92
and bone, 92
and depression, 197
and exercise, 257, 261, 288, 292-293
and fat deposition, 195
and growth hormone, 10, 197, 329
and hydration, 130-131
and immunity, 92, 197
and insulin resistance, 92
and meal frequency, 162
and muscle, 92
and overtraining, 250
and sex hormone suppression, 256
and sex, 216
and sleep deprivation, 200-201
and stress response, 196
and testosterone, 197, 328-329
evolutionary function, 198
cottage cheese, 193
crash dieting, 114
creatine phosphate, 237, 245, 338
Crete, 46, 54, 172
Crist, Douglas, 240
Cushing's syndrome, 17
deca-durabolin, see "anabolic steroids"
dehydration, 94, 130-131
dehydroepiandrosterone, 47, 324
delta 5 desaturase, 171, 178-180
delta 6 desaturase, 179-180

345

Futrex-5000, 113
Galapagos tortoise, 1
Galileo, 38
Galloway, Jeff, 250
garlic, 328
gastric inhibitory polypeptide, 80
genome, 25
Gironda, Vince, 136
glucagon, 15, 76, 91
   active release vs. passive release, 81
   and serum cholesterol/triglyceride, 47
   and eicosanoids, 171, 178
   and evolution, 25
   and fat burning, 79
   and protein, 80, 156
   and body weight regulation, 67
   catabolic, 79, 91
   function, 78
gluconeogenesis, 88, 91
glucose, 79, 81, 83, 117, 145, 166, 245 (see also "sugar")
glycemic index, 145, 239
glycogen, 77, 81, 83, 92, 117, 119
   and detraining, 283
   and exercise performance, 139, 241
   and energy production during exercise, 237
   and fat storage/burning, 78-79, 81
   liver vs. muscle, 145
   loading, 82
   sparing effect, 93, 241
   storage capacity/rate of depletion, 78
glycogen synthase, 81-82
glycolysis, 237, 245
gonadotropins, 11 (see also "follicle-stimulating hormone", "luteinizing hormone")
gorging, 162
Gould, Lance K., 49
grains, 27
growth hormone,
   anabolic, 5
   and alcohol, 212
   and atherosclerosis, 5
   and blood sugar, 201, 239
   and bodyfat, 87
   and bone, 248
   and serum cholesterol/triglyceride, 5
   and cortisol, 11, 197, 329
   and estrogen/progesterone, 12
   and exercise, see Chapter 21
   and gonadotropins, 11
   and immunity, 5, 304
   and insulin, 87, 90
   and muscle, 5-6

   and personal relationships, 217
   and protein, 156
   and sleep, 200-202
   and testosterone, 11, 287
   and the pre-workout meal, 240
   anti-aging, 16
   decline with aging, 11, 14
   history of use, 5-6
   lipolytic, 5
gynecomastia, 213
heart disease, see "cardiovascular disease"
heart rate, 305
HIFWAC fruits, 151
hippocampus, 197
Holyfield, Evander, 114, 339
Holyfield Principle, 339
hominids, 24
Homo erectus, 24
Homo hablis, 24
Homo sapiens (origin of), 24
homocysteine, 39-40
homosexual men, 197, 203
Hormonal Health, 13, 92
hormonal hunger, 45, 70-71, 99-104
hormonal synergy, 11, 14-15
hunter-gatherers, 27
hydration, 130-131
hydrogenation, 174, (see also "trans fatty acids")
hydrostatic weighing, 111
hyperadaptive period, 281-284
hypogonadism, 324
hypohydration, 131 (see also "hydration", "dehydration"
hypothalamus, 70, 98, 195, 203
IGF-1, see "insulin-like growth factor I"
immunity,
   and cancer, 303-304
   and cortisol, 92, 197, 304
   and depression, 197
   and dietary fat, 170
   and exercise, 303-304
   and growth hormone, 5, 304
   and stress, 196
impotence, 323-324, 215
incandescent light, 208
Industrial Revolution, 28, 52, 162
informercials, 273
insulin, 17 (see also "insulin resistance")
   anabolic, 78
   and alcohol, 211-212
   and body weight regulation, 67
   and bodyfat, 76-77, 82, 101
   and cancer, 77

347

and carb-load meals, 139-140
and serum cholesterol, 47-48
and cigarette smoking, 215
and coronary risk, 47
and dietary fiber, 28
and eicosanoids, 171
and energy levels, 82-83
and evolution, 25
and exercise, 257, 276
and food cravings/appetite, 70-71, 99-102
and growth hormone, 87, 90
and meal frequency, 161-161
and protein, 80, 160-161
and saturated fat, 55, 101
and serotonin, 83-84, 102
and serum triglyceride, 47-48
and sleep deprivation, 200
and stress, 197
and testosterone, 326, 331
and the post-workout meal, 243
and the pre-workout meal, 238-239
anti-lipolytic effect, 101, 238-239
function, 77
insulin resistance, 87, 100-101, 145
insulin-like growth factor I
    and carb-load meals, 139
    and estrogen, 12
    and growth hormone, 12, 90
    and insulin, 76, 78, 90-91
    and progesterone, 12
    and protein, 91, 156
    anti-aging, 16
intensity, see "exercise variables"
intensity/volume ratio, 257-259, 262-263, 267-268, 284, 288, 290-291
interval training, 251, 267-269
ions, 130
isoflavones, 328
Japanese diet, 159
jogging, 250-251 (see also "long-distance running")
Jordan, Michael, 340
juicing, 129
Kavanaugh, James, 176
ketogenic diet, 96 (see also "Atkins Diet")
ketones, 68, 129
Kevorkian, Jack, 50
Klatz, Ronald, 19
kidneys, 156-157
Kuwait, 207
lactate threshold, 238
lactic acid, 236-238, 261
Laron dwarfism, 90
Leonard, Sugar Ray, 340

leptin, 65
leukemia, 206 (see also "cancer")
life expectancy, 25, 52-53
Life Extension, 174
lipases, 167, 247
lipids, 129 (see also "fat")
lipogenesis (defined), 17
lipogenic enzymes, 145, 167
lipolysis (defined), 18
lipoprotein lipase, 65-66
liquor, see "alcohol"
liver, 12, 90, 213
load, see "exercise variables"
localized overtraining, 294, 298
Lombardi, Vince, 343
long-distance running, 246, 258, 262 (see also "jogging")
L-tryptophan, 34
Lunch meats, 153
luteinizing hormone, 197, 256, 324, 329
lycopene, 328
lysine, 80
macronutrient cycling, 117, 122
malic, 167
maltodextrin, 166, 243
mammals, 25
margarine, 174-176
McCulley, Kilmer, 39
meat, 153-154, 156, 188, 192
    and hunter-gatherer diet, 27
    domestic vs. wild, 169
    during the metabolic shift period, 118
Medewar, P.B., 304
Mediterranean diet, 172
melanoma, 205-206, 208
melatonin, 200, 203
menopause, 12-14
menstrual cycles (and exercise), 256, 293
metabolic rate
    and aging, 19
    and exercise, 244-245, 247
    and muscle mass, 19, 245-246
mind-muscle connection, 282, 287, 291, 305, 338-341
mineral, 96, 94
mitochondria, 245
moles, 206
mood, 198, 208 (see also "depression")
motor unit, 282
multiple sclerosis, 204
muscle, (see also "muscle fibers", "mind-muscle connection")
    and ATP/CP, 237

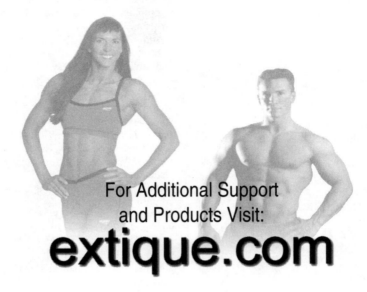

For Additional Support
and Products Visit:
extique.com